Pediatric Neurology

ESSENTIALS FOR GENERAL PRACTICE

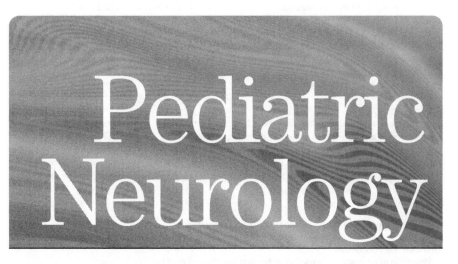

Pediatric Neurology

ESSENTIALS FOR GENERAL PRACTICE

Peter L. Heilbroner, MD, PhD

Attending Pediatric Neurologist
Department of Neuroscience
The Valley Hospital
Ridgewood, New Jersey

Glenn Y. Castaneda, MD

Attending Child Neurologist
Department of Neurology
Vassar Brothers Hospital
Poughkeepsie, New York

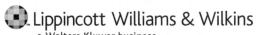 Lippincott Williams & Wilkins
a Wolters Kluwer business

Philadelphia · Baltimore · New York · London
Buenos Aires · Hong Kong · Sydney · Tokyo

Acquisitions Editor: Frances DeStefano
Managing Editor: Lauren Aquino
Project Manager: Frances Gunning
Senior Manufacturing Manager: Benjamin
Rivera

Marketing Manager: Kim Schonberger
Cover Designer: Christine Jenny
Production Service: GGS Book Services
Printer: R.R. Donnelley

Library of Congress Cataloging-in-Publication Data

Heilbroner, Peter Louis.
    Pediatric neurology : essentials for general practice / Peter L.
Heilbroner, Glenn Y. Castaneda.
        p. ; cm.
    Includes bibliographical references and index.
    ISBN 13: 978-0-7817-6945-7
    ISBN 10: 0-7817-6945-0
    1. Pediatric neurology.   I. Castaneda, Glenn.   II. Title.
    [DNLM: 1. Nervous System Diseases. 2. Child. 3. Family Practice. 4. Infant.
WS340H466p2007]
    RJ486.H438 2007
    618.92'8—dc22

                                                                2006024803

Care has been taken to confirm the accuracy of the information presented and to describe
generally accepted practices. However, the authors, editors, and publisher are not responsible
for errors or omissions or for any consequences from application of the information in this
book and make no warranty, expressed or implied, with respect to the currency, completeness,
or accuracy of the contents of the publication. Application of the information in a particular
situation remains the professional responsibility of the practitioner.

The authors, editors, and publisher have exerted every effort to ensure that drug selection
and dosage set forth in this text are in accordance with current recommendations and practice
at the time of publication. However, in view of ongoing research, changes in government
regulations, and the constant flow of information relating to drug therapy and drug reactions,
the reader is urged to check the package insert for each drug for any change in indications and
dosage and for added warnings and precautions. This is particularly important when the
recommended agent is a new or infrequently employed drug.

Some drugs and medical devices presented in the publication have Food and Drug
Administration (FDA) clearance for limited use in restricted research settings. It is the
responsibility of the health care provider to ascertain the FDA status of each drug or device
planned for use in their clinical practice.

To purchase additional copies of this book, call our customer service department at (800)
638-3030 or fax orders to (301) 223-2320. International customers should call (301) 223-2300.

Visit Lippincott Williams & Wilkins on the Internet: at LWW.com. Lippincott Williams & Wilkins
customer service representatives are available from 8:30 am to 6 pm, EST.

*To Irving Fish, MD, who showed us that
clinical sense does not preclude common sense;
to our patients; and to our families, without whom
this book would not have been possible.*

Introduction

Many physicians feel uneasy approaching a young patient who has a complaint suggesting a disorder of the nervous system. The most obvious and oft-cited reason stems from their training, when they did not have an opportunity to evaluate or treat a large enough number of pediatric patients with a neurological problem. In addition, we have found that many physicians were not taught practical concepts that would enable them to feel more confident when seeing pediatric neurological cases.

Physicians in other fields who try to learn more about child neurology from textbooks generally do not find the approach they are seeking. These authoritative sources, indispensable for the pediatric neurologist, are too detailed and devote too much space to uncommon diseases to make it easy to learn the concepts and skills needed to treat the common disorders.

Pediatric neurology textbooks also are not designed to quickly answer the non-pediatric neurologist's questions: When should (MRI) be ordered—or repeated—to evaluate a child's headaches? How concerned should I be about the arachnoid cyst noted in the MRI report? What should I do when a child diagnosed with attention-deficit/hyperactivity disorder (ADHD) is not responding to medication? And what does it really mean when his mother tells me that he has a "processing problem"? In a case of developmental delay, when should I suspect a degenerative disorder? And which tests should I order? Is an electroencephalogram (EEG) useful in evaluating a child who has frequent behavioral outbursts? What do I tell a parent who wants to know if her son's tics will lead to Tourette syndrome? A major reason for writing this book was to provide readily accessible answers to everyday questions.

WHY LEARN PEDIATRIC NEUROLOGY?

Pediatric patients with headaches, suspected seizures, fainting spells, tics and head injuries are often evaluated in the office or emergency room. The parents of children with school-related and behavioral problems or suspected ADHD often seek medical guidance, as do parents of infants who are delayed in attaining motor or language milestones. Other patients will, occasionally, present with signs or symptoms of a more serious neurological disorder such as Guillain-Barre syndrome, transverse myelitis, or a central nervous system tumor that must be promptly diagnosed and appropriately treated.

Unless all of these patients can be quickly seen by a pediatric neurologist – something not possible in many places in the United States, and in many other countries – the physician responsible for their care must know how to proceed. He should recognize the differential diagnosis suggested by the history, use the physical examination to explore possibilities suggested by the differential diagnosis, know which tests will provide the most useful information, and be able to offer effective initial and when possible definitive treatment.

Pediatric neurological referral will ultimately be necessary for difficult or serious cases, and most parents would like their pediatrician to understand the neurologist's approach and perspective. To many parents, neurological problems are mysterious and frightening; therefore it is important that the primary care physician clearly understand these disorders and their treatment. Throughout this book we address the questions that parents most often ask. We also review a number of subjects that tend to cause confusion and impede communication with the family: the purpose and interpretation of the EEG, the terms used to characterize learning disabilities, and what causes headaches.

THE SCOPE OF THIS BOOK

Pediatric Neurology: Essentials for General Practice does not replace a traditional textbook. Our primary purpose is to teach useful clinical skills and thoroughly review the diagnosis and treatment of the more common disorders seen in the office or clinic. We also suggest an approach to neurological syndromes encountered in the emergency room. Such syndromes include the child with an altered mental status or whose gait has acutely deteriorated. Also included are overviews of the surgical management of epilepsy and the treatment of brain tumors that may be helpful for the pediatric resident caring for hospitalized patients.

We do not include some rare diseases, and we discuss other disorders generically (e.g., "Mucopolysaccharidoses," rather than separate sections each devoted to a specific kind of mucopolysaccharidosis). Our approach is not intended to minimize the importance of rare diseases. To the children and families affected by a rare disorder, their condition is overwhelmingly important, and the physician who cares for these patients provides an invaluable service. That having been said, a heavy emphasis on rare diseases in an introductory book is distracting to the physician who needs to learn about the conditions he will see on a regular basis.

This book briefly discusses the management of neurological conditions encountered in the intensive care unit, such as coma, spinal cord injury and elevated intracranial pressure. If a more comprehensive discussion of ICU neurology is sought, the reader may consult definitive pediatric, medical and neurosurgical reviews and textbooks.

Chapter 1 presents guidelines intended to help the physician take the history of a neurological complaint. We then offer suggestions for a physical examination guided by the differential diagnosis suggested by the history. The doctor who seeks a general overview should start by reading through Chapter 1. The same chapter may also serve as a general reference for the physician who has more neurological experience. The remainder of the book is devoted to specific syndromes and disorders.

Acknowledgments

The authors would like to recognize our teachers in the Department of Neurology, New York University Medical Center: Edwin H. Kolodny, MD, Ruth D. Nass, MD, Sandra L. Forem, MD, John T. Wells, MD, Jeffrey C. Allen, MD, and Irving Fish, MD (to whom we dedicate this book). We fondly remember Richard N. Reuben, MD. We are also indebted to the faculty of the NYU Department of Pediatrics, and to the many adult neurologists with whom we trained in the NYU Department of Neurology. Dr. Heilbroner would like to thank the faculty of the Department of Pediatrics, Long Island College Hospital and the members of the Departments of Pediatrics and Neuroscience, The Valley Hospital.

We greatly appreciate the generosity of Eliot Lerner, MD, Howard Seigerman, MD (both of The Valley Hospital), and especially Ajax George, MD (New York University Medical Center) who donated many MRI and CT images from their collections for reproduction in this book.

Dr. Heilbroner would also like to thank the many physicians who took the time to look over chapters, make suggestions, and contribute material for this book. All of my colleagues and friends at Neurology Group of Bergen County, P.A. provided advice and encouragement. John Nasr, MD, and Jennifer Cope, MD made valuable contributions to the chapter on epilepsy. Susan Molinari, MD reviewed the chapter on movement disorders and offered thoughtful suggestions. Reed Perron, MD and Daniel Van Engel, MD reviewed many chapters and provided valued criticism. Robert Pancza, PhD and Lois Hochberg, PhD made useful suggestions for the chapter covering learning disabilities and ADHD. Thanks also to Mitchell Steinschneider, MD, PhD, Lisa Nalven, MD, Daniel Adler, MD, Frank Mangianello, MD, David Namerow, MD, and Irwin Berkowitz, MD. Special thanks and appreciation to Ralph L. Holloway, PhD, Thomas L. Kemper, MD, Giles F. Whalen, MD, Leonard Scherlis, MD, James Meltzer, PhD, and Pi Hoffman.

Dr. Castaneda would like to thank the doctors and staff of eRiver Neurology of New York, and the doctors, residents, staff and medical students at Albany Medical College, Neuroscience Division.

Finally, we would like to thank our families for their love and support during the long course of our medical training, and our subsequent careers.

Contents

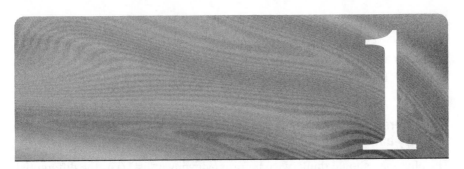

SUGGESTIONS FOR HISTORY
AND PHYSICAL EXAMINATION

APPROACH TO THE FAMILY

Parents may be frightened when their child develops a neurological symptom. The worst possibility—that their child has a life-threatening or disabling disease—is feared, since everyone knows that the brain is a critically important, intimidatingly complicated, mysterious organ. Advice from "expert" friends, the overdramatic tone of medical reporting on television, and the Internet tend only to exacerbate the parents' anxiety, and as a result, they may arrive in the office in a state of great consternation, expecting the worst.

Assuming that the *physician* does not suspect a serious condition based on his evaluation, his most important role often becomes one of *reassurance*. It is important to remember that *a neurological symptom is not by definition a serious symptom!* Just as a typical case of fever is far more likely to result from a benign viral infection than from tuberculosis, a child's tremor is far more likely to be a sign of neurological immaturity than an early sign of Wilson disease, and a headache is much more often a migraine headache than a symptom of a brain tumor. Therefore, we should not jump to order invasive, expensive tests because a symptom happens to be neurological, just as we do not reflexively order a computed tomography (CT) scan of the abdomen for every child with a stomachache.

A calm manner and nontechnical language will usually help relax the family. It is helpful to directly address unspoken fears (i.e., "It's normal to worry about a brain tumor when your child has migraines. You'll be glad to know that a tumor virtually never causes migraine headaches.").

The physician often can make parents feel better by *demystifying medical terms*. When a parent learns that epilepsy is defined as a history of two or more unprovoked seizures, or that Tourette syndrome is defined as history of motor and vocal tics of more than 1 year in duration, or that cerebral palsy is a general term that means a history of delayed motor development (in many cases, relatively mild), the parent is given perspective and will relax, even if the parent suspects that the child's problem may be significant.

The differential diagnosis is not for the parents to worry about

The physician should think twice before reviewing a "list" (i.e., the differential diagnosis) with the family. He should be especially wary when the differential diagnosis is long and complicated, such as when a patient is being evaluated for a first seizure or for markedly delayed development. It is best to give the family a general sense of the diagnostic possibilities, order appropriate tests, and say that more will be known when the test results come back. Giving the family a long list of possible diagnoses will only exacerbate their anxiety. Every new medical term they hear will lead to 10 more questions, the answers to most of which will be of no concern to them once the diagnosis has been made.

Tell the family to beware of the Internet

The Internet can be a good source of information for families, but websites are inconsistent in quality and often misleading. Parents should try to stay off the Internet until a diagnosis has been made or at least until the differential diagnosis has been narrowed. Like hospital dramas on television, many websites distort the significance of medical symptoms and signs. For example, if the parent of a mildly hypotonic child enters the word "hypotonia" into an Internet search engine, she may be directed to sites devoted exclusively to serious neurological conditions such as spinal muscular atrophy, Rett syndrome, and muscular dystrophy. The fact that the great majority of mildly hypotonic children have *no* serious underlying disorder may not even be mentioned.

Explaining the cause, not using jargon, and acknowledging the limits of our understanding

We often must explain to parents that many neurological diagnoses [e.g., migraine, attention-deficit hyperactivity disorder (ADHD), and tic] are made primarily on the basis of *recognizing a characteristic pattern of symptoms and signs*, rather than by laboratory and diagnostic test [magnetic resonance imaging (MRI), electroencephalogram (EEG), etc.] results. A primary focus on the clinical presentation is disorienting to many people, who are used to relying on test results (e.g., a positive or negative throat culture) and who will persist in asking about the exact cause of their child's problem. When the cause is known, it should, of course, be shared with the family. Our understanding of the cause of many neurological disorders is incomplete, however, and this fact should not be disguised.

Pseudoscientific terms ("a processing problem" in a case of learning disability or "a chemical imbalance" in a case of depression) should generally be avoided in these conversations. These terms do not explain the child's condition to parents and, therefore, only lead to more questions ("What *kind* of processing problem?" "Can you test my child for a chemical imbalance?"). It is better to simply say, with respect to the previous two examples, that educational testing reveals that your child comprehends information that she reads better than information that she hears or that your child appears depressed. Theories about the underlying cause can then be presented, as long as they are characterized as theories.

When the parents ask why the exact cause of their child's problem cannot be demonstrated, it can be explained, if need be, that we obviously do not biopsy the human nervous system except in the most serious cases (and even if we could, the results would reveal little about the working brain). In this respect, neurology is different from many other medical specialties whose practitioners routinely obtain tissue for diagnosis, and this leads to a somewhat abstract quality to neurological diagnosis making. We cannot definitively demonstrate to a parent that the language area of the brain of their child with a learning disability has a pattern of synaptic connections that differs from some other children; that the brain of their child with a primary generalized seizure disorder contains neurons that discharge abnormally; or that their depressed son's raphe nucleus may not release enough serotonin. (Functional imaging technologies are potentially useful in this regard and one day may be more widely available.) Once again, this limitation does not prevent us from diagnosing our patients accurately and treating their condition to everyone's satisfaction.

TAKING THE HISTORY OF A NEUROLOGICAL PROBLEM

Red flags

Many pediatric patients who come to the office or clinic with a neurological complaint are ultimately diagnosed with a condition, such as benign developmental motor delay, tic disorder, migraine, or concussion, that is either treatable or, if left untreated, does not have grave implications for the patient's health. Intermixed with these cases, however, will be some patients whose condition is potentially much more serious. **Although we emphasize that this list does not include every serious disorder and there is no simple formula that can be used to quickly determine that a patient has a serious problem, the following six clinical syndromes should always merit extra attention and prompt diagnostic testing (Table 1.1).**

TABLE 1.1

"Red flags": serious syndromes in child neurology

Unexplained focal neurological symptoms or signs
Developmental regression or marked stagnation
Symptoms and signs of elevated intracranial pressure and hydrocephalus
Seizures with implications for the patient's development, such as infantile spasms
Symptoms and signs of meningitis
Unexplained, persistent loss of a neurological function (e.g., marked change in mental status, loss of the ability to walk)

Unexplained focal neurological symptoms or signs

A *symptom* (such as a headache) is a *complaint*. The *doctor* or *another individual observes* a *sign* (e.g., "the patient's reflexes are abnormally brisk" or "my 2-year-old child is falling down a lot").

A disease process affecting a *localized region of the nervous system* usually causes one or more *focal neurological symptoms or signs*. Focal neurological symptoms and signs, especially if not transient, should always be regarded as abnormal. Focal neurological signs and symptoms are often *unilateral* (noted on only one side of the body). Two classic syndromes are hemiparesis (weakness of the upper and lower extremity on one side) and hemianopsia (loss of a visual field). *A lesion within the opposite cerebral hemisphere* is the usual cause. Infarction (stroke) in the left hemisphere, for example, often causes weakness of the right arm and leg or a right visual field deficit. However, the physician must keep in mind that *brainstem, cerebellar,* and *spinal cord lesions* often cause *ipsilateral* (on the same side as the lesion) or *bilateral* symptoms. For example, weakness of both legs might be caused by a tethered spinal cord, incoordination of the right hand might be caused by a right cerebellar tumor, and loss of ability to move the eyes to the right might be caused by demyelination in the right half of the pons.

A majority of pediatric neurological complaints, such as headache, learning problems, fainting spells, tremor, tic, delayed fine motor skills, and behavioral problems *do not result from a localized disease process in the nervous system*. Table 1.2 lists some typical pediatric neurological problems and suggests the likelihood that the problem is the result of a lesion in a specific area of the nervous system.

Transient focal neurological symptoms

Transient focal neurological symptoms lasting only a few seconds or minutes are differentiated from *persistent* focal neurological symptoms. *Concussion, migraine, and partial seizure* are the most common causes of transient

TABLE 1.2

Various pediatric neurological syndromes and likelihood of a focal disturbance in the nervous system as the cause

Problem	Caused by a focal lesion?
Headache	Relatively unlikely but always must be considered
Learning disability	Possible in cases of previous brain injury; otherwise, almost never
Attention-deficit hyperactivity disorder	Virtually never
Mildly delayed gross or fine motor development with otherwise normal neurological examination	Virtually never
Autism	Virtually never
Blurred vision	Possible; other causes more common
Seizure	Must be considered in the case of a focal-onset or poorly characterized seizure
Hemiparesis	Likely
Ataxia	Likely (but can be caused by medication, migraine, other nonstructural causes)
Double vision	Likely

neurological symptoms. Concussion and migraine do not result from a structural lesion in the brain, and if the history suggests migraine or concussion, the chances are good that the patient does not have a serious underlying disorder. However, partial seizures *can* be caused by a structural lesion and should be evaluated promptly with MRI and EEG if they were not febrile seizures.

Chronic focal neurological symptoms

The physician must also differentiate a focal deficit of *recent* onset from a *chronic* focal deficit. A chronic focal neurological deficit (such as chronic right hemiparesis) is usually the result of a previously diagnosed problem (for example, a brain injury many years in the past), whereas a recent-onset focal symptom or sign suggests a new problem warranting investigation.

Developmental regression or stagnation after normal development

A *mild delay* in attaining infantile and early childhood developmental milestones (especially motor milestones) is frequently reported and is not usually caused by a serious underlying disorder. However, a history of *lost, previously attained developmental milestones, severe developmental delay,* or *marked stagnation of development* is *always* cause for concern. Autism, a degenerative or neuromuscular disease, chronic infection (e.g., congenital human immunodeficiency virus), or a brain tumor may present with developmental stagnation or regression.

Symptoms and signs of elevated intracranial pressure and hydrocephalus

Signs and symptoms of elevated intracranial pressure (ICP) are reviewed below (see exam of patient with headaches) and in Chapter 2. Brain tumor, pseudotumor cerebri, and hydrocephalus are important conditions that cause an elevation of the ICP in a child or adolescent. Hydrocephalus in a neonate and infant does not result in elevated ICP because the cranial sutures are not yet closed and, instead, causes *progressive macrocephaly*.

Seizure disorders with serious implications

Infantile spasms in particular must be recognized.

Symptoms and signs of meningitis

A child or adolescent with a *headache, a stiff neck or a Kernig or Brudzinski sign, and fever* should be assumed to have *meningitis* and should promptly be sent for a lumbar puncture. *Meningitis in an infant or toddler* may present less dramatically. These patients may not have a stiff neck or exhibit other signs of meningeal irritation. The most characteristic signs of meningitis in very young patients are *fever and altered mental status* (decreased alertness, lethargy, or irritability).

A headache and a stiff neck *unaccompanied* by fever suggests *cervical disease* (the most common cause) or, although seen rarely in the pediatric population, a *subarachnoid hemorrhage*.

Marked, unexplained loss of neurological function

The patient who is rapidly losing the ability to walk, for example, must be immediately evaluated. Unexplained mental status changes always warrant close attention.

SUGGESTIONS FOR TAKING THE HISTORY

1   The *rate of onset* of a patient's symptoms often helps define the differential diagnosis (Table 1.3). For example, if a patient has lost the ability to walk over a period of *a few seconds or minutes*, a traumatic injury, ischemic stroke (brain or spinal cord), or a hemorrhage is the most likely cause. If this problem has developed over the course of *hours or days*, an immunologically

TABLE 1.3
Time course of neurological disorders

Acute onset (seconds to minutes)	Subacute onset (hours to days)	Gradual onset (weeks to months)	Progression over months to years	Stable for years	Intermittent
Trauma Infarction Hemorrhage	Infection Inflammation Demyelination Toxin/drug	Tumors Some degenerative disorders Smoldering infection (abscess)	Degenerative disorders Some tumors Chronic infection (e.g., human immunodeficiency virus)	Previous neurological injury/disease (prior stroke, cerebral palsy, spina bifida, etc.)	Migraine Seizure Vasovagal syncope Breath-holding spells Panic attacks

mediated disorder such as Guillain-Barré syndrome, transverse myelitis, or an infection in the nervous system (e.g., a brain abscess) should be suspected. The patient who has become unable to walk over a period of *weeks to months* may have a spinal tumor. If the patient's gait has been deteriorating over a period of *years*, a degenerative neuromuscular disease may be the cause. Finally, if the patient has *never* walked, the cause is probably a nonprogressive condition such as spina bifida or cerebral palsy. In addition, it is important to recognize that *migraine, vasovagal syncope, breath-holding spells, seizures, and panic attacks* are the most common causes of *transient or intermittent neurological symptoms.*

2 The physician should always inquire about *nonneurological symptoms.* For example, a patient may come to the office because of headaches, but it is only after she is asked if she has been feeling excessively fatigued or has a rash, arthralgias, or a sore throat that the cause of the headaches (Lyme disease, mononucleosis, or another viral syndrome) is suggested.

3 The physician should always ask if the patient is *currently taking a prescription medication* that could cause the presenting complaint. The patient with a tremor may be taking an antidepressant, a stimulant drug for ADHD, or a beta-agonist drug for asthma. The ataxic patient may be taking an antiepileptic drug or a sedative-hypnotic. The patient with headaches may be taking methylphenidate, a vitamin supplement, or an antibiotic. Seizures can be provoked by several medications (see Chapter 6).

4 The *family history* is important in neurological and psychiatric cases. Common conditions that often "run in the family" include ADHD, learning disability, migraine, tic/Tourette syndrome, mood and anxiety disorders, syncope, tremor, and several forms of epilepsy. In the much rarer case of a metabolic or degenerative disorder, the family history is often very important.

5 *Psychogenic disorders are common.* Indeed, the primary problem turns out to *be* psychogenic, or at least exacerbated by psychological factors, in an appreciable number of cases that, at first glance, suggested an organic disorder. A clue suggesting a psychogenic cause for the patient's apparently neurological problem is the occurrence of that problem *only in a particular situation or setting.* Some examples include headaches that bother a patient at one divorced parent's house but never at the other parent's house, bizarre behavior at home that is never noticed by a child's teacher, or trouble walking that started immediately after an emotionally traumatic event. Another clue suggesting a nonorganic problem is *inconsistency of physical findings,* such as a patient's inability to raise a lower extremity off of the examination table despite intact ability to support weight on the same extremity while standing. *Some diagnostic testing is generally indicated, but the doctor should not continue to order tests if the results are normal and he strongly suspects a psychogenic disorder.*

We should be comfortable talking about psychogenic problems with our patients and their families. When a doctor does not honestly identify a patient's problem as stress or anxiety related, it is confusing to the family and contributes to the stigma associated with behavioral disorders. It should also be explained that saying that a psychiatric/psychological etiology exists for a patient's symptoms does not necessarily mean that the patient is not experiencing real symptoms.

ROLE OF EEG AND MRI

MRI and EEG are helpful in making the diagnosis of some, but by no means all, neurological disorders. These tests are often inappropriately ordered (for example, in cases of ADHD, tic disorder, and typical vasovagal spells). The usefulness of these tests is discussed throughout this book. Table 1.4 provides examples of appropriate and inappropriate clinical situations in which to order these tests.

PHYSICAL EXAMINATION
Focus on the differential diagnosis suggested by the history

Many physicians make the mistake of performing the same physical examination when evaluating a patient with a neurological problem of any kind. We would recommend a more individualized approach. A history of a fainting spell, a history of back pain, and a history of a school-related problem are entirely different complaints, and each suggests a unique differential diagnosis and particular aspects of the examination that should be emphasized. **A focused neurological examination is much more likely to provide useful information than a boilerplate examination.**

TABLE 1.4

Magnetic resonance imaging (MRI) and electroencephalogram (EEG) in common pediatric neurological cases

Condition	MRI	EEG
Headache	Ordered to exclude a mass lesion or arteriovenous malformation. Most causes of headache are *not* diagnosable by MRI.	Not indicated.
Learning disability, attention-deficit hyperactivity disorder	Not indicated in typical cases.	Not indicated.
Tic	Not indicated unless a different kind of movement disorder is suspected.	Not indicated unless a focal seizure is suspected.
Seizure (nonfebrile)	Usually indicated, other than in cases of idiopathic primary generalized epilepsy (see Chapter 6).	Generally indicated.
Syncope	Very low yield.	Not indicated unless seizure suspected.
Autism	May show nonspecific abnormalities; no value in making the diagnosis of autism.	Indicated if history of seizures (*not* tantrums/ outbursts) or in *rare* cases of suspected Landau-Kleffner syndrome (see Chapter 9).
Unexplained focal neurological signs/symptoms	Usually indicated (except in clear cases of peripheral nerve injury).	Indicated if patient has a history of seizures.
Developmental delay	In cases of mild/moderate motor delay, yield is low. Consider in cases of global (motor and cognitive) delay and especially developmental regression.	Indicated only if patient has a history of seizures.

TABLE 1.5

Suggestions for focused neurological examination

Complaint	Emphasis of examination
Headache/head injury	Inspect the cranium in cases of trauma, in particular for signs of a basilar skull fracture. Evaluate neck for stiffness, tenderness, and adenopathy; assess tenderness to percussion of sinuses. Examine optic fundi for papilledema or hemorrhage. Perform full assessment of mental status in cases of head injury. If no specific neurological complaints, a concise examination of cranial nerves, motor system, and cerebellar function is often adequate.
School and behavioral problems	Behavioral and cognitive assessment is stressed; screen for learning disability. Look for behaviors suggestive of attention-deficit hyperactivity disorder (ADHD), anxiety, or depression. Check for "soft signs."
Tic/movement disorder	Behavioral assessment should be included given comorbid disorders (ADHD, etc.). Observe abnormal movements. Assess tone for evidence of rigidity. In cases of tic disorder (most common), concise motor and cranial nerve exam is sufficient. In cases of other movement disorders, a comprehensive motor examination is required.
Seizures	Examine skin for signs of a neurocutaneous disorder. Observe for hyperventilation if absence seizures are suspected. Especially in cases of focal-onset seizures when no brain imaging study has yet been completed, a comprehensive neurological examination is recommended to search for focal signs.
Syncope	Take orthostatic blood pressure readings; examine skin, thyroid gland, heart, and lymph nodes. Concise cranial nerve, motor, and cerebellar assessment.
Hemiparesis	*Comprehensive* cranial nerve, motor, sensory, reflex, and cerebellar examination.
Ataxia	*Comprehensive* cranial nerve, motor, sensory, reflex, and cerebellar examination.
Neck or back pain (especially if accompanied by complaints of weakness or numbness)	Range of motion of neck, neck and back tenderness, straight leg-raising test; and *comprehensive* motor, reflex, and sensory examination.

The examination of a child with a school-related problem should include screening for a learning disability and a careful assessment of behavior looking for signs of ADHD, anxiety, or depression. The examination of the patient who has fainted should include orthostatic blood pressure readings, cardiac auscultation, and evaluation of the skin, thyroid gland, and lymph nodes looking for signs of a nonneurological medical problem (e.g., hypothyroidism, mononucleosis) that might cause the patient to faint or feel lightheaded. The examination of a patient with back pain should include an assessment of strength, gait, sensation, and deep tendon reflexes in the lower extremities; spinal tenderness; and the straight leg-raising test to assess nerve root irritability. Conversely, it is generally unnecessary to spend 20 minutes testing the power of every muscle group of a child who was referred for a school or behavioral problem, to perform a comprehensive sensory examination if the patient has a history of a typical fainting spell, or to perform a lengthy cognitive evaluation when the primary complaint is back pain, assuming that the history does not suggest any additional concerns.

Am I going to miss something important?

We also suggest *a concise examination of all neurological systems*, which is described in the following sections, that should always be performed to make certain that no important physical findings or occult problems are missed. In cases that seem unusual or atypical or when standard therapy does not appear to be effective, we also urge that the physician "step back" and perform (or repeat) a comprehensive examination that may reveal evidence of a more unusual disorder.

Table 1.5 includes examples of common complaints and aspects of the physical examination to be emphasized.

GENERAL EXAMINATION

This section reviews aspects of the **general physical examination that are particularly important in neurological cases**. An approach to the neurological part of the examination follows. Once again, we emphasize that *the entire examination is rarely necessary*. A sense of the likely differential diagnosis should guide the examiner.

1 **Vital signs** should always be recorded. **Fever** suggests an infection either directly involving the nervous system or, more often, resulting in a secondary neurological complaint, such as the headache associated with a nonspecific viral syndrome. Low blood pressure may explain fainting.

2 The **head circumference** of **neonates, infants, and toddlers** should be measured. The head circumference should also be measured in cases of **premature birth, perinatal complications, and delayed development, or when the patient's head appears large, small, or unusually shaped.**

Measurement of the head circumference is always from glabella (between the eyebrows) through inion (external occipital protuberance). Poor measurement technique is among the most common causes of a "large" or "increasing" head circumference (see Chapter 11 and Fig. 11.1).

3 The patient's **general appearance** should be noted. Obesity often causes sleep apnea, which can lead to fatigue, headaches, and difficulty concentrating. Obesity may also suggest a behavioral or genetic disorder (e.g., Prader-Willi syndrome or an eating disorder). An emaciated appearance may result from a large number of underlying medical and psychiatric disorders.

4 The **skin always must be examined**. Café-au-lait spots, melanotic whorls, port wine stains, and hypopigmented macules are often signs of a *neurocutaneous disorder* (Figs. 1.1–1.3; see Chapter 14) associated with seizures, tumors of the nervous system, developmental delay, and behavioral problems.

5 **Dysmorphic facial features**, including hyper- or hypotelorism, low nasal bridge, and deformities of the face, ears, mandible, teeth, or palate, suggest a *syndrome of congenital malformation*. Other physical features suggestive of a congenital syndrome include an unusual appearance or distribution of scalp

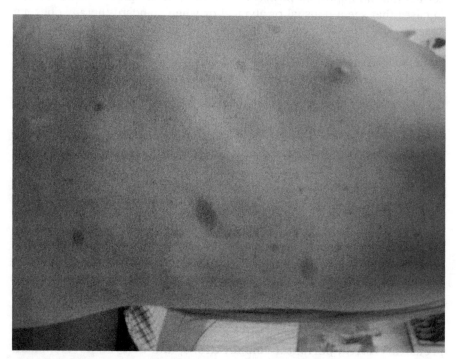

Figure 1.1 Neurofibromatosis type I: café-au-lait spots and axillary freckling.

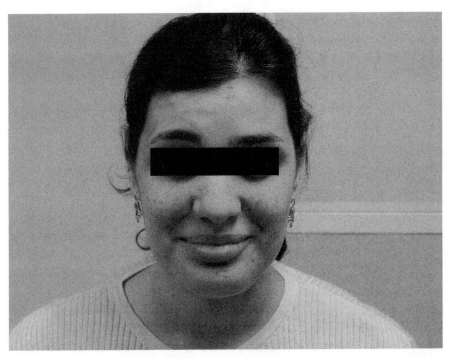

Figure 1.2 Tuberous sclerosis: adenoma sebaceum.

hair; small, malformed, extra, or too few digits; simian crease; and abnormally formed limbs. Other patients will have a history of malformed internal organs. Such children often have a history of delayed motor and language development, cognitive impairments, and behavioral problems.

6 The **heart, lungs, and abdomen** must always be examined. A cardiac murmur, while often "innocent," may result from a congenital heart defect that is associated with neurological or behavioral problems (in cases of Williams syndrome, for example) or could be a source for cerebral emboli predisposing to stroke. Hepatosplenomegaly is a rare but important finding that, to a pediatric neurologist, suggests a lysosomal storage disease.

7 **Signs of a congenital spinal defect** (tuft of hair, lipoma, and sacral dimple) are especially important if the presenting complaint is an abnormal gait or loss of sphincter control. These *external stigmata of spina bifida* are also often noted in asymptomatic patients, and an approach to diagnostic testing is suggested in Chapter 11.

8 **Orthopedic abnormalities** (e.g., scoliosis, lordosis, or pes cavus) can be an early sign of a *spinal tumor* or a *progressive neuromuscular disease* such as Charcot-Marie-Tooth disease. Spinal deformities also develop in the later stages of Rett syndrome, muscular dystrophy, and other degenerative disorders.

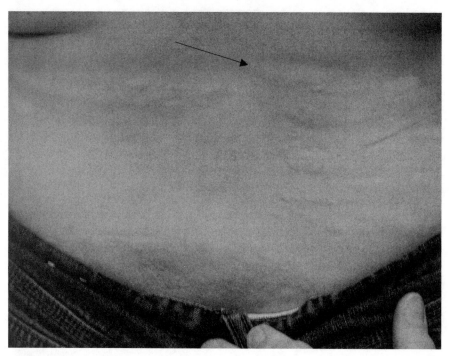

Figure 1.3 Tuberous sclerosis: large hyperpigmented lumbar shagreen patches and hypopigmented macules (*arrow*).

9 **Asymmetrical development of the extremities** can be a sign of an underlying neurodevelopmental or acquired disorder. Potentially significant signs include leg-length discrepancy, atrophy of muscles in one extremity or on one side of the body, and asymmetry of digits.

10 **Nuchal rigidity** is assessed in cases of headache. If the neck of an older child, teenager, or adult flexes easily and without pain, meningitis or subarachnoid hemorrhage is *unlikely* to be the diagnosis. If there is resistance to neck flexion, however, other *tests of meningeal irritation* should be performed. *Kernig sign* is a reflexive *flexion of the thigh* by the *patient* to relieve pain caused by *flexion of the neck* by the *examiner*, and *Brudzinski sign* is *pain* elicited by *extension of the leg* after the *thigh is first flexed* to 45 degrees above the horizontal (all by the examiner).

It is important to be aware that *these signs of meningeal irritation often cannot be elicited from infants less than 1 year of age, when neck and axial muscles are not well developed. Therefore, the diagnosis of meningitis in an infant cannot be excluded by the finding of a supple neck.*

11 The examination of the patient with a **history of headaches** must always include **inspection of the optic fundi** to make certain that there is not papilledema. In cases of headache, maxillary sinus (and frontal sinus, in adolescents) *tenderness to percussion* also should be assessed. The examiner may listen over the orbits and mastoids for a *cranial bruit* caused by an arteriovenous malformation (AVM). In many cases, however, cranial bruits are benign.

12 If the patient has had a **head injury**, the cranium should be palpated for signs of a skull fracture (marked tenderness, swelling, step-off). The examiner should recognize the **signs of a basilar skull fracture**: purplish *"raccoon eyes,"* discoloration over the mastoids (*Battle sign*), and *blood behind the tympanic membrane.* A *cerebrospinal fluid leak* is suggested by a complaint of fluid dripping from the nose or ears. Cerebrospinal fluid, and not nasal mucus, will give a positive result for glucose when tested with a urine dipstick.

13 In cases of **back injury** or **back pain**, the *straight leg-raising test* is used to help determine whether there is nerve root involvement (*radiculopathy*). With the patient supine, the lower extremity is passively elevated to 45 degrees above the horizontal. An increase in pain, especially pain radiating to the lower extremity, caused by this maneuver suggests nerve root involvement. In contrast, a fracture of a lumbar vertebra will often cause pain or tenderness that is exaggerated by *spinal percussion* and that often does not radiate to the thigh or leg.

NEUROLOGICAL EXAMINATION

The standard neurological examination is divided into six parts: *behavioral/ mental status, cranial nerves, motor system, reflexes, sensory system, and cerebellar system* (1).

The neurological examination should be a useful means of exploring the differential diagnosis and not a tedious chore. Therefore, we suggest a **concise version of the examination**, which is adequate for many situations, as well as (in some cases in later chapters) suggestions and indications for a more **comprehensive assessment**. We suggest that the examiner think carefully about the differential diagnosis, **use parts of the concise examination to evaluate aspects of the nervous system unlikely to be involved, and perform a comprehensive examination when appropriate.**

BEHAVIOR

Concise assessment

The patient's **level of consciousness** (alert, drowsy, lethargic, obtunded, unresponsive), **affect** (calm, agitated, distractible, hyperactive, depressed, anxious, hostile, etc.), **social interactiveness** (presence of eye contact, quality of interaction with the examiner and parents), and **language skills** (direction following ability; comprehension; speech quantity, content, and articulation) are always assessed. Observation and conversation are often an adequate assessment, especially if the parent or patient has no specific complaint of a cognitive or behavioral problem.

More comprehensive assessment

A more comprehensive behavioral/cognitive assessment is necessary in the case of a patient referred for a **developmental, behavioral, or school-related problem**. In cases of **head injury** or **change in mental status** and if there has been general neurological deterioration, the patient's cognitive status is of primary importance. Chapters 3, 5, 9, and 12 offer guidelines for a cognitive, learning, and mental status assessment.

If the examiner suspects that a toddler is *late to develop speech*, the child's *hearing* must be assessed. This must be done by means of formal audiometric testing. In many other cases, delayed speech is an *early sign of autism*. *Speech apraxia* is a general term for difficulty articulating sounds. It is a fairly common developmental problem that is often associated with other neurodevelopmental delays and sometimes behavioral problems. *Dysarthric* (uncoordinated) speech is noted in cases of cerebellar disease; it is an *acquired* problem in most cases. *Aphasia* is an acquired language disorder that is caused by an injury to the cerebral cortex, usually in the left hemisphere, and that is rarely diagnosed in children and adolescents.

CRANIAL NERVES

Concise assessment for children and adolescents

For patients who appear generally well and have no focal neurological complaints or signs, the cranial nerve examination can be limited to **pupillary reaction to light, the optic fundus, eye movements through all gaze positions, and assessment of facial, palatal, and tongue movement**. This series of tests should take only a few moments for the experienced doctor. However, the funduscopic examination may require practice before it can be done quickly and accurately. At a minimum, the physician should learn to assess the optic disc and vessels for signs of papilledema, identify a macular cherry red spot, and recognize retinal hemorrhages. Until the physician has become proficient, it is suggested that a funduscopic examination be practiced in every case, even if the patient is being evaluated for a nonneurological complaint.

More comprehensive cranial nerve assessment

If the presenting complaint involves **vision, facial weakness, or swallowing**; if any **focal neurological signs are noted during the rest of the examination**; or if there has been **general neurological deterioration**, a more comprehensive assessment of the cranial nerves becomes necessary.

The visual fields are evaluated by confrontation testing, and visual acuity is assessed with a vision card ("near card") held at about 14 inches from the patient. The near card tests the integrity of the *neurological systems* underlying vision (pathway leading from the retina to the occipital lobes) and not the patient's visual acuity. If the patient complains of *double vision* but the extraocular movements appear normal, the *reflection of a pocket light off the right and left cornea* should be checked for symmetry in all gaze positions. *Double vision always results from misalignment of the two eyes.* The reflection of the light should be symmetrical (with respect to the midpoint of the pupils) in all gaze positions. **Double vision is one of the more potentially serious symptoms in neurology and always merits close attention. If the extraocular movements appear disconjugate or the corneal light reflex is asymmetric, an MRI should be ordered to look for a brainstem, cranial nerve, or orbital tumor unless an ophthalmological cause has been established.**

If there is a recent history of weakness of *all the muscles of one side of the face, Bell palsy* is almost always the cause. The patient with Bell palsy *should not be able to raise her eyebrow* on the side of the palsy. A cerebral hemispheric lesion, in contrast to Bell palsy, causes *paresis of only the lower half of the face* (see Chapter 14) as well as, in the majority of cases, *weakness of the hand or arm* on the same side as facial weakness.

Asymmetric movements of the palate and tongue are rarely noted in children. When present, these findings suggest a brainstem lesion and are an indication for MRI.

In the older child or teenager, hearing is tested if there is a complaint of *hearing loss, ringing in the ears, or vertigo.* Office tests that may better define the hearing problem are reviewed in Chapter 14. In cases of suspected hearing loss, formal audiometric testing is necessary. Unilateral hearing loss is rare but should raise the possibility of a vestibular neuroma, usually a manifestation of neurofibromatosis type II (see Chapter 14).

Cranial nerve examination in younger patients

The cranial nerve examination of infants, toddlers, and young or uncooperative children primarily relies on **observation.** The physician can assess the extraocular movements as the child looks about the room or follows a light and the movements of the face, tongue, and uvula when the child smiles or cries. When it is difficult to observe how the pupils react to light (as when the patient has dark irises), examination with a flashlight in a dark room is often successful. Visual fields can be assessed by bringing novel objects slowly from behind the patient's head across the child's field of vision, first on one side and then the other. Another method may be by simultaneously bringing similar objects in each of the examiner's hands into the child's peripheral field of vision. A child with intact visual fields would look at one and then the other object.

The examiner must possess considerable skill if he wishes to properly examine the optic fundus of an infant or toddler. In practice, the "funduscopic" examination of these patients is often limited to checking for the red reflex. If the examiner is lucky, he will glimpse the optic disc. The patient should be referred to an ophthalmologist for a dilated funduscopic examination if the presence of a macular cherry red spot needs to be determined (as in the case of a degenerative disorder), if retinal hemorrhages are suspected, or if the infant has a problem involving vision.

MOTOR SYSTEM

Concise assessment for children and adolescents

A thorough motor examination is always indicated if the presenting complaint involves strength, coordination, or gait; if focal neurological symptoms are reported or focal signs are noted on examination; or in cases of general neurological deterioration.

In many other cases, however, such as when the patient comes to the office because of a school or behavioral problem, syncope, or migraine, the motor examination is *unlikely* to contribute to the diagnosis. In such cases, it is reasonable to make the motor examination concise, concentrate on more relevant aspect of the examination, and leave plenty of time for a talk with the family.

A **concise motor examination** should include **biceps and grip strength**; ability to **stand, walk, toe and heel walk, jump or hop, and run**; and observation for abnormal posturing. Resistance to passive limb movement, or **muscle tone**, should also be noted. An adequate evaluation of *fine motor ability* in such cases is accomplished by asking the patient to wiggle the fingers of both hands ("play the piano"), rapidly touch the index finger and thumb together, and "walk" his or her hand rapidly across the table top using the index and middle fingers. The young patient should be asked to perform these movements with both hands simultaneously and each hand independently. Fine motor testing often will demonstrate "soft signs" (see Soft Signs section) in developmentally delayed children. *Pencil skills* are evaluated, when necessary, by asking the patient to write a few sentences about a subject of her or the examiner's choice. *Left handedness* is often relevant to the diagnosis of learning disability and should be noted.

If there is no complaint of weakness or incoordination and these tests reveal no abnormality, further testing of the motor system is often unnecessary, and the examiner may feel comfortable moving to the next phase of the examination.

More comprehensive motor assessment

If the primary complaint is weakness, a problem walking, or incoordination or if there are focal complaints or signs, a more comprehensive motor evaluation becomes necessary. In these cases, the power of the trapezius (shoulder shrug), sternocleidomastoid (turning of the head), deltoid (abduction of the arm at the shoulder), biceps (flexion of the forearm), triceps (extension of the forearm), wrist flexors and extensors, and hand intrinsic muscles should be tested. In the *pronator drift test*, the patient is asked to extend both arms with palms facing upwards and eyes closed. If one arm drifts downward and pronates, weakness on that side is suggested. Asking the patient to shake his head from side to side as if saying "no" may elicit pronator drift if it does not occur with eye closure alone.

Power of the psoas (hip flexion) and gluteus (hip extension), hamstrings (leg flexion) and quadriceps (leg extension), tibialis anterior (dorsiflexion of the foot) and gastrocnemius (plantar flexion), and the extensors and inverters and everters of the foot should be assessed with the patient lying in the supine position.

The standard grading scale for muscle power is:

0/5—no movement of the muscle tested
1/5—trace movement of the muscle
2/5—insufficient power to overcome gravity
3/5—power sufficient to overcome gravity but not resistance from the examiner
4/5—power that can overcome gravity and some resistance from the examiner
5/5—full power

Pluses and minuses (e.g., 4+, 5−) are often added for the sake of nuance but are of little value unless an examiner is doing serial assessments for his own record and comparison.

Testing for a *Gower sign*, suggesting *hip and thigh muscle weakness* typical in cases of *myopathy*, should be included if there is a history of a delay in or regression of motor development. A *Gower sign* means that a patient can only transition from a sitting position on the floor to a standing position by *using his arms* to help push off the floor and straighten his torso. **As a general rule, *diseases of muscle produce proximal weakness* (of the shoulders, hips, and thighs), whereas *diseases of the nerve cause distal weakness* (of the hands, legs, and feet).**

Soft signs

A pediatric neurologist always keeps an eye out for **"soft signs"** when he examines young children. The finding of a soft sign *never identifies a specific disorder* but does suggest general neurodevelopmental delay or immaturity. Children exhibiting soft signs often have a history of premature birth, delayed motor or language milestones, or neurobehavioral problems. Commonly noted soft signs include: (a) *clumsy fine finger movements*; (b) *spread* (e.g., the entire upper extremity moves during an attempted movement of only the hand); (c) *mirror movement* (unintentional movement of the opposite hand or arm when the child makes a hand or arm movement, such as waving goodbye); (d) *overflow* (an unrelated body part, such as the tongue, moves during a hand movement); and (e) *clumsiness while hopping or running*. Marked *asymmetry* of soft signs, although rare, should be noted because this finding is equivalent to a focal neurological sign and may suggest a structural abnormality in the brain.

Gait

The assessment of gait is a very important part of the neurological examination. A normal gait usually is evidence of adequate lower extremity strength and coordination, although subtle lower extremity weakness may only be evident when the patient rises from a chair, climbs stairs, or tries to jump or hop. Typical **pathological gait patterns** should be recognized. A *circumducting gait* often accompanies *spastic hemiparesis or paraparesis* (as in cases of cerebral palsy or prior stroke); a *slap-foot gait* is usually caused by *neuropathy* (e.g., Charcot-Marie-Tooth disease); a *waddling gait* is a sign of *myopathy* (e.g., muscular dystrophy); and an *ataxic gait* suggests a *disease of the cerebellum*.

A *clumsy gait* in a young child is often a sign of nonspecific and ultimately benign developmental motor delay; this diagnosis should be suspected if the child's gait has always been clumsy and there is no history of regression of motor skills. An *antalgic* gait refers to gait or posture assumed in order to lessen or avoid pain due to muscle, joint, bone, or other organ disease. In a toddler or young child, this may not clearly appear as a limp. The child will try movements that will minimize the weight applied to the affected limb or joint and the amount of time that weight is placed on the limb. This is often mistaken as a sign of weakness rather than of pain.

An odd-appearing gait that does not correspond to one of the previously mentioned patterns is often *psychogenic (hysterical gait)*. *Ataxia abasia (lunging from side to side)*, a psychogenic gait, is often mistaken for true ataxia.

The *tightness of the heel cords* should be checked if a toddler walks clumsily or frequently falls. The examiner should be able to dorsiflex the foot to about *10 degrees above the horizontal*. Tight heel cords, preventing dorsiflexion of the foot, are commonly noted in cases of cerebral palsy (see Chapter 10) and can be the only abnormal finding in mild cases. Tight heel cords also can result from muscular dystrophy and other neuromuscular disorders (e.g., Charcot-Marie-Tooth disease) but are not an early sign of these diseases, and unlike in cerebral palsy, the deep tendon reflexes are often decreased rather than increased.

Children with tight heel cords often *walk on their tiptoes. Toe walking not caused by tight heel cords* is a common *habit* of children with *autism*, but it is also often a habit of normal children.

Motor assessment of the infant and toddler

The evaluation of the motor system in infants and very young children is, again, largely based on observation. The young infant should move all four extremities equally and, when older, should use either hand to reach for and manipulate objects. The gait of young children should be symmetrical, and

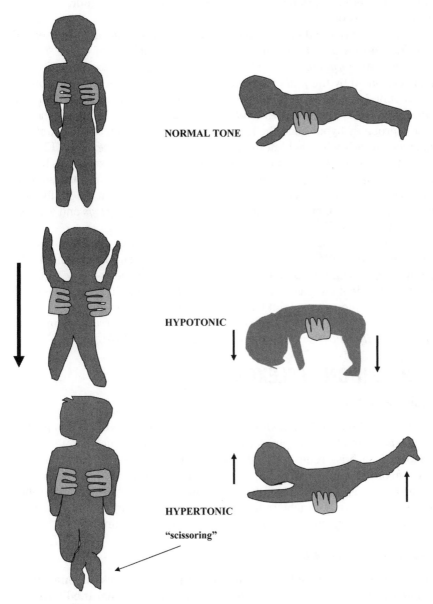

Figure 1.4 Vertical and horizontal suspension tests.

use of the hands should be symmetrical as well, although preferential use of the right hand often develops by about 3 years of age.

The history of infants should always include a *developmental assessment* of the age at which head control and ability to roll over, sit, and pull to a standing position were achieved. The toddler should learn to walk by 16 months of age and to run by 2–3 years of age. However, it is important to recognize that there is considerable variability in the ages at which normal children achieve their motor milestones.

Both axial (truncal) and extremity muscle tone should be assessed in the neonate and infant. The examiner seeks evidence of either *"floppiness,"* suggesting *hypotonia*, or *stiffness*, suggesting *hypertonicity*. Truncal tone is evaluated by the *pull-to-sit* maneuver, in which the infant lying on his back is pulled gently by his hands so that his back and head no longer rest on the table. If this demonstrates *head-lag* at an age of more than 2 months, the infant is probably hypotonic. The hypotonic infant will often *slip through the examiner's hands* when held in the position of *vertical suspension* (Fig. 1.4; the infant is held in a vertical position, supported only by the examiner's fingers under the axillae) or *"drape"* when held in *horizontal suspension* (the infant is supported only by the examiner's hand under the abdomen). In cases of hypertonicity, the same maneuvers often produce *scissoring of the legs* and *arching of the neck and back*.

Passive movements of the limbs evaluate *muscle tone in the extremities*. Hypotonic limbs offer decreased resistance to movement; hypertonic limbs are stiff. *Spasticity*, which is noted in most cases of hypertonicity, refers to velocity-dependent increased muscle tone and a "clasp-knife" response when an extremity is moved at a joint (for example, during elbow flexion).

The examiner should be aware that *extremity tone and truncal tone may differ markedly in the same patient* (see Chapters 8 and 10).

DEEP TENDON REFLEXES

Concise assessment

A brisk or diminished deep tendon reflex is rarely the only sign of a neurological disease. Therefore, the physician should not fret too much about a single hard-to-elicit or brisk reflex when the patient does not describe and/or has no other sign of a motor, sensory, gait, or balance problem. The reflex examination also can be concise in these cases; the examiner may test one deep tendon reflex in each extremity (e.g., brachioradialis in the upper extremity and quadriceps in the lower extremity) and move to another phase of the examination.

More comprehensive assessment

In the case of a patient with a focal motor deficit or marked generalized weakness, the examination of deep tendon reflexes combined with the motor examination helps to localize the disorder to the brain; cervical, thoracic or lumbar spinal cord; nerve; or muscle. The biceps, triceps, brachioradialis, quadriceps, ankle, and plantar reflexes should be tested in these cases. A *crossed adductor reflex* (percussion of the medial thigh causing adduction of the opposite thigh) is sometimes elicited in cases of a lesion in the brainstem or cervical or thoracic spinal cord. *Clonus* is a self-sustaining deep tendon reflex, most often obtained at the ankle, suggesting spasticity or an upper motor neuron lesion (see next section).

The standard grading scale for deep tendon reflexes is:

0—no obtainable reflex.
Tr.—trace reflex
1—low normal reflex
2—normal reflex
3—brisk reflex
4—clonus
5—sustained clonus (not always used)

Once again, pluses and minuses are often added (e.g., 1+) but are of limited usefulness.

A *Babinski sign* (upgoing toe and fanning of the other toes on one foot elicited by gently stroking the sole) suggests an upper motor neuron disease (see next section) but is a normal finding in a young infant.

Primitive reflexes (Moro, grasp, tonic neck, stepping, placing, and parachute reflexes) should be assessed in the infant. It is often easier to elicit a grasp reflex or an asymmetric or obligate tonic neck reflex than to elicit deep tendon reflexes in a crying inconsolable infant or toddler. *Asymmetry* of a primitive reflex, especially the Moro reflex, suggests focal weakness, as in the case of a hemispheric lesion or Erb palsy. The *delayed appearance* of a primitive reflex or the *persistence* of a primitive reflex as an infant grows older is associated with syndromes of *developmental delay or regression.*

PUTTING THE EXAMINATION TOGETHER: UPPER AND LOWER MOTOR NEURON SYNDROMES

The cell body of an *upper motor neuron* is a tiny part of the *motor cortex* of a cerebral hemisphere (Fig. 1.5). The axon of this cell travels caudally (downwards) through the cerebral white matter into the brainstem, *crosses the midline* in the medulla, and joins the *corticospinal tract*. The distal end of the axon synapses on a spinal *anterior horn cell*. The anterior horn cell, or *lower motor neuron*, sends its axon, as part of a *motor nerve* that does not cross the midline, to supply a *muscle*. *Cervical* anterior horn cells project

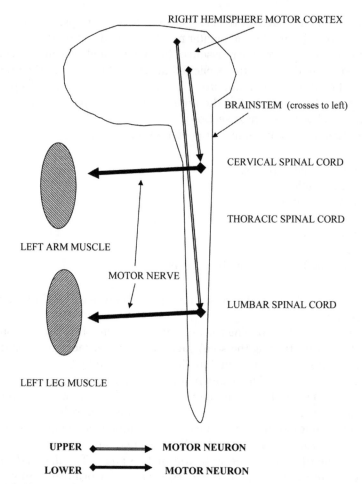

Figure 1.5 Upper and lower motor neurons.

to muscles in the *upper extremity,* and *lumbar* anterior horn cells project to muscles in the *lower extremity.*

Diseases (e.g., stroke, cervical or thoracic tumor) affecting the **upper motor neuron ultimately cause weakness, spasticity, and exaggerated deep tendon reflexes**. Examples would include the paretic, spastic, and hyperreflexic left arm and leg of a patient who has a history of a stroke or tumor in the right cerebral hemisphere (Fig. 1.6) and the paretic, spastic, and hyperreflexic left leg of a patient who has a tumor compressing the left side of the thoracic spinal cord (Fig. 1.7). (Note that these signs are contralateral in cases of a lesion above the brainstem and ipsilateral in cases of a spinal cord lesion. This is because the upper motor neuron crosses the midline in the medulla.)

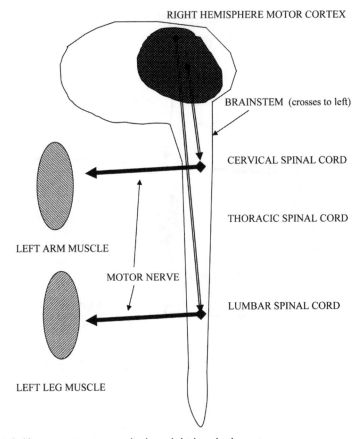

RIGHT HEMISPHERE MOTOR CORTEX

BRAINSTEM (crosses to left)

CERVICAL SPINAL CORD

THORACIC SPINAL CORD

LEFT ARM MUSCLE

MOTOR NERVE

LUMBAR SPINAL CORD

LEFT LEG MUSCLE

Figure 1.6 Upper motor neuron lesion: right hemisphere tumor.
Patient has left hemiparesis (arm and leg) with spasticity and brisk deep tendon reflexes.

The physician should be aware that **an upper motor neuron syndrome usually takes several weeks to develop following an acute neurologic event**; in the interim, there may be *decreased* tone and *diminished* reflexes in the affected limb. For example, a patient with a stroke may initially present with flaccid left hemiparesis, which evolves over the course of a month into spastic left hemiparesis.

In contrast, diseases of the **lower motor neuron** cause **weakness, decreased muscle tone, and diminished reflexes.** These signs are **present immediately following an injury and persist indefinitely**. The site of the lesion may be the anterior horn cell body (i.e., the spinal cord), the motor nerve root, the nerve, or the neuromuscular junction. Typical presentations would include the flaccid lower extremities of a child with a history of lumbar meningomyelocele (Fig. 1.8), the weakness and areflexia associated with Guillain-Barré syndrome (Fig. 1.9), and the flaccid arm of a baby born with a brachial plexus injury (Erb palsy; Fig. 1.10).

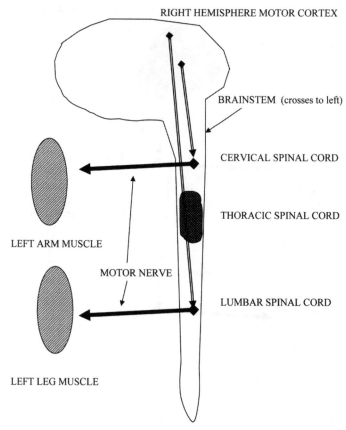

Figure 1.7 Upper motor neuron lesion: tumor compressing left side of spinal cord.
Patient has weakness of left lower extremity with spasticity, brisk reflexes. Upper extremity unaffected.

SENSORY EXAMINATION

In many cases, the sensory portion of the neurological examination can simply be omitted. Certainly, a time-consuming sensory examination is almost never a necessary part of the evaluation of a patient who has a nonfocal disorder such as tension-type headaches and ADHD. In such cases, the physician's time is better spent obtaining a more complete history, concentrating on more relevant aspects of the physical examination, and discussing the diagnosis with the family and answering their questions.

When and how to perform a sensory examination

When a child or adolescent patient reports persistent sensory loss or paresthesias (tingling or burning), these symptoms should be taken seriously because they are relatively unusual complaints at this age. *Persistent sensory complaints often are caused by neuropathy; less often, they are the result*

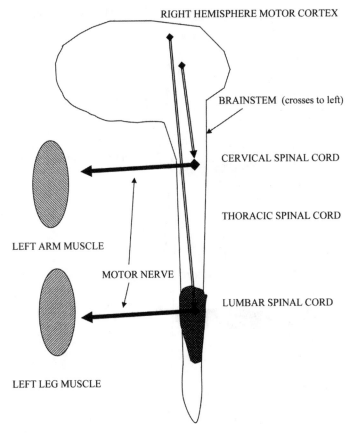

Figure 1.8 Lower motor neuron lesion: meningomyelocele.
Patient has flaccid weakness of lower extremities and diminished reflexes.

of a mass lesion or demyelination in the brain or spinal cord. (Transient sensory symptoms are often related to migraine headaches and, less often, to focal seizures.) Other complaints that suggest the need for a sensory examination include unexplained focal or generalized weakness, loss of the ability to walk, incontinence, and pain that radiates to an upper or lower extremity.

The physician should test pin sensitivity (perception of a mildly painful stimulus such as the sharp edge of a broken tongue depressor), light touch sensitivity, and vibration sensitivity in the area in which the patient reports an abnormal sensation. The patient's perception of the same stimulus is then assessed in areas in which he or she reports no abnormal symptoms. A *"sensory level"* (dermatome below which sensory changes are noted) should be sought and, if identified, suggests a disease of the *spinal cord*; the sensory level will help localize where along the length of the spinal cord the etiologic lesion may be. Diseases of the *peripheral nerves* are associated with a *stocking-glove* pattern of sensory loss. Sensory loss *in one arm or leg suggests* a localized peripheral nerve injury or disease (*mononeuropathy*) or *nerve root involvement,*

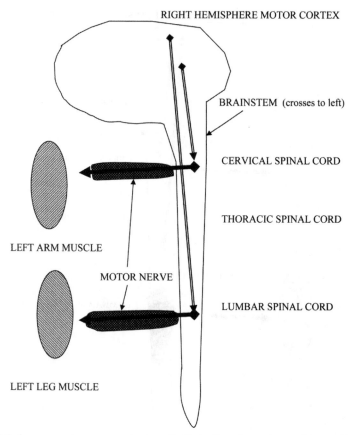

RIGHT HEMISPHERE MOTOR CORTEX

BRAINSTEM (crosses to left)

CERVICAL SPINAL CORD

THORACIC SPINAL CORD

LEFT ARM MUSCLE

MOTOR NERVE

LUMBAR SPINAL CORD

LEFT LEG MUSCLE

Figure 1.9 Lower motor neuron lesion: Guillain-Barré syndrome (demyelination of motor nerves).
Patient has flaccid weakness of arms and legs and diminished reflexes.

especially if accompanied by *pain in the same limb. Hemisensory loss* (decreased sensation on one side of the body) is a rare complaint in children, suggesting a *thalamic or spinal cord lesion.*

A *positive Romberg sign* means that a patient cannot maintain balance when standing with his or her eyes closed and arms outstretched in front. The Romberg sign is a sign of *a sensory deficit (loss of proprioception), not of a cerebellar disease.* It is sometimes noted in cases of neuropathy or spinal cord disease.

CEREBELLAR TESTS

The primary function of the cerebellum is to coordinate movements of the body. Basic clinical tests of coordination include the *finger-to-nose-to-finger test* (the patient is asked to touch his nose, then the examiner's finger,

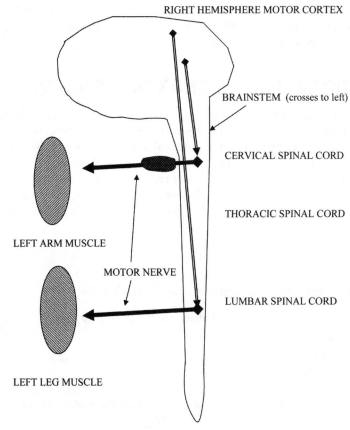

RIGHT HEMISPHERE MOTOR CORTEX

BRAINSTEM (crosses to left)

CERVICAL SPINAL CORD

THORACIC SPINAL CORD

LEFT ARM MUSCLE

MOTOR NERVE

LUMBAR SPINAL CORD

LEFT LEG MUSCLE

Figure 1.10 Lower motor neuron lesion: Erb palsy.
Patient has flaccid weakness of left arm with diminished reflexes caused by injury to left brachial plexus.

and then his nose again) and *tandem gait assessment* (heel-toe walk), both of which should be included in the evaluation of all patients old enough to cooperate. A test of *rapid alternating movement* (tapping the back and palm of the hand, alternately, against the thigh) also evaluates coordination. The *heel-to-shin test* (the patient, seated or lying on his back, glides his heel along his shin from the knee to the ankle, keeping the heel along the midline) is often added in cases of suspected cerebellar disease.

Abnormal cerebellar findings include *intention tremor, ataxia (uncoordinated arm movements or unsteady gait)*, and *nystagmus*. Nystagmus (varieties of which are discussed in Chapter 14) is an involuntary rhythmic movement of the eyes that may result from ocular, cerebellar, vestibular, and brainstem disease, as well as *drug toxicity* (the most common cause). A few beats of *end-gaze nystagmus* (noted on full abduction of the eye) are a normal finding.

Observation of gait, posture, coordination of the hands during play and eye movements generally suffice to evaluate cerebellar function in toddlers and uncooperative young children.

FUNCTIONAL LOCALIZATION IN THE BRAIN

Many children seen for a neurological complaint do not have a localizable neurological lesion. In more serious cases, however, an understanding of patients' conditions is often enhanced by a practical knowledge of neuroanatomy and functional localization (Table 1.6). A brief summary follows.

The two *cerebral hemispheres* comprise the *cerebral cortex* or outer *gray matter*, the underlying cerebral *white matter*, and the deep gray matter nuclei of the *limbic system* and the *basal ganglia*. The *cell bodies of neurons lie in*

TABLE 1.6

Common terms for and causes of motor and speech impairment

Term	Definition and most common causes[a]
-paresis (as in hemiparesis, monoparesis, etc.)	Weakness
-plegia (as in hemiplegia, monoplegia, etc.)	Paralysis
Monoparesis/monoplegia	Weakness/paralysis of one extremity; *brain lesion, spinal cord lesion, peripheral nerve injury*
Hemiparesis/hemiplegia	Weakness/paralysis of both extremities on one side of the body; *brain or cervical spinal lesion*
Diparesis/diplegia	Weakness/paralysis of both legs (usually) or both arms (rare); spastic diplegia from infancy is usually caused by *bilateral cerebral white matter injury* (see Chapter 10); acquired diplegia is usually a sign of *spinal cord disease*
Apraxia/dyspraxia	Difficulty planning/conceptualizing movements or speech; *usually developmental in young children and often improves over time*
Dysarthria	Incoordinated or slurred speech, usually acquired; *cerebellar disease*
Aphasia	Acquired speech disorder; *cerebral cortex lesion*; rare in children
Ataxia	Motor incoordination; *cerebellar or spinal cord lesion, peripheral nerve disease, drug intoxication, or medication overdose*

[a] Most common causes are italicized.

the gray matter, and their *axons and dendrites, together with supporting cells, make up the white matter.*

The *frontal lobes* primarily are responsible for *voluntary movements* and the *planning and initiation of movements.* The *basal ganglia* are a group of deep gray matter structures found primarily in the frontal lobes that play a critical role in the *execution and refinement of voluntary movements.* The left frontal lobe (in right-handed people) contains *Broca's speech area.* The most anterior parts of the frontal lobes (prefrontal lobes) are thought to mediate *motivation, inhibition,* and other important aspects of *behavior.* The *temporal lobes* contain the primary *auditory areas* of the cortex; the left temporal lobe is especially important for *receptive language* (auditory comprehension). The temporal lobes also contain many parts of the *limbic system* that are important for *emotional responses* and *memory.* The *parietal lobes* contain the *somatosensory areas* of the cortex. The left parietal lobe also plays an important role in *comprehension and speech formulation,* whereas the right parietal lobe mediates *visual-perceptual functions* such as shape and pattern recognition and spatial orientation. The *occipital lobes* contain the primary visual areas of the brain and are almost exclusively devoted to visual processing.

The *cerebral white matter* is made up of axons and dendrites, which is the "wiring" that interconnects areas of the cortex and also connects these areas to deeper brain structures, including the basal ganglia, limbic system, thalamus, brainstem, and spinal cord. The white matter is "white" because of the presence of *myelin,* which is the fatty coating on axons that allows for efficient neural transmission. The *corpus callosum* is the white matter pathway that allows for communication between the two cerebral hemispheres.

The *thalamus* functions as a *relay station* linking the brain, brainstem, cerebellum, and spinal cord. It is subdivided into a number of *thalamic nuclei,* each with a specific set of connections. The nearby *hypothalamus* is a smaller group of nuclei that are important for *body temperature regulation, thirst,* and *hunger* and that make *releasing factors,* which regulate the functions of the *pituitary gland.*

The *brainstem, including the midbrain, pons, and medulla,* contains the nuclei of most of the *cranial nerves.* The *midbrain* contains the nuclei of cranial nerve III, which mediate *pupillary constriction* and *vertical eye movements. Horizontal eye movements* are synchronized in the *pons.* Therefore, *midbrain lesions* tend to cause a disruption of *vertical eye movements,* whereas *pontine lesions* disrupt *horizontal eye movements.* The nuclei of cranial nerve V (facial sensation, jaw movements) are distributed widely from the midbrain through the pons and medulla. The nuclei of cranial nerves VI (abduction of the eye) and VII (facial muscles, taste, salivation, other functions) lie mostly in the pons. Cranial nerve nuclei (VIII) mediating *hearing and balance* are found in the rostral portion of the *medulla.* The caudal medulla contains the nuclei of cranial nerves IX, X, XI, and XII, which primarily mediate *taste, salivation, tongue and palatal movements,* and the movements of muscles within the *larynx.*

TABLE 1.7
Localization of function in the brain

Brain region(s)	Primary functions	Most common result of lesion
Frontal lobes	Planning, inhibition, execution of voluntary *movements*; in left hemisphere, contains Broca's *speech* area; prefrontal lobes important in *personality*	*Hemiparesis* on opposite side; expressive *aphasia* (left frontal lesion); *changes in personality* (disinhibited or "flat affect"); focal motor *seizures*
Parietal lobes	*Somatic sensation*; left hemisphere lobe important for *language*, right hemisphere lobe important for *visual-spatial* skills; visual fibers pass through both parietal lobes	*Sensory loss* (usually subtle); *aphasia* (left parietal lesion); loss of visual-spatial abilities (right hemisphere lesion); visual field loss due to interruption of tracts to occipital lobe; sensory *seizures*
Temporal lobes	*Auditory* function; left hemisphere lobe important for receptive language; temporal lobes contain limbic system structures (*emotion and memory*); visual fibers pass through temporal lobes	Receptive *aphasia* (left temporal lesion); changes in *emotion, personality, and memory*; visual field loss due to interruption of tracts to occipital lobe; complex partial *seizures*
Occipital lobes	*Visual* cortex	*Loss of a visual field*; partial *seizures* with visual symptoms
Cerebral white matter	Myelinated connections between cortical areas, to thalamus and other subcortical nuclei, and to the spinal cord	*Spasticity* and *cognitive slowing* are most common, but signs and symptoms are variable; *seizures do not occur*
Basal ganglia	Initiation and refinement of *movements*	*Movement disorders*: parkinsonism, rigidity, tremor, chorea, and dystonia; *seizures do not occur*
Brainstem	Contains *cranial nerve nuclei*; respiratory center; many long tracts pass through or synapse; reticular formation	Double vision, difficulty swallowing, facial weakness or sensory loss, ataxia, spasticity, hemiparesis; respiratory arrest; *seizures do not occur*

Brain region(s)	Primary functions	Most common result of lesion
Thalamus	*Relay station* for ascending, descending, and intracerebral pathways; involved in maintenance of alertness	Variable depending on part affected; large lesions often cause obtundation or coma; *seizures do not occur*
Cerebellum	*Coordination* of movements and gait	Gait and limb *ataxia*; nystagmus; *seizures do not occur*

The brainstem also contains the *reticular formation*, which is important for maintaining general *alertness*, and nuclei that secrete the neurotransmitter serotonin (*raphe nucleus*) and norepinephrine (*locus ceruleus*). The *pons and medulla* together initiate and coordinate *respiration*. Many *long tracts* to and from the cerebral cortex, thalamus, cerebellum, and spinal cord pass through or synapse in the brainstem.

The *cerebellum* is primarily responsible for *motor coordination*. It has connections to the spinal cord and many other parts of the brain, including the brainstem, thalamus, and cerebral hemispheres.

The effect of a lesion in each of these areas of the brain is summarized in Table 1.7. It is also useful to know which of these parts of the brain, when injured, may give rise to an epileptic seizure, and this is also noted in Table 1.7. Finally, it should be kept in mind that young children tend to recover from brain injuries better than older children, adolescents, and adults and that focal symptoms and signs are often less pronounced in the younger age group, especially months or years after a stroke or neurological trauma.

REFERENCES

1. Haerer AF. *DeJong's The Neurological Examination*. Philadelphia: Lippincott; 1992.
2. Pincus JH. Neurologic meaning of soft signs. In: Lewis M, ed. *Child and Adolescent Psychiatry*. Philadelphia: Lippincott; 2002:573–581.

2

HEADACHE

Many children and teenagers suffer from headaches that also cause their parents and doctor to worry. Parents may fear a serious cause because they do not know how common headaches are in the pediatric population. Doctors tend to worry because, during their residency, they saw many patients with headaches caused by a brain tumor or an equally serious disease.

Although headaches cause a great deal of suffering and disrupt our patients' lives, they fortunately result from a serious underlying condition in a relatively small percentage of cases. *Migraine headaches, tension-type headaches, medication-overuse headaches, headaches following a head*

TABLE 2.1

General frequency of causes and types of headache in children and adolescents

Common	Uncommon to rare
Tension-type headache	Sinusitis
Migraine and variants	Viral meningitis
General medical condition (infection, postviral syndrome, etc.)	Bacterial meningitis
	Lyme meningitis
Medication-overuse headache	Postlumbar puncture headache
Concussion, neck sprain, and postconcussive syndrome	Brain tumor and other malignancies
	Brain abscess
	Pseudotumor cerebri
	Subarachnoid hemorrhage
	Arteriovenous malformation
	Chiari I malformation
	Cluster headache
	Temporomandibular joint syndrome
	Hypertension
	Venous sinus thrombosis

Case 2.1

An 8-year-old girl is brought to the doctor's office because of headaches. For the last year she has been complaining of a headache several times a week. Her headaches mostly occur on school days but have not been severe enough to cause her to miss school. She rarely mentions having a headache during weekends or vacations. She has never had a headache that awakened her from sleep. When asked, she does not recall where her head usually hurts.

There is no history of nausea, vomiting, photophobia, visual distortions, or any other unusual symptoms. The patient's general health has been good. Her parents do mention that she is anxious about her schoolwork and has had trouble learning mathematics.

She presents as quiet and shy. The general physical examination reveals a supple neck and normal-appearing optic fundi. No rash, sinus tenderness, evidence of joint swelling, or adenopathy is noted. Her neurological examination reveals no focal deficits.

An office cognitive assessment demonstrates grade-level reading ability. However, the patient has trouble interpreting complex sentences, solving simple word problems, and subtracting two-digit numbers.

Diagnosis: *Tension-type headaches*; possible learning disability as an exacerbating factor.

Outcome: MRI was discussed with the parents but was deemed unnecessary since their daughter's headaches only occur when she is feeling stressed. She was referred for a psychoeducational evaluation and to a learning consultant. Her parents were told to treat the more severe headaches with ibuprofen, not to be given more than two to three times per week so as to prevent the development of medication-overuse headaches. At follow-up 3 months later, the child reports only occasional headaches. She in now in a special math and language class and making better progress.

injury, and *headaches due to a viral or postinfectious syndrome* account for the great majority of the headaches evaluated in the office and clinic (1,2). Pediatricians who want to manage headaches effectively should become well acquainted with these common syndromes and their treatment, while still remaining aware of the warning signs of more serious, rarer causes (Table 2.1).

WHAT CAUSES HEADACHES?

There are no sensory nerve endings in the brain. Therefore, brain tumors cause headaches only when they grow large enough to stretch the pain-sensitive cerebral blood vessels and meninges or when they obstruct the normal flow of cerebrospinal fluid and cause hydrocephalus. Many doctors nevertheless continue to send headache sufferers for a yearly magnetic resonance imaging (MRI) or computed tomography (CT) scan to search for a small brain tumor (thought to have been missed by a previous imaging study) that they believe has been causing the patient's headaches "all along." This practice is not based on a good understanding of the pathogenesis of headaches and, given the high cost of brain imaging studies as well as the possibility of unnecessary radiation exposure, should be discouraged.

The pathophysiology of the common headache syndromes remains less than satisfactorily elucidated. Migraine has been attributed to depression of cortical neuronal activity, the effect of neuropeptides within cerebral vasculature, cerebral arterial dilatation and spasm, and sporadic brainstem release of serotonin and norepinephrine (3,4). Branches of the trigeminal nerve mediate headache pain, and therefore, some theories suggest that trigeminal inflammation or excessive activity causes migraine (4). It is possible that the pathophysiology of migraine is not the same for all patients. The reader may wish to consult Ramadan's review of current theories (5). Other common headache syndromes are also not well understood. Cranial muscle contraction, which generations of neurology residents were taught causes tension-type headaches, is no longer considered to be of primary importance (6), and the pathophysiology of tension-type headache, a very common syndrome, remains largely unknown. Headaches often occur in association with common, self-limited infectious illnesses (viral syndromes), but despite their frequency, these headaches also have not been well explained.

ROLE OF IMAGING STUDIES

CT and MRI are useful to exclude the possibility that an intracranial mass lesion is causing a patient's headaches but are of little value in making the diagnosis of the more common headache syndromes. *The diagnosis of most causes of headache relies primarily on a **good history*** and is usually confirmed (often by an absence of abnormal findings) by the physical/neurologic examination.

THREE QUESTIONS TO ASK

The most important questions to ask while taking the history concern: (a) *when and how frequently the headaches occur;* (b) *how severe the headaches are;* and (c) *what symptoms accompany the headaches.* In many cases, the answers yield enough information to enable the physician to make the diagnosis (Table 2.2).

How often and when?

The ***pattern of occurrence*** of the headaches is important to note. *Episodic* headaches separated by periods of complete relief are usually *migraine* headaches. *Headaches accompanying the menstrual period* are also usually migrainous. Headaches reported by older children and adolescents *on school days, but not weekends or vacations* are almost always *tension-type headaches* exacerbated by stress. This is also generally true for young children, but unfortunately, these patients often cannot be relied upon to accurately report their symptoms and may be less aware of their headaches when they are playing than when they are in more stressful situations.

Headaches after a head injury are almost always a manifestation of *postconcussive syndrome. Chronic daily headaches* are often caused by *stress, overuse of an analgesic medication,* or a *general medical illness.* A *viral syndrome* often causes a complaint of *new-onset but persistent headaches* from a patient who never previously had headaches and may be suspected if the patient reports having had general medical symptoms (sore throat, myalgias, or generalized fatigue) before the headache appeared. Headaches that *awaken the patient from sleep* are often migrainous. However, *causes of raised intracranial pressure (tumor, etc.) must always be considered in the case of new-onset and nighttime-awakening or sleep-associated headaches.* Careful funduscopy should always be performed, and MRI or CT should be ordered if another cause cannot be determined.

The parent should be asked to keep a **headache diary** *if there is uncertainty about when and how often the headaches occur.*

How severe?

Asking a child to grade the severity of his headaches on a scale of 1 to 10 is asking for trouble. Few children (fortunately) know what really severe pain is like, and consequently, all headaches will be labeled as a "10." It is better to judge the severity of the headaches by **asking if the child misses enjoyable activities** because of his headaches. The young child who complains, "I have a headache" but continues to play happily can be safely assumed not to be in great distress. Most patients with a *tension-type headache recover after a brief period of rest* and are typically *able to participate in activities* even if they still have a headache. Headaches from increased intracranial pressure (ICP; pseudotumor cerebri and space-occupying lesions) also tend to be low grade and are typically chronic, although they usually gradually worsen and are associated with other neurological symptoms. In contrast, patients suffering from a *migraine* headache *usually need to sleep for hours to make their headache go away* and are forced to *miss even the most enjoyable activities.*

What symptoms accompany the headaches and persist between headaches?

Nausea, vomiting, sensitivity to bright light, and a variety of *transient neurological phenomena* (paresthesias, slurred speech, scotoma) are symptoms characteristic of *migraine* headaches. Headaches caused by a *systemic (usually infectious) illness* are associated with fatigue, malaise, myalgias, joint pain, fever, rash, and other *constitutional symptoms. Tension-type headaches and medication-overuse headaches* are typically *not* associated with other physical symptoms.

Headaches accompanied by one or more *persistent focal neurological symptoms*, a *stiff neck*, or a *change in the patient's personality or behavior* are cause for concern and are usually an indication for *MRI or lumbar puncture.*

Whether or not the *patient returns to "normal" between headaches* without any lingering complaints or signs is an important detail of the history. The patient with lingering complaints (of nausea, visual auras, paresthesias, etc., albeit milder) whose personality or behavior has changed or whose academic performance has inexplicably deteriorated should be given careful attention.

TWO LESS IMPORTANT QUESTIONS: WHERE DOES IT HURT, AND WHAT DOES IT FEEL LIKE?

The patient should of course be asked where his or her head usually hurts. However, the location of the headaches often is not that diagnostically important. Most children's migraine headaches are bilateral, generalized, or variable in location (in contrast to the classically one-sided migraine headaches reported by adults). Tension headaches, postconcussive headaches and viral illness–associated headaches are also usually bilateral, generalized, or migratory. Many children cannot even recall the location of their headaches and rarely are able to describe the quality of their headaches in terms adult neurologists like to use ("throbbing," "band-like," "ice-pick," etc.); they just smile shyly and shrug their shoulders when asked what their headaches feel like.

WHEN IS THE LOCATION OF THE HEADACHE IMPORTANT?

The location of the headache *is* diagnostically important in a significant minority of cases. *Sinusitis* is suggested by *pain in the maxillary region* and *tenderness to percussion. Temporomandibular joint syndrome* is suggested by a history of bitemporal pain that is exacerbated by jaw movement. Cluster headaches, which are uncommon in adults and rare in the pediatric population, present as *brief but excruciating bouts of unilateral orbital pain. Pain in the back of the head* that worsens with neck movement is often a clue that the pain originates in the *cervical spine.* A *mass lesion in the posterior fossa* or a *Chiari I malformation* can also cause occipital headaches. Since typical migraine and tension headaches rarely are occipital in location, headaches in this location deserve special attention.

PHYSICAL EXAMINATION

The physical examination should follow the guidelines outlined in Chapter 1. The optic fundi must be examined to make certain that there is no papilledema, or if that is not possible due to the child's age and raised intracranial pressure is suspected, the child may be referred to an ophthalmologist. The neck is evaluated for stiffness, tenderness, and range of motion. If the patient has a headache accompanied by a *stiff neck*, maneuvers to elicit *Kernig sign and Brudzinski sign* (see Chapter 1) should be performed. Percussion of the maxillary, and in older children and adolescents, frontal sinuses may elicit tenderness, suggesting sinusitis. In rare cases, a *cranial bruit* from an *arteriovenous malformation* is detected by auscultation over the mastoids or orbits. If the patient's pain is primarily in the temporal area, he may be asked to open and close the mandible while the temporomandibular joint is palpated to feel for a *jaw click* (a sign of temporomandibular joint syndrome). If the patient has general complaints such as fever, fatigue, or malaise, the examiner should look for signs of infection (rash, redness of the pharynx, joint swelling, adenopathy, etc.).

The assessment of mental status, cranial nerves, motor system, reflexes, and gait may follow the guidelines for a concise examination (see Chapter 1) if

TABLE 2.2

Clues to the diagnosis of common headache syndromes

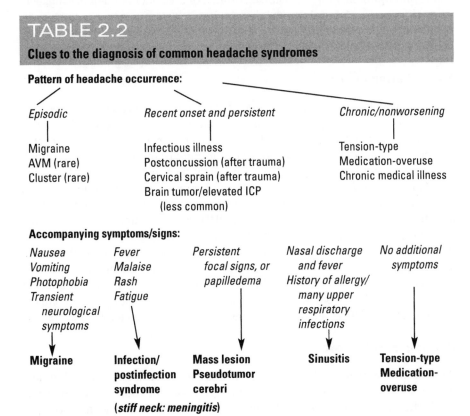

Pattern of headache occurrence:

Episodic	Recent onset and persistent	Chronic/nonworsening
Migraine AVM (rare) Cluster (rare)	Infectious illness Postconcussion (after trauma) Cervical sprain (after trauma) Brain tumor/elevated ICP (less common)	Tension-type Medication-overuse Chronic medical illness

Accompanying symptoms/signs:

Nausea Vomiting Photophobia Transient neurological symptoms	Fever Malaise Rash Fatigue	Persistent focal signs, or papilledema	Nasal discharge and fever History of allergy/ many upper respiratory infections	No additional symptoms
Migraine	**Infection/ postinfection syndrome** (*stiff neck: meningitis*)	**Mass lesion Pseudotumor cerebri**	**Sinusitis**	**Tension-type Medication- overuse**

the patient is alert and has no specific neurological complaints. If persistent focal neurological symptoms are reported, a more comprehensive cranial nerve, motor, and cerebellar examination is always necessary. Once again, *transient* focal complaints in association with headache generally suggest migraine.

COMMON HEADACHE SYNDROMES

Tension-type headache

The patient with a history of *tension-type headaches* typically complains of headaches that occur *frequently* or even *daily*. Exacerbation of the headaches during the school day and in other *stressful situations* is common. The patient may describe the headaches as being mild, moderate, or even severe, but the interview usually reveals that the headaches *do not prevent participation in enjoyable activities*. Relief after a *brief period of rest* is consistent with the diagnosis of tension-type headache, whereas a need to sleep for hours to relieve the pain is more suggestive of migraine.

The patient with a history of tension-type headaches usually *does not describe other symptoms*. A history of *vomiting* or of *transient visual symptoms* (photophobia, blurred vision, scotoma, or a visual field defect) suggests *migraine* and not tension-type headaches. *Systemic symptoms* (fever, fatigue, myalgias, and malaise) suggest that the headaches result from a non-neurological (usually infectious or postinfectious) illness and not stress.

Exacerbating factors

Children and adolescents with a history of chronic tension headaches are usually experiencing a great deal of stress, and the cause needs to be explored. In many cases, the problem is school. The patient may be an overachiever who has trouble unwinding or may have an undiagnosed learning disability that makes schoolwork stressful and discouraging. Not surprisingly, these patients' headaches *occur mostly on school days and go away during weekends and vacations*, although they may mysteriously reappear on Sunday nights. [Headaches in children with attention-deficit hyperactivity disorder (ADHD) are also rather common during school days but are often a side effect of stimulant medication.] In other cases, there is a *problem affecting the family* such as an impending divorce, the loss of a parent's job, or a relative who has a serious illness. The patient may have difficulty getting along with other children or may have recently moved and left friends behind. Teenagers are likely to experience stress as a result of conflicts with parents, anxiety about school and the future, and personal relationships.

Common misdiagnoses

Patients with a history of tension-type headaches are often suspected of having an allergy, a sinus condition, or an "eye problem" that is causing their headaches. Many have been to the allergist, ear/nose/throat specialist, or ophthalmologist prior to coming for neurologic evaluation.

None of these suspected causes is usually the real cause. *Allergies do not generally cause headaches* and are even less likely to be the cause if no typical allergic symptoms (rhinitis, rash, wheezing, etc.) are reported. Signs and symptoms of sinusitis are discussed in the following section; *sinusitis is unlikely if there is no history of chronic nasal discharge, fevers, or frequent upper respiratory infections.*

Headaches in a nonorbital location are rarely, if ever, caused by an ophthalmological problem. Even when a patient's headaches localize to the orbit, migraine, not an ophthalmological problem, is the usual cause. *Eyestrain headaches* occur only *while the patient is reading* and should *disappear as soon as he or she stops reading.*

Physical examination and diagnostic studies

The patient with a history of tension-type headaches often appears tense, anxious, or unhappy. The physical examination should be unremarkable. Any abnormal finding may suggest a different diagnosis.

CT or MRI of the brain is not necessary when an older child or teenager has headaches that completely disappear during weekends and vacations or occur only in stressful situations. If the headaches occur all the time or in an unpredictable pattern or if the child is young, a brain imaging study is often ordered, mostly to reassure the parents that there is no brain tumor. *MRI very rarely reveals an intracranial lesion in cases of chronic headache when there are no focal neurological complaints and the neurological examination is within normal limits* (7). When MRI does turn out to be abnormal, an incidental finding (e.g., an arachnoid cyst) is usually the abnormality reported. The finding usually has nothing at all to do with the patient's headaches and has no serious implications, but it may be very worrisome to the family, which may be a good reason to think twice before ordering MRI in the first place.

Behavioral treatment

Chronic headache can be a debilitating condition. As physicians taking care of these patients, we are given a unique opportunity to help these children and adolescents minimize the occurrence of headaches. To begin with, they should be taught habits and lifestyles that they can carry with them to adulthood that will reduce the frequency of these headaches.

In treating patients with recurrent or chronic headaches, an emphasis should initially be placed on nonpharmacological management (i.e., the identification and avoidance of triggers or exacerbating factors). Stress reduction, emotional self-awareness, regular sleep habits, regular exercise, and a reasonable diet can all be helpful. Avoidance of caffeinated beverages is often helpful in particular, as rebound from caffeine often causes a headache. In many cases, these modifications decrease the frequency of tension headaches without the need for prescription medication.

The treatment of chronic tension-type headaches should always *address the source of the patient's stress*. Biofeedback sessions, as well as the teaching of stress reduction and pain management techniques, may be helpful. Assistance in school or psychotherapy is often appropriate.

Basic symptomatic treatment

If the child's headaches are mild, conservative treatment is suggested. It is reasonable not to give any medication to the child who says, "I have a headache" but continues to play happily.

Headaches of moderate severity may be treated with an appropriate dose, based on body weight, of acetaminophen or ibuprofen. The physician should be aware that parents tend to make two mistakes when treating their child's headaches with nonprescription drugs. The first is administering *too small a dose*, resulting in no relief. The second is administering the medication *every day for weeks or months*, which often results in the syndrome of medication-overuse headache. Therefore, parents must be told that a sufficient dose of an analgesic medication should be administered but also that the *medication should not be given daily for more than 2 weeks*. If headaches continue, a preventive medication may be helpful. The patient should also be medically re-evaluated to make certain that a more serious cause of the headaches has not been missed.

Medication-overuse headache

Medication-overuse (rebound) headache is a common problem (8). In many cases, the patient has a history suggestive of tension-type headaches that have become more frequent despite the fact that he or she has been taking ibuprofen or another analgesic drug every day for several months. In other cases, there is a history of migraine headaches or postconcussion headaches that have been treated with an analgesic (prescription or nonprescription) taken for symptomatic relief too regularly. Many people are unaware that *if they take an analgesic medication daily for a long period of time, their headaches may become frequent and severe* (9). Treatment relies primarily on the patient discontinuing the overused medication, which may result in an increase in the headache frequency over the short term but, ultimately, should produce a significant improvement. If the patient is unwilling to "go cold turkey," a headache-preventive drug can be prescribed to the patient. After a few weeks, it should be possible for the patient to stop taking the analgesic.

Medications for headache prevention

Patients with a history of frequent tension-type headaches often respond well to a medication for headache prophylaxis. A *tricyclic antidepressant* (TCA) (10,11) is often effective. A TCA is also useful in many cases of medication-overuse headache, allowing patients to discontinue an overused analgesic without experiencing severe rebound headaches. *Amitriptyline* and *nortriptyline* are the TCA medications most widely prescribed for tension headache prevention. Of these two drugs, nortriptyline causes less sedation and is better tolerated. The usual initial dose of nortriptyline is 10 mg every night before bed. If no improvement or limited improvement in the frequency of the patient's headaches after 2 weeks is reported, the dosage may be increased to 20 mg. The dose can be further increased to 30 or 40 mg for adolescents, if necessary, but a consistent benefit has not been noted. Adverse effects, which are relatively uncommon and usually mild, include sedation, dry mouth, tachycardia, agitation, anxiety, and nausea. Theoretical risks include cardiac arrhythmia and seizures, which very rarely occur and usually only occur at the much higher doses used to treat depression. If a dose greater than 30 mg is prescribed, monitoring with electrocardiogram (EKG) every 6 months is suggested. A TCA should not be prescribed to any patient with a history of epilepsy since it may provoke a seizure.

Other medications that may decrease the frequency of tension-type headaches include gabapentin, cyproheptadine, valproate, and topiramate (12,13) (see migraine prophylaxis).

If the patient's headaches become less frequent (at least 70% improvement) as a result of taking a preventive drug, the patient should continue to take the drug for 3 to 6 months, at which point it may be tapered off. In many cases, the headaches will remain infrequent. Some patients may require a longer course of treatment. Attempts at stress reduction, biofeedback, or psychotherapy must also continue.

Headaches caused by a nonneurological illness

Clinical presentation

A history of *fatigue, malaise, myalgias, joint pain, rash, or fever* accompanying headaches suggests that the *headaches are just one symptom of a nonneurological illness*. Often, however, the patient and parents focus only on the headache, and it is not until they are asked about other symptoms that they are brought up. The most common cause of this clinical picture is an *infection or a postinfection syndrome*. Mononucleosis, *Mycoplasma pneumoniae* infection, enterovirus infection, streptococcal pharyngitis, and Lyme disease can present in this manner. In many cases, no specific diagnosis is made, and the headaches are attributed to a nonspecific viral infection. If *neck stiffness* is noted, *meningitis* should be suspected. Less common causes of headache accompanied by constitutional symptoms include other infectious diseases, hyper- or hypothyroidism, malignancy, and autoimmune diseases.

Laboratory studies may include a complete blood count (CBC) with erythrocyte sedimentation rate (ESR), Lyme titer, antinuclear antibody, Epstein-Barr virus (EBV) titers, Mycoplasma titers, and thyroid stimulating hormone. All of these tests are not necessary to order in every case and also do not preclude the need for other tests. The history and physical examination will often suggest which tests are most appropriate. Brain MRI is often ordered but rarely reveals a significant abnormality. An infectious disease consultation may be appropriate.

Treatment

If a treatable cause for the patient's condition, such as Lyme disease or *Mycoplasma pneumoniae* infection, is diagnosed, an appropriate antibiotic should be prescribed. However, in most cases, no specific diagnosis is made, or a condition for which there is no specific treatment, such as mononucleosis, is diagnosed. A nonprescription analgesic is suggested as the first-line therapy for headache relief in all these cases. *Acetaminophen with codeine* may be effective if the headaches are severe. A short course (less than 1 week) of a *corticosteroid* (if not contraindicated for medical reasons) sometimes relieves a severe headache associated with viral infections and postviral syndromes, but the headache may recur once the corticosteroid is tapered off. *Gabapentin* or *nortriptyline* is sometimes effective. In most cases, the headaches eventually remit regardless of the drug prescribed.

Chronic fatigue syndrome

Patients with *chronic fatigue syndrome* (CFS) often report severe headaches. CFS is not uncommon in children and adolescents (14). Other symptoms include *persistent, debilitating fatigue, lightheadedness, myalgias, photophobia, abdominal pain, diarrhea, rash, and difficulty sleeping.* Criteria for CFS published in 1994 by the Centers for Disease Control suggest that symptoms must have been present for at least 6 months and are not attributable to another medical cause. The fatigue associated with CFS markedly *worsens after exercise. Fibromyalgia,* possibly a variant form of CFS, primarily is diagnosed in female patients and is characterized by severe migratory musculoskeletal pain.

CFS is a debilitating illness and is not caused by depression or malingering. Many patients have been misdiagnosed with either depression or another disorder (e.g., "chronic Lyme disease").

In cases of suspected CFS, the history, physical examination, and laboratory and diagnostic tests should not suggest another diagnosis. The EBV IgG titer is sometimes elevated, which is a nonspecific finding only suggesting prior exposure to EBV. CFS is no longer attributed to chronic EBV infection. MRI yields no significant information. All this is frustrating to the patient and tends to reinforce many physicians' skepticism about the validity of CFS. However, the *tilt-table test* often reveals *orthostatic hypotension,* suggesting that CFS may be associated with or even caused by a disorder of the autonomic nervous system (15,16).

Amitriptyline, nortriptyline, sertraline, and methylphenidate have been used to treat the symptoms of CFS. The headaches are usually refractory (preventive drugs may be tried) but eventually gradually stop occurring. Rest and a gradual return to physical exercise may help promote recovery, which is still often very prolonged, taking years for many adults with CFS. The prognosis for children and adolescents, many of whom report significant improvement in their symptoms after 1 to 2 years, tends to be better (14).

Migraine

Clinical features

Many children and adolescents have *migraine headaches* (1,2). In children, migraine headaches often first present during middle childhood (in boys) or adolescence (in girls). However, children as young as 2 years of age may have migraine headaches or a history suggesting a migraine variant syndrome (cyclic vomiting, benign paroxysmal vertigo).

Migraine is often a hereditary condition, and a *family history of migraine* may be mentioned during the interview.

Migraine headaches are typically *severe enough to prevent the patient from attending school and participating in other activities*. Indeed, if the patient is generally able to function well during his headaches and does not report nausea, vomiting, photophobia, or other typical symptoms, his headaches should not be labeled as migraines.

Women and teenage girls often report that their migraine headaches occur *shortly before or during their menstrual period*. Migraine may also first present after an episode of even minor head injury in a person genetically predisposed to migraine. Otherwise, however, migraine headaches *occur sporadically and unpredictably*. In contrast to many patients' tension-type headaches, migraine headaches usually occur during weekends and vacations as well as school days.

The frequency of the headaches varies. Some people experience a migraine headache only once or twice a year; other people experience migraines several times a week. Still other patients may have a bout of headaches that lasts for several days and then are headache-free for several months before having another bout. This phenomenon, sometimes called "cluster migraine," should not be confused with cluster headache, which is a distinct and much rarer disorder.

Adult patients classically describe migraine headaches that are *unilateral* (the word migraine is derived from the French "hemicrain," or half the head) and *pounding*. Children and adolescents do not consistently report either of these characteristics; their headaches are variable in location, and the pain is not of a typical quality.

Nausea, vomiting (after which the headache may disappear), and *sensitivity to bright light and loud noise* suggest migraine. The patient often needs to *lie down in a dark room* and reports *improvement after sleep. Scotomas*—illusions of flashing lights, black spots and zigzag lines—are often reported. Between headaches, the patient may be prone to *motion sickness* that may result from mildly abnormal brainstem and cerebellar activity (17).

Transient focal neurological symptoms, such as unilateral paresthesias, loss of part of or all of a visual field, and slurred speech, often accompany migraine headache. During the prodromal period (aura), these may be the only symptoms noted by the patient. Some patients who experience these transient neurological symptoms never develop a headache (*acephalgic migraine*). The neurological manifestations of migraine are often frightening to parents and patients, who may fear that they were caused by a stroke. They may be reassured that these symptoms are characteristic of migraine.

Hemiplegic migraine is a relatively uncommon familial condition, linked to genes on chromosomes 1 and 19 (18,19). Patients present with *hemiplegia or hemiparesis accompanying migrainous headaches*. MRI is usually ordered in these cases but is usually normal. In very rare cases, a hemiplegic migraine headache can develop into a cerebral infarction (stroke).

Physical examination and role of imaging studies

The *diagnosis of migraine is based primarily on the history*. A *family history of migraine* supports the diagnosis. During the headache, the patient usually appears in pain, is sensitive to bright light, and may be nauseated or vomiting. Rarely, a visual field deficit, aphasia, or hemiparesis may be noted during an acute attack, but in a new patient, this should motivate the clinician to search for other possible etiologies. ***Between episodes, the general physical and neurological examination of the migraine sufferer should yield no abnormal findings that could explain headaches.***

There is, at most, a limited role for MRI in the diagnosis of migraine. *Brain tumors do not cause severe headaches separated by long periods of complete relief.* If the headaches are associated with focal neurological signs or symptoms, especially hemiparesis or hemiplegia, MRI may be ordered to search for an *arteriovenous malformation (AVM; see following section)*, but the yield is very low.

Many patients with a history suggestive of migraine are sent for MRI anyway. Parental anxiety, uncertainty about the diagnosis, misdiagnosis, and medicolegal fears are the usual reasons and are understandable. *Repeat* MRI studies, however, are not justifiable unless the patient's headaches dramatically change in quality.

Migraine "triggers"

Many patients have a migraine headache when they are sleep deprived or under stress. Other patients say that they get a headache after prolonged exposure to sunlight or when the weather changes. Lack of sleep is the most easily remediable of these factors. Stress reduction is as important for the migraine sufferer as it is for the patient with a history of tension-type headaches.

Some patients report that, after they eat a *particular kind of food*, they consistently get a migraine headache. *Tyramine*-containing foods, such as chocolate, cheddar cheese, soy products, beans, monosodium glutamate, smoked meats that contain nitrites, yeast, red wine, and beer, are especially likely to provoke a headache. However, each of these foods is a "trigger" *for only a small percentage of all patients who have migraine headaches*. Many physicians have nevertheless been trained to give the migraine sufferer a list of all of these and many other tyramine-containing foods to avoid. The list is long and includes many common foods, making it difficult to maintain this diet. A more practical approach is either to *eliminate one type of food at a time* from the diet or to ask the parents to *keep a diary* of the food that their child ate prior to every headache. If these measures implicate a particular food, it may be removed from the diet. If no food trigger is identified, dietary modification, other than the suggestion that the patient should eat regular meals and avoid caffeinated beverages (withdrawal from caffeine being a common cause of headache), is unlikely to be very helpful.

Symptomatic pharmacological treatment of migraines

The initial treatment for patients who have infrequent migraine headaches (no more than two headaches a month) is acetaminophen or ibuprofen (Table 2.3). The medication should be given at an *adequate dose* at the *first sign* of a

TABLE 2.3
Treatment of migraine headaches

Nonpharmacological: adequate sleep and diet, avoid caffeinated beverages; stress reduction, headache diary to identify food triggers

Nonprescription drugs: acetaminophen or ibuprofen taken at first sign of headache; avoid chronic use to prevent rebound headaches

Prescription drugs for treatment of acute attack: Butalbital/caffeine/acetaminophen (Fioricet); sumatriptan and other triptans for adolescents (NOT for hemiplegic or basilar migraine)

Preventive drugs (if patient has >2 severe headaches per month): nortriptyline, cyproheptadine, topiramate, valproate, and others

Drugs for intractable migraine: short course of a corticosteroid, single dose of haloperidol; AVOID OPIATE ANALGESICS!

headache. Younger children need to be reminded to go to their parents or the school nurse as soon as they feel a headache coming on, and parents need to be vigilant about giving the medicine promptly.

Patients whose headaches do not respond to a nonprescription analgesic may be prescribed an *acetaminophen/caffeine/butalbital*–containing drug (Esgic, Forest; Fioricet, Novartis; or generic equivalent). One-half tablet is administered to young children (less than approximately 8 years of age), and a full tablet is administered to older children and teenagers. A single dose usually terminates the headache, but the medication can be given every 6 hours if the headache persists. Butalbital often causes drowsiness, and therefore, the drug should not be given to a child in school. (In some cases, particularly for those who do not chronically consume caffeinated beverages, ibuprofen or acetaminophen taken with a can of caffeinated beverage is also effective.)

During the last decade, *sumatriptan* (Imitrex, GlaxoSmithKline) and several pharmacologically similar medications have become more and more widely prescribed to patients with a history of migraine headaches. These drugs are collectively known as *triptans*. Although FDA approval of all triptans currently is limited to adult patients, these drugs are often prescribed to adolescents, and a recent study (20) demonstrated safety and efficacy of sumatriptan for children as young as 8 years of age.

Sumatriptan is available as 25-, 50-, or 100-mg tablets or as a single-dose 5- or 20-mg nasal spray that is often used by patients whose migraines are accompanied by vomiting. An injectable form is available but less often used. Sumatriptan and other triptans may be taken at any point during a migraine headache but are most effective if taken immediately after the onset of symptoms. If necessary, a second dose can be taken in 2 hours, but a triptan should not be taken more than three times in a 24-hour period.

Flushing and heart palpitations are common adverse effects of triptans. Because of their vasoconstricting effect, triptans are *contraindicated in cases of hemiplegic migraine* and for patients with a *history of cardiac or cerebrovascular* disease. A family history of one of these conditions may also be a reason not to prescribe a triptan. Triptans are *not used to treat basilar migraine.*

Preventive treatment of migraine

Patients who experience *frequent migraine headaches (more than two severe headaches a month)* should consider taking a *migraine preventive medication.* Unfortunately, many patients who might benefit from migraine prophylaxis are not offered preventive therapy and come to rely exclusively on medications taken to abort their headaches when they occur. Medication-overuse headaches often develop as a result.

Currently, five drugs (methysergide, divalproex sodium, propranolol, timolol, and topiramate) are Food and Drug Administration (FDA) approved for migraine prophylaxis. Approval is limited to adults, however, and clinical experience suggests that some of these drugs may work better for adult than pediatric patients.

There are also a number of clinically proven and widely used medications for migraine prophylaxis that work well for children and teenagers. *Nortriptyline*, discussed earlier, is effective and has a mild side effect profile. The dosage is the same as for the patient with chronic tension-type headaches. *Cyproheptadine* (Periactin, Merck) is an antihistaminic medication with serotonin-blocking activity that is taken at a dose of 2 to 4 mg two to three times daily. Adverse effects may include sedation, increased appetite, and occasionally, in longer term therapy, depression caused by serotonin blockade. Extended-release *divalproex sodium* (Depakote ER, Abbott) is approved for use in the pediatric population for the control of epileptic seizures and is also approved for adults as a migraine preventive. The dosage for adults is 500 to 1000 mg taken once daily, which is also appropriate for adolescents; 250 to 500 mg can be prescribed to younger children. Adverse effects of valproate are discussed in Chapter 6; CBC and liver function tests are periodically drawn. *Topiramate* (Topamax, Ortho-McNeill), another antiepileptic drug approved for children, is an effective migraine prevention medication. The dosage range for migraine prevention is 15 to 50 mg once to twice daily. Topiramate can cause fatigue and drowsiness and, therefore, should be started at a low dose. Appetite suppression is a common side effect of topiramate. *Gabapentin* (100 to 300 mg twice to three times daily) is also an antiepileptic medication and may be useful as a migraine prevention medication. *Propranolol* has long been prescribed for the prophylaxis of migraine headaches. However, adverse effects, including bradycardia, hypotension, syncope, exacerbation of asthma, fatigue and depression, limit this drug's usefulness. Some physicians prescribe a *calcium channel-blocking drug* (e.g., nifedipine). *Riboflavin* is said to be effective for some patients. A recent study (21) demonstrated efficacy for *coenzyme Q10* taken at a dose of 100 mg three times daily.

Patients taking a prophylactic drug should notice a significant decrease in the frequency and severity of their headaches. If there is no improvement after 1 to 2 weeks, the dose may be gradually increased within the range specified. If there is no improvement after two titrations or if adverse effects occur, the medication should be tapered off and a different drug tried. The process is always trial and error, but in most cases, an effective and well-tolerated medication is eventually found. Once shown to be effective, the medication should be continued for 3 to 6 months. At this point, the headache cycle often has been interrupted long enough to taper the drug with a good result. Longer term therapy may be necessary for some patients.

Patients taking a medication for migraine prophylaxis may experience occasional breakthrough headaches that can be treated with any of the medications (acetaminophen, ibuprofen, butalbital/acetaminophen/caffeine, and triptans) listed earlier.

Intractable migraine

Physicians will occasionally need to treat a patient who is having a *severe migraine headache that has not responded to several drugs*. An opiate analgesic (morphine, meperidine, oxycodone, etc.) is often *and inappropriately* prescribed in this situation. Although the opiate may provide temporary relief, the headache will typically return and worsen after the drug wears off in a few hours. *Opiate analgesic medications are not recommended for the treatment of an intractable migraine headache.*

There are better options. A short course of a *corticosteroid* (Medrol dosepak, Pharmacia/Upjohn; or prednisone, 60 mg daily for 5 days) should be prescribed and proves to be effective within 24 hours in most cases. For the patient in the emergency room, a bolus of intravenous dexamethasone (4 to 10 mg) can be given, followed by an oral corticosteroid to be taken after the patient leaves the hospital. In refractory cases, a single dose of *haloperidol* (1 to 5 mg) or metoclopramide (22) often stops the headache. If the patient must be hospitalized, treatment should include continuation of a corticosteroid, butalbital/caffeine/acetaminophen, and an antiemetic drug, if needed.

Migraine variants

The syndrome of episodic vertigo, ataxia, vomiting, and occipital headache is called *basilar migraine*. Patients with basilar migraine usually also have a history of more typical migraine headaches; in other cases, family members have been diagnosed with migraine. In cases of basilar migraine, MRI is usually ordered to examine the brainstem and cerebellum, although it may not be necessary if the patient also has a history of typical migraine headaches and the symptoms of vertigo completely disappear between episodes. The treatment of basilar migraine is directed primarily at alleviating vertigo with meclizine (12.5 mg every 6 hours). A butalbital/caffeine/acetaminophen medication can be taken for pain relief. *Triptans should not be used to treat basilar migraine.*

Exercise-induced headaches occur immediately after vigorous physical activity. Vomiting and visual disturbances are not typically reported. In theory, an intracranial abnormality, such as a tumor, arteriovenous malformation, aneurysm, or Chiari I malformation, could cause this kind of headache, although is rarely discovered. MRI may be indicated in some cases. Patients may take ibuprofen or indomethacin prior to strenuous activity to prevent the headaches.

Abdominal migraine (cyclic vomiting) is a syndrome characterized by *unexplained, recurrent bouts of intractable vomiting*. These patients do not usually complaint of headaches. A gastrointestinal cause should be excluded. A family history of migraine tends to support the diagnosis of abdominal migraine. Treatment is difficult since orally administered medication often cannot be tolerated while the child is vomiting. A rectally administered antiemetic medication (chlorpromazine or other drugs) may be helpful. A migraine-preventive drug is sometimes useful; some success has also been achieved with topiramate. The bouts of vomiting usually gradually diminish in frequency and eventually stop occurring altogether.

Patients with *acute confusional migraine* present with *altered mental status*, with or without headache. The diagnosis of this rare syndrome *requires exclusion of other causes of altered mental status* (see Chapter 13). A history of migraine headaches is not essential but helps to support the diagnosis.

The condition once called *ophthalmoplegic migraine* is no longer considered a migraine variant and is now thought to occur as a result of inflammation of structures within the orbit. Symptoms and signs include orbital pain and *partial or complete paralysis of extraocular movements and pupillary responses*. Vision may be affected. There are often permanent sequelae such as extraocular paresis. A corticosteroid is often prescribed and may be beneficial.

Headache following a head injury

Concussion and postconcussive syndrome are common causes of headache that are discussed in Chapter 12.

LESS COMMON CAUSES OF HEADACHE
Sinusitis

Many patients use the term "sinus headaches" to describe what are, in fact, tension-type or migrainous headaches. Sinusitis usually is associated with *fever, heavy or persistent nasal discharge, conjunctival injection, or periorbital swelling*. Vertigo is occasionally reported. There is often a history of frequent upper respiratory infections. Pain is usually worst in the maxillary or periorbital area.

The physical examination classically reveals *tenderness to percussion* of the maxillary area or the frontal area (in teenagers and adults). CT or MRI demonstrates *marked mucosal thickening* (mild thickening is a common and nonspecific finding) in one of more of the facial sinuses, a *retention cyst,* or an *air-fluid level* (Fig. 2.1). Diagnostic features of sinusitis headaches are further reviewed in a recent publication (23). Treatment usually consists of an antibiotic and a nasal decongestant. In chronic or refractory cases, the patient should be referred for ear, nose, and throat (ENT) consultation. Sinus surgery is sometimes beneficial for patients with a history of chronic or recurrent episodes of sinusitis.

Sphenoid sinusitis may cause generalized headaches that do not correspond to the clinical profile of one of the more common headache

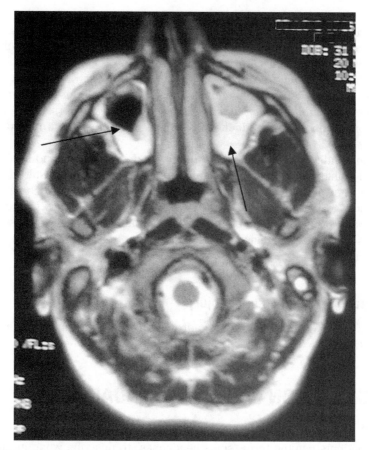

Figure 2.1 MRI demonstrates marked mucosal thickening (*right*) and air-fluid level (*left*) in case of **maxillary sinusitis.**
(Courtesy Howard Seigerman, MD and Eliot Lerner, MD, The Valley Hospital.)

syndromes. In other words, there is no history of migrainous features, psychological stress, focal neurological symptoms, or systemic medical complaints. The neurological examination is normal, and maxillary or frontal sinus tenderness is not noted. The radiological finding (CT or MRI) of an *air-fluid level or opacification of the sphenoid sinus* is diagnostic. Treatment is usually the same as for other forms of sinusitis. ENT consultation is recommended.

Meningitis

If a child or adolescent presents with symptoms of *fever and headache and looks ill* and the physical examination reveals signs of *meningeal irritation* (stiff neck, positive Kernig or Brudzinski sign), the patient should be *assumed to have bacterial meningitis and sent directly to the emergency room for a lumbar puncture* (LP). In the case of an infant or toddler, the clinical presentation may be one of *lethargy, irritability, poor appetite, and fever*; meningeal signs are often not present.

When a patient is suspected of having meningitis and needs an LP, many neurologists order a CT scan first because of the possibility of herniation if an LP is performed on a patient with an undiagnosed intracranial mass lesion. The risk of this actually occurring is small, and the first priority must be to diagnose and treat meningitis. However, if funduscopy reveals *papilledema*, a CT scan should certainly be ordered. Some neurologists recommend that, if CT is unavailable and funduscopy is inconclusive, the patient should be given an intravenous dose of a corticosteroid and antibiotic, and LP should be deferred until imaging can be performed. This is a conservative approach. Ideally, LP is performed prior to the administration of the antibiotic and corticosteroid so as not to affect the results of the cerebrospinal fluid (CSF) culture.

Analysis of the CSF, in typical cases of bacterial meningitis, should reveal pleocytosis with a predominance of neutrophils, elevated protein, and decreased glucose. The Gram stain or culture may reveal the bacterium. In exceptional cases, the culture reveals evidence of tuberculous or fungal meningitis, which are conditions usually associated with a more chronic course and a predominance of lymphocytes or mononuclear cells.

The patient with bacterial meningitis should be admitted to the intensive care unit. MRI of the brain should be ordered to look for evidence of an abscess, cerebritis, empyema, or ventriculitis. Supportive measures include elevation of the head of the patient's bed to 30 degrees, fluid restriction, and, in some cases, a corticosteroid, mannitol, or mechanical hyperventilation to decrease cerebral edema and perfusion pressure. Septicemia resulting in shock and multiple organ failure is common in cases of bacterial meningitis. Mortality and morbidity are high even with the best care. Important short- and long-term neurological complications are stroke, cognitive impairment, cranial nerve palsies, hearing loss, and epilepsy.

Viral Meningitis

Viral meningitis typically presents with fever, headache, and meningeal signs on examination. Patients with viral meningitis tend to look less ill than patients with bacterial meningitis, but the two conditions cannot be reliably distinguished clinically. In cases of viral meningitis, the CSF culture result by definition is negative. The CSF glucose should be normal, protein is typically elevated, and a lymphocytic pleocytosis is noted. Lyme titer should be ordered in cases of presumed viral meningitis. Viral meningitis is a very unpleasant but self-limited disease. Headaches may persist for a few weeks and can be treated with ibuprofen or acetaminophen with codeine. Gabapentin sometimes effectively alleviates refractory postmeningitis headaches.

If the Lyme titer and Western blot suggest a recent infection and LP reveals a lymphocytic pleocytosis, the patient is assumed to have *Lyme meningitis*. An elevated CSF Lyme titer is not required to confirm the diagnosis. An appropriate course (14 to 28 days) of an intravenous antibiotic, such as ceftriaxone or penicillin, is prescribed to treat Lyme meningitis.

Post-LP headaches

A headache is commonly reported after LP but should not occur more than 48 hours after the procedure. Recurrent headaches after 48 hours are often caused by a *persistent CSF leak*. The headaches are usually most severe and accompanied by vomiting when the patient *sits upright*. Maintaining a supine position for several days usually stops the headaches. Caffeine-containing medications (e.g., Fioricet) are sometimes helpful. In refractory cases, a "blood patch" (epidural injection of the patient's blood near the site of the lumbar puncture) performed by an anesthesiologist, neurologist, or another physician trained in this procedure is the definitive treatment.

Cluster headache

Cluster headache is generally an uncommon disorder that is even rarer in childhood. Young men are most often afflicted. Cluster headaches present as *recurrent daily bouts of excruciating pain in the orbital/maxillary area*, lasting for *1 hour or less*, with the bouts *continuing to occur for several weeks* (the "cluster"). Only one side of the face is affected. *Conjunctival injection, Horner's syndrome*, and *nasal stuffiness* may accompany the headaches. The patient is then typically headache-free for months before experiencing another cluster. Cluster headaches are not normally a familial trait, but there is often a family history of *migraine* headaches.

A medication to prevent recurrence, often *carbamazepine, oxcarbazepine,* or *divalproex sodium,* is taken daily (see Chapter 6). A bout in progress is effectively treated with a short course of a *corticosteroid,* as for intractable migraine. Other treatments include inhaled *100% oxygen* administered in the emergency room and *sumatriptan.*

Subarachnoid hemorrhage

A *subarachnoid hemorrhage* (SAH) from a ruptured cerebral arterial aneurysm is a very rare disorder in the pediatric population. In most pediatric cases that initially suggest SAH, the patient's symptoms are eventually attributed to exercise-induced migraine or cervical muscle spasm. However, when any patient complains of an excruciating headache ("*the worst headache of my life*") of abrupt onset, SAH must be seriously considered. *Signs of meningeal irritation in an afebrile patient* further suggest SAH.

The patient should be sent to the emergency room, and a *noncontrast CT scan* of the head should be promptly ordered. In cases of SAH, CT usually reveals blood (white) outlining cerebral sulci or the brainstem (Fig. 2.2). However, CT may not detect a small hemorrhage, and therefore, *LP must be performed if the CT scan is read as normal.* In cases of SAH, the CSF is either pink or *xanthochromic* (yellow-tinged due to the presence of bilirubin) in appearance.

Any patient with an SAH must be admitted to the intensive care unit. A neurosurgeon should see the patient as soon as possible. Nimodipine,

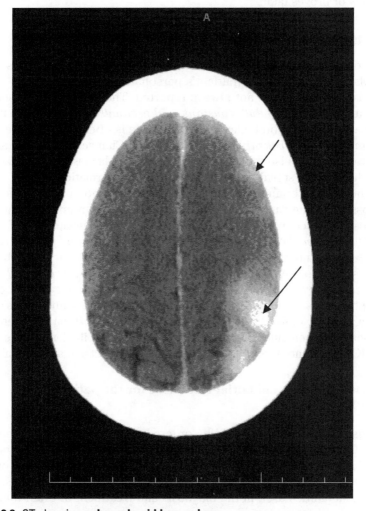

Figure 2.2 CT showing **subarachnoid hemorrhage.**
Note blood (hyperdense material) overlaying and outlining cerebral sulci. (Courtesy of Howard Seigerman, MD and Eliot Lerner, MD, The Valley Hospital.)

60 mg orally every 4 hours, is prescribed to reduce the risk of vasospasm and stroke. Usually the patient is treated as a case of elevated ICP. Magnetic resonance angiography (MRA) or cerebral angiography is ordered to visualize the aneurysm, which usually is found at the point of anastomosis of a major cerebral artery and the circle of Willis.

The aneurysm is occluded by a metal clip placed by the neurosurgeon, or a coil is placed within the aneurysm by means of an endovascular catheter promote thrombosis. These procedures are usually performed as soon as possible in an effort to prevent rebleeding from the aneurysm. Many patients recover completely, but a large SAH often causes permanent neurological disability or proves fatal.

Brain tumor

Incoordination, ataxia, double vision, hemiparesis, focal seizures, or an unexplained change in the patient's personality suggests a *brain tumor*. A headache is often but not always reported. The headaches caused by a brain tumor are usually *dull, constant, and gradually worsen.* Since lying in bed exacerbates cerebral edema, the headache is often *worst in the morning.* V*omiting on awakening* is often reported. Changes in position and the Valsalva maneuver also tend to exacerbate the headaches. Severe headaches and lethargy suggest hydrocephalus or impending herniation.

A majority of brain tumors in the pediatric population arise in the posterior fossa, causing gait ataxia, spasticity resulting from involvement of the corticospinal tract or another motor pathway, or disconjugate gaze. *A history of double vision should always alert the clinician to the possibility of a brain tumor.* Tumors of the *pons* cause double vision characterized by *horizontal* separation of images, whereas tumors of the *midbrain and pineal gland* cause *vertical separation.* If the tumor involves one of the cerebral hemispheres (as is more common in infants, adolescents, and adults), there may be a history of *focal seizures* or *contralateral deficits* such as hemiparesis, aphasia, or hemianopsia (a visual field deficit). Papilledema suggests elevated ICP or a tumor large enough to cause mass effect and anatomical shifts.

Diagnostic studies and initial treatment for the patient with a Brain Tumor

Contrast-enhanced MRI should be ordered in all cases of suspected brain tumor. Contrast-enhanced CT is an acceptable initial test if MRI is not available. If a brain tumor is diagnosed, MRI of the spinal cord is usually ordered since many pediatric brain tumors metastasize within the neuraxis. Other imaging modalities used in the diagnosis and treatment of brain tumor are reviewed in Chapter 14.

A brain tumor causing an elevation of ICP is a medical emergency. A neurosurgeon must see the patient immediately. Dexamethasone, given at a loading dose of 1 to 2 mg/kg followed by a maintenance dose of 1 mg/kg every 6 hours, should be started. The head of the patient's bed is elevated to 30 degrees above the horizontal, and fluid intake is restricted (usually to two thirds of maintenance). If herniation appears to be impending based on the clinical picture (diminished consciousness, pupillary changes) or an imaging study, mannitol is often administered, and hyperventilation is started to decrease cerebral perfusion pressure.

Large tumors are usually grossly resected (debulked). A ventriculoperitoneal shunt (see Chapter 11) is placed if the tumor has caused hydrocephalus. Smaller lesions are completely resected when possible. It is important to realize that *the margins of the tumor visible by MRI often do not correspond to the pathological margins. In many cases, tumor cells have migrated into surrounding, normal-appearing brain tissue, so that gross resection is often not curative.*

The importance of surrounding brain tissue is also always considered in the decision to operate. If the tumor is of a less aggressive type and situated within a critical area (e.g., left-hemisphere speech area), nonsurgical treatment may be more appropriate. In some cases, the tumor may respond to radiation therapy, chemotherapy, or radiosurgical ablation (gamma-knife).

A stereotactic biopsy is usually performed to enable pathological diagnosis of tumors not amenable to gross resection. In other cases, such as when there is uncertainty about whether a small abnormality shown by MRI is in fact a tumor, the patient is closely followed with serial MRI before any surgical intervention is considered. Functional imaging (see Chapter 14) may be helpful in this situation.

Following tissue diagnosis, an oncologist with experience in the treatment of pediatric brain tumors is consulted to recommend further treatment. Chemotherapy, radiation therapy, both, or neither may be appropriate depending on the pathology of the tumor.

Some brain tumors, such as *cerebellar pilocytic astrocytoma* (Fig. 2.3), are curable by gross resection. *Oligodendrogliomas* and *neuronal tumors* also may be surgically curable. *Medulloblastoma*, the most common pediatric brain tumor, is often curable by surgery combined with radiation therapy and sometimes chemotherapy. The prognosis for *astrocytoma* (Fig. 2.4) and *ependymoma* (Fig. 2.5) is more guarded and varies depending on the patient's age and the location and histological characteristics of the tumor. The prognosis is poorest for high-grade hemispheric gliomas (*glioblastoma multiforme*) and *diffuse pontine gliomas* (Fig. 2.6). The latter are virtually untreatable and almost always result in death within 6 months to 2 years (24–26).

Pseudotumor cerebri

Pseudotumor cerebri (PTC) is a syndrome of *raised intracranial pressure* not caused by a space-occupying lesion. The underlying pathophysiology is not well understood. PTC often is diagnosed in *obese female patients*, usually

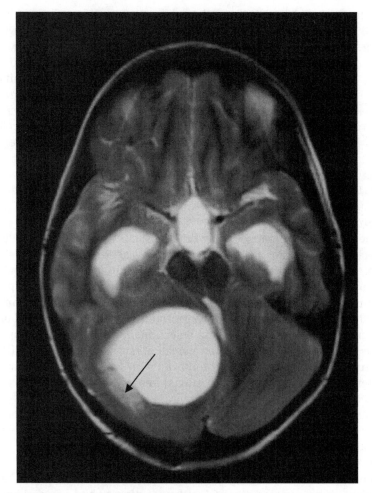

Figure 2.3 MRI showing **cerebellar astrocytoma** in 13-year-old adolescent male.
Note Large Cyst with Small Mural Tumor (*arrow*). (Courtesy of Ajax George, MD,
New York University School of Medicine.)

adolescents and young adults. In other cases, a *medication* (especially vitamin
A and its derivatives, tetracycline, oral contraceptives, and corticosteroids)
causes PTC. Other associations include otitis media, mastoiditis, sinusitis,
autoimmune disorders, diseases of the thyroid gland, and polycystic ovarian
syndrome (27,28). Many cases remain idiopathic, although a recent study (29)
documents that many patients diagnosed with PTC were found to have a congenital stenosis of an intracranial venous sinus.

Patients usually complain of a *headache* that is typically worst upon
awakening and, in most cases, *blurred vision, double vision,* or *partial loss
of vision. Sixth-nerve palsy* or *gaze-evoked nystagmus* (see Chapter 14) is

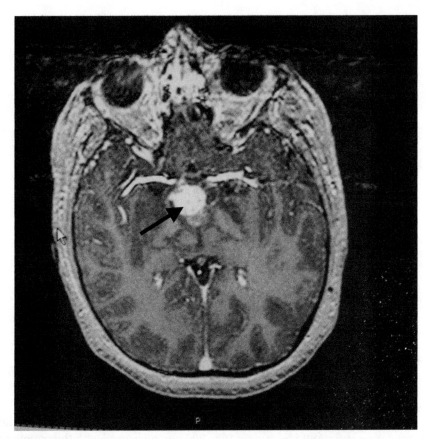

Figure 2.4 MRI showing **hypothalamic astrocytoma** in a 12-year-old boy.
(Courtesy of Ajax George, MD, New York University School of Medicine.)

often noted on examination. *Papilledema* is considered a necessary finding for diagnosis by most neurologists but may not have developed when patients are examined in the earliest stages of the disease. In some cases, papilledema is the first sign of the disease, noted by an alert optometrist who then sends the patient for neurological evaluation.

These patients are usually thought to have a brain tumor, and contrast-enhanced MRI is therefore ordered. No evidence of a tumor is revealed, but in many cases, slit-like ventricles and a subtle fluid transudate in the periventricular white matter are noted by the radiologist. Images of the cerebral venous sinuses must be carefully examined for evidence of *venous sinus thrombosis* ("empty delta sign"). *Magnetic resonance venography* (MRV), if available, may demonstrate *venous sinus stenosis.* Laboratory tests for an underlying endocrinological or autoimmune disorder should be ordered if no other cause for elevated ICP is discovered.

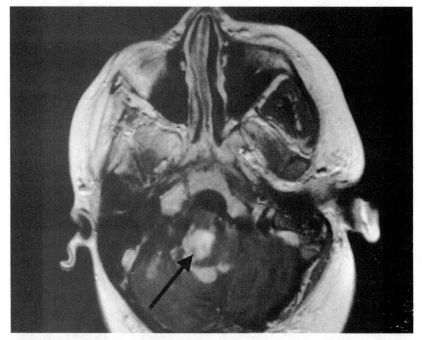

Figure 2.5 MRI showing brainstem **ependymoma** in a 7-year-old girl.
(Courtesy of Ajax George, MD, New York University School of Medicine.)

The diagnosis of PTC must be confirmed by LP. In cases of PTC, the opening pressure should be greater than 200 mm measured with the patient in the *lateral decubitus* (not sitting) position. Much higher readings (>300 mm) are common. LP often is both diagnostic and therapeutic, often providing immediate relief of long-standing daily headaches.

Treatment

The greatest danger of untreated PTC is *loss of vision*. The patient should be referred to an ophthalmologist for visual field mapping and periodic re-examinations. Obese patients must be strongly encouraged to lose weight. Any medication known to cause PTC must be discontinued, and any potentially contributing medical condition must be treated.

Acetazolamide, at a dose of 250 mg twice daily, is usually started. If the headaches do not improve, the dose may be increased to 500 mg twice daily. Topiramate, with its carbonic anhydrase action, may also be effective and may be particularly useful for obese patients because of its tendency to cause weight loss. Furosemide is also used to treat PTC. Corticosteroids are sometimes effective but tend to promote weight gain.

Treatment with medication should result in improvement of headaches and vision, resolution of papilledema, and a decrease in ICP measured by LP.

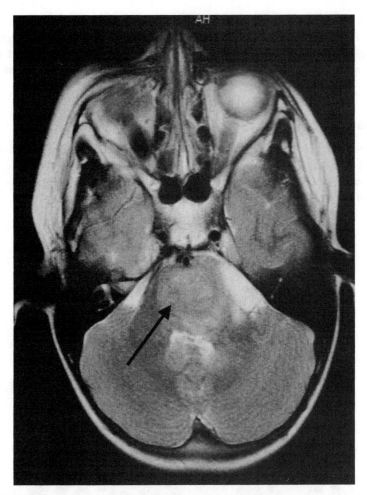

Figure 2.6 MRI showing a **diffuse pontine glioma** (*arrow*) in a 6-year-old girl.
(Courtesy of Ajax George, MD, New York University School of Medicine.)

In cases of PTC that do not respond to medication, removal of up to 50 cc of CSF once a week by means of LP will alleviate the patient's symptoms and sometimes appears to cure the disorder. Surgical procedures (CSF shunting, optic nerve fenestration) are performed in the most refractory cases.

Brain abscess

A bacterial embolus from a sinus, middle ear, or endocardial focus of infection may give rise to a *brain abscess*. Symptoms usually include headache, lethargy, and low-grade fever. Seizures may occur, or focal neurological signs may be noted depending on the location of the abscess. Papilledema is not typically found on examination. MRI during the earliest stage of abscess formation may suggest a localized area of infected brain tissue (*cerebritis*). Cerebritis rapidly progresses to liquefaction and capsule formation, at which point contrast-enhanced MRI will usually reveal a *ring-enhancing lesion*. Treatment entails one or more antibiotics, a corticosteroid, and surgical drainage of the abscess. Focal neurological deficits and seizures may persist after treatment.

Arteriovenous malformation

An *arteriovenous malformation* (AVM) (Fig. 2.7) is a cluster of abnormally formed blood vessels that presumably forms during fetal development. An AVM may be found in any location in the central nervous system as well as in other organs.

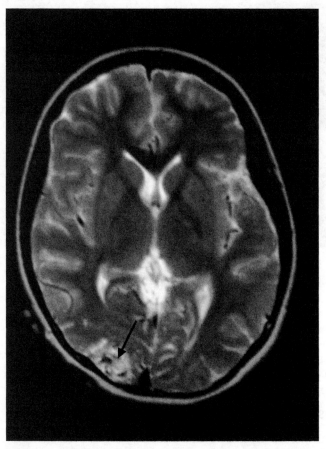

Figure 2.7 MRI showing a **arteriovenous malformation** (*arrow*) in a 14-year-old adolescent male.
(Courtesy of Ajax George, MD, New York University School of Medicine.)

The patient with an AVM usually is brought to medical attention because of (a) *seizures*; (b) *transient episodes of aphasia, ataxia, or hemiparesis*; or (c) *an intracerebral hemorrhage*. Headaches may occur but are almost never the only symptom of the AVM. The neurological examination is usually unremarkable. A *cranial bruit* is a classic although unusual physical finding.

Contrast-enhanced MRI (see Fig. 2.1) or CT typically reveals a serpiginous cluster of partially calcified blood vessels. Treatment with an antiepileptic drug is initiated if there is a history of seizures or if the AVM involves the cerebral cortex. Surgical resection, endovascular coagulation, and radiofrequency ablation (Gamma-knife) (30) are the definitive treatments; a combination of these treatments may be necessary in some cases.

INCIDENTALLY REPORTED INTRACRANIAL ABNORMALITIES

MRI of the brain often reveals an incidental finding or anatomical variant. Incidental findings are noted in more than 10% of MRI studies ordered for evaluation of headache, both in adults and children (31,32). These findings are almost always of no clinical significance but may be disconcerting to the family. Parents should be made aware *at the time MRI is ordered* that there is a reasonable likelihood that an incidental abnormality will be reported.

An *arachnoid cyst* (Fig. 2.8) is a trapped collection of cerebrospinal fluid within the meninges. Arachnoid cysts cause no problem of any kind for the vast majority of patients in whom they are incidentally discovered. Migraine headaches, syncopal episodes, school problems, autism, developmental delay, and virtually all other neurological problems should NOT be attributed to the arachnoid cyst. In very rare cases, the arachnoid cyst will progressively enlarge and compress the brain, in which case it is sometimes repaired surgically. In all other cases, the cyst should simply be ignored. It is not necessary to order follow-up MRI except in cases of a very large cyst that is causing mass effect.

An *enlarged CSF cistern* adjacent to the midbrain or cerebellum (Fig. 2.9) is a normal variant with no clinical significance. The finding of *dilated Virchow-Robin spaces* means that the radiologist has noted extra space between the cerebral blood vessels and surrounding brain tissue. This finding is also of no clinical significance.

A cyst in the pineal gland (*pineal cyst*) results from trapped endogenous hormone (Fig. 2.10). Pineal cysts are *not* pineal gland tumors, cause no symptoms, and require no intervention. Some radiologists advise follow-up MRI in 6 months, but the follow-up study rarely reveals a change in the appearance of the cyst.

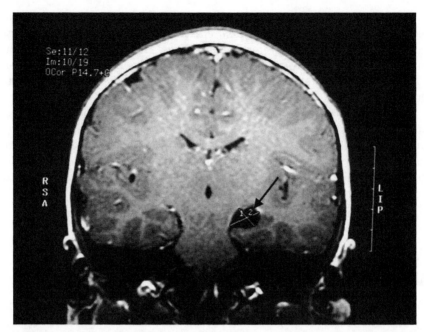

Figure 2.8 MRI showing a **arachnoid cyst** (*arrow*) in a 15-year-old adolescent female. (Courtesy of Ajax George, MD, New York University School of Medicine.)

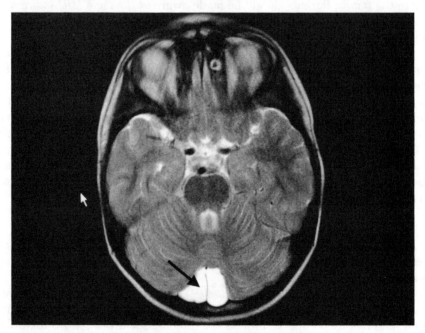

Figure 2.9 MRI showing **enlargement of the cerebellar cistern.** (Courtesy of Ajax George, MD, New York University School of Medicine.)

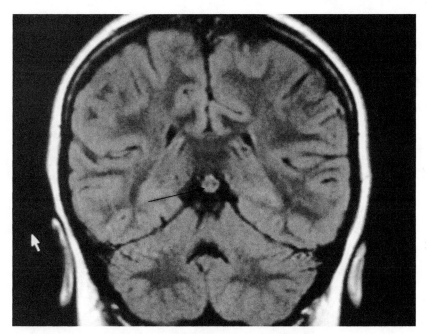

Figure 2.10 MRI showing a **pineal cyst** (*arrow*) in a 7-year-old girl.
(Courtesy of Ajax George, MD, New York University School of Medicine.)

Venous angiomas are presumably of developmental origin and do not generally cause neurological problems. If the angioma is found in an area of the brain thought to be giving rise to seizures, a neurosurgeon may be consulted, although resection of the angioma would be very unusual.

The radiological finding of a *Chiari I malformation* means that the caudal brainstem and cerebellar tonsils protrude through the foramen magnum. The clinical presentation of a symptomatic Chiari I malformation includes *occipital* headaches and intermittent episodes of ataxia, diplopia, and other *symptoms or signs of brainstem or cerebellar dysfunction* (33,34). These symptoms generally only occur when the cerebellar tonsils protrude more than 1 cm and are so compressed that they cause entrapment of the fourth ventricle. A symptomatic Chiari I malformation is shown in Figure 2.11.

The great majority of patients whose MRI report includes the radiological diagnosis of a Chiari I malformation do not have a history of occipital headaches or brainstem symptoms, and their Chiari malformation was incidentally discovered by MRI that was ordered for another reason. Surgery is never indicated in such cases. Only in symptomatic cases is surgery to enlarge the posterior fossa performed, since the operation (posterior fossa craniotomy) is associated with a substantial risk of complications.

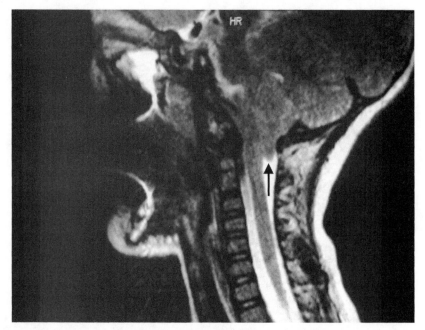

Figure 2.11 MRI showing symptomatic **Chiari I malformation** in a 13-year-old adolescent female.

Note Marked Protrusion of Cerebellar Tonsil into Foramen Magnum with Entrapment. (Courtesy of Ajax George, MD, New York University School of Medicine.)

WHEN AND WHEN NOT TO ORDER A BRAIN IMAGING STUDY

A headache of recent onset accompanied by one or more **unexplained persistent focal neurological symptoms or neurological deficits** is **always** an indication for a brain imaging study (Table 2.4). A brain imaging study is also **always** indicated in cases of a new-onset headache accompanied by an **unexplained change in mental status, a seizure, or papilledema** and is **always** indicated when **the history suggests a subarachnoid hemorrhage**.

An imaging study **is often ordered but not always indicated** to evaluate (a) headaches that *are not of a clearly recognizable type* (are not typical migraines, tension-type headaches, etc.); (b) other *headaches of recent onset*; (c) *headaches causing nighttime awakening*; (d) *headaches in young children* (because of unreliability in the history); and (e) *occipital headaches*. The entire clinical picture must be taken into consideration in these cases.

A brain imaging should *not* be ordered to evaluate:

1. **Headaches in an otherwise asymptomatic older child or adolescent that occur only during periods of psychological stress** (only on school days, directly after a traumatic event, etc.)

2. **Migraine headaches that are not associated with focal neurological symptoms**
3. **Headaches accompanying a mild or identifiable febrile illness** (viral syndrome, streptococcal pharyngitis, etc.) assuming the examination reveals **no signs of meningitis or elevated intracranial pressure** and the neurological examination is normal
4. **Headaches that have not changed in character or frequency, and an imaging study in the past was normal**

TABLE 2.4

When to order a brain imaging study

Characteristics of headache	Need for imaging
Accompanied by persistent focal neurological signs or symptoms, seizures, or a change in mental status	Always necessary
Papilledema noted on examination	Always necessary
Abrupt, "worst headache of my life"	CT necessary to exclude subarachnoid hemorrhage (lumbar puncture necessary if result normal)
Headache in a young child (<6 years)	Often ordered due to unreliability in the history
Headache causing awakening from sleep	Often ordered; however, usually migrainous or the result of medication overuse
Occipital headache or headache always in the same location	Often ordered; consider MRI of cervical spine in cases of occipital headache
Unexplained headaches of recent onset or that do not fit a recognizable clinical syndrome	Often ordered
Headaches only occurring during times of psychological/emotional stress in patient >6 years old	Not indicated
Typical migraine, especially if positive family history of migraine	Not indicated
Mild or well-characterized febrile illness with headache (viral syndrome, streptococcal pharyngitis, mononucleosis, etc.), assuming mental status is normal, patient does not have meningeal signs, and the neurological examination is normal	Not indicated
No significant change in headache location, quality, or pattern of occurrence; previously normal brain imaging study	Not indicated

TABLE 2.5
Comparison of CT and MRI for brain imaging

CT	MRI
Can be performed quickly (often in less than 5 minutes); useful in emergency room setting	Often takes 30 minutes or longer
Conscious sedation rarely required; claustrophobia rare	Conscious sedation required for infants and young children; many patients of all ages become claustrophobic
Entails radiation exposure	No radiation exposure
Enables quick diagnosis of intracranial bleeding; better than MRI for revealing some bone pathology (osteophyte, fracture, etc.); shows a cerebral parenchymal abnormality of moderate to large size; artifact limits view of brainstem	Not good for examining bone; intracranial bleeding is easier to see by CT; much better resolution of gray and white matter structures than CT and far superior images of the posterior fossa and brainstem
Often takes 24 hours or more to demonstrate infarction (stroke)	Diffusion-weighted MRI sensitive almost immediately to ischemic changes
Intravenous contrast often causes an allergic reaction	Intravenous contrast rarely causes an allergic reaction

CT AND MRI

CT and MRI each have clinical and practical advantages and shortcomings. Table 2.5 provides a summary (Table 2.5).

Since blood and bone are better visualized by CT than by MRI, CT is recommended when intracranial bleeding or a skull fracture is suspected and, therefore, is often ordered in cases of suspected intracranial bleeding or trauma. Many abnormalities of the brain parenchyma—for example, tumors of moderate to large size—can be seen using CT, making CT an adequate screening test when MRI cannot be performed quickly. However, MRI provides a much more detailed view of the cerebral gray and white matter and is also superior to CT for examining the brainstem, since the dense bone surrounding the posterior fossa causes artifact in CT images. If a physician wants to examine the brainstem or search for a small cortical malformation or tumor that might have caused a focal seizure, he should order an MRI. MRI can detect an ischemic stroke almost immediately after the onset of symptoms, whereas CT may not reveal any abnormality for more than 24 hours.

CT usually does not require sedation, and the CT scanner rarely makes patients feel claustrophobic. Infants and young children usually require conscious sedation before MRI due to the length of the procedure. Patients of all ages may become claustrophobic in the MRI machine. However, "open" MRI is less intimidating, and the images produced by the newer open MRI machines are approaching the quality of traditional machines. MRI does not expose the patient to radiation.

Contrast

A contrast material intravenously administered before an imaging study allows for *visualization of the arterial circulation* and demonstrates any *disruption of the blood–brain barrier*. A contrast-enhanced imaging study, therefore, should be ordered when the physician strongly suspects a *tumor, AVM, abscess, or intracranial infection* or when the noncontrast study shows a suspicious abnormality. Noncontrast imaging is adequate in cases of *trauma, bleeding, and suspected stroke and to look for static anatomical abnormalities* (congenital malformations). With respect to headaches, contrast should be ordered when focal signs, papilledema, or other neurological abnormalities are noted.

The contrast material used for CT often causes an allergic reaction, whereas the contrast material (gadolinium) used for MRI rarely does.

REFERENCES

1. Moore A, Shevell M. Chronic daily headaches in pediatric neurology practice. *J Child Neurol.* 2004;19:925–929.
2. Lewis DW, Gozzo YF, Avner MT. The "other:" primary headaches in children and adolescents. *Pediatr Neurol.* 2005;33:303–313.
3. Silberstein SD, Lipton RB, Goadsby PJ. *Headache in Clinical Practice.* London: Martin Dunitz; 2002:47–65.
4. Welch KM, Cutrer FM, Goadsby PJ. Migraine pathogenesis: neural and vascular mechanisms. *Neurology.* 2003;60(suppl 2):S9–S14.
5. Ramadan NM. Targeting therapy for migraine: what to treat? *Neurology.* 2005;64 (suppl 2):S4–S8.
6. Silberstein SD, Lipton RB, Goadsby PJ. *Headache in Clinical Practice.* London: Martin Dunitz; 2002:116–117.
7. Lewis DW, Dorbad D. The utility of neuroimaging the evaluation of children with migraine or chronic daily headache who have normal neurological examinations. *Headache.* 2000;40:629–632.
8. Katsarava Z, Fritche G, Muessig M, et al. Clinical features of withdrawal headache following overuse of triptans and other headache drugs. *Neurology.* 2001;57:1694–1698.
9. Zwart JA, Dyb G, Hagen K, et al. Analgesic use: a predictor of chronic pain and medication overuse headache. The Head-HUNT study. *Neurology.* 2003;61:160–164.
10. Silberstein SD, Freitag FG. Preventive treatment of migraine. *Neurology.* 2003;60 (suppl 2):S38–S44.
11. Holroyd KA, O'Donnell FJ, Stensland M, et al: Management of chronic tension-type headache with tricyclic antidepressant medication, stress management therapy, and their combination: a randomized controlled trial. *JAMA.* 2001;285:2208–2215.
12. Mathew NT, Hulihan JF, Rothrock JF. Anticonvulsants in migraine prophylaxis. *Neurology.* 2003;60(suppl 2):S45–S49.
13. Spira PJ, Beran RG. Gabapentin in the prophylaxis of chronic daily headache: a randomized, placebo-controlled study. *Neurology* 2003;61:1753–1759.

14. Krilov LR, Fisher M. Chronic fatigue syndrome in youth: maybe not so chronic after all. *Contemp Pediatr.* 2002;19:61.

15. Stewart J, Gewitz MH, Weldon A, et al. Patterns of orthostatic intolerance: The orthostatic tachycardia syndrome and chronic fatigue. *J Pediatr.* 1999;135:218–225.

16. Stewart J, Gewitz MH, Weldon A, et al. Orthostatic intolerance in adolescent chronic fatigue syndrome. *Pediatrics.* 1999;103:116–121.

17. Harno H, Hirovenen T, Kaunisto MA, et al. Subclinical vestibulocerebellar dysfunction in migraine with and without aura. *Neurology.* 2003;61:1748–1752.

18. Ahmed MAS, Reid E, Cooke A, et al. Familial hemiplegic migraine in the west of Scotland: a clinical and genetic study of seven families. *J Neurol Neurosurg Psychiatry.* 1996;61:616–620.

19. Ducros A, Joutel A, Vahedi K, et al. Mapping of a second locus for familial hemiplegic migraine to 1q21-23 and evidence for further heterogeneity. *Ann Neurol.* 1997;42:885–890.

20. Ahonen K, Hamalainen ML, Rantala H, et al. Nasal sumatriptan is effective in treatment of migraine attacks in children: a randomized trial. *Neurology.* 2004;62:883–887.

21. Sandor PS, DiClemente L, Coppola G, et al. Efficacy of coenzyme Q10 in migraine prophylaxis: a randomized controlled trial. *Neurology.* 2005;64:713–715.

22. Friedman BW, Corbo J, Lipton RB, et al. Metoclopramide as effective as sumatriptan for ER migraine treatment. *Neurology.* 2005;64:463–468.

23. Cady RK, Dodick DW, Levine HL, et al. Sinus headache: a neurology, otolaryngology, allergy, and primary care consensus on diagnosis and treatment. *Mayo Clin Proc.* 2005;80:908–916.

24. Levy AS. Brain tumors in children: evaluation and management. *Curr Probl Pediatr Adolesc Health Care.* 2005;35:230–245.

25. Jallo GI, Biser-Rohrbaugh A, Freed D. Brainstem gliomas. *Childs Nerv Syst.* 2004;20:143–153.

26. Kaatsch P, Rickert CH, Kuhl J, et al. Population-based epidemiologic data on brain tumors in German children. *Cancer.* 2001;92:3155–3164.

27. Glucek CJ, Aregawi D, Goldenberg N, et al. Idiopathic intracranial hypertension, polycystic-ovary syndrome, and thrombophilia. *J Lab Clin Med.* 2005;145:72–82.

28. Fenichel G. *Clinical Pediatric Neurology.* Philadelphia: Saunders; 2001:115.

29. Farb RI, Vanek I, Scott JN, et al. Idiopathic intracranial hypertension: the prevalence and morphology of sinovenous stenosis. *Neurology.* 2003;60:1418–1424.

30. Schauble B, Cascino GD, Pollock BE, et al. Seizure outcomes after stereotactic radiosurgery for cerebral arteriovenous malformations. *Neurology.* 2004;63:683–687.

31. Illes J, Desmond JE, Huang LF, et al. Ethical and practical considerations in managing incidental findings in functional magnetic resonance imaging. *Brain Cogn.* 2002;50:358–365.

32. Lewis DW, Ashwal S, Dahl G, et al. Practice parameter: evaluation of children and adolescents with recurrent headaches: report of the Quality Standards Subcommittee of the American Academy of Neurology and the Practice Committee of the Child Neurology Society. *Neurology.* 2002;59:490–498.

33. Osborne AG. *Diagnostic Neuroradiology.* St. Louis: Mosby; 1994;16–17.

34. Adams RD, Victor M, Ropper AH. *Principles of Neurology.* New York: McGraw Hill; 1997:1006–1007.

3

SCHOOL PROBLEMS AND ATTENTION-DEFICIT HYPERACTIVITY DISORDER

Many children and teenagers are brought to their pediatrician's office because of poor grades, failure to acquire academic skills, or because they are behaving inappropriately in the classroom. The teacher of a prekindergarten age child may have told the parents that their child has not yet learned to recognize letters and numbers, that he has trouble comprehending verbal directions, or that he is hyperactive. Grade-school age children are often referred because of delayed reading skills or because of a history of restlessness and distractibility in class. Teenagers are usually brought for evaluation because of poor grades, poor study habits, and disruptive or oppositional behavior in school. The physician should also consider the possibility of a school-related problem in the case of a child or adolescent who "hates school"; is angry, anxious, or depressed for unclear reasons; or has unexplained physical symptoms (headaches and stomachaches) on school days.

"NOT FOCUSING"

In many cases, a teacher has complained that the child is not focusing in class. Although this observation usually implies that the teacher suspects attention-deficit hyperactivity disorder (ADHD), the physician should not make the mistake of automatically assuming that ADHD is the appropriate diagnosis for every child with a "focusing problem." **"Not focusing" is a behavior, not a diagnosis.** ADHD is always a potential cause of poor concentration, but the child's inattentiveness also might result from a learning disability, depression or anxiety, a sleep disorder, a medical disorder, or a problem in the home. Anything less than a careful history and examination, evaluation of the child's academic abilities, and exploration of social/psychological factors does a disservice to a child referred for "not focusing" and to any patient who has a problem in school.

Questions to ask the family

1. At what age was a problem first suspected? Did the child do well in kindergarten, first grade, etc.? When did teachers begin to be concerned about the child's academic performance? When did the child's grades start to decline?
2. How severe is the problem? Are the child's grades just mediocre or in the failing range? In how many and which subjects is the child doing poorly? Is there a possibility that the child will not be promoted to the next grade, or has that already occurred?
3. Was the child late to learn to read? Is the child now reading at grade level? Is reading comprehension (ask about social studies), listening comprehension (ask about ability to follow multistep directions), or calculation ability an area of weakness?
4. Is there a history of delayed language milestones or a speech problem?
5. Did the parents complete high school? Do they read for enjoyment? Has anyone in the family been diagnosed with a learning disability, ADHD, or a language disorder?
6. Is the child distractible, inattentive, restless, fidgety, impulsive, or hyperactive? Can he or she maintain concentration for more than a brief period of time during a variety of quiet activities (*other than* watching television and playing video games)? For example, does the child enjoy reading, playing a musical instrument, playing with building toys, drawing, board games, chess, woodworking, crafts, or putting puzzles together?
7. Does the child fail to bring homework home or hand it in? Is getting the child to do homework a nightly battle? Is he or she generally disorganized or forgetful?
8. Are appropriate limits to encourage studying set at home? Are competing distractions, such as television and video games, permitted to take over on school nights? Is the child's schedule so full of extracurricular activities (football practice, dance lessons, etc.) that he has little time left to do his homework?
9. Does the child often seem anxious, depressed, or angry? Does he or she get along with the parents, siblings, and other children? Is life in the family unhappy or stressful for some reason?

LEARNING DISABILITY

General concepts

During their years in grade school, children are expected to acquire age-appropriate reading, writing, comprehension, and mathematical skills as well as a considerable amount of basic knowledge about the world. More advanced analytical skills are required for junior high school, high school, and college, when students are expected to learn much more specialized and detailed information.

In a general sense, a person of normal intelligence with a reasonable education, who has no medical or behavioral problem impacting academic performance, and who has been trying hard to learn can be said to have a *learning disability* (LD) when his academic progress is slower than expected. The prevalence of LD in the United States is high, approaching 5% (1,2).

An LD refers to a *specific, definable* cognitive deficit and is thus distinguished from *mental retardation* (see Chapter 9), which implies *globally subnormal intelligence* as measured by a standardized intelligence test. Thus, many educational psychologists diagnose an LD on the basis of a discrepancy between *ability* (as measured by a test of *intelligence*) and *achievement* (meaning skills acquired) in a particular academic area. However, this definition fails to account for poor achievement caused by other factors (such as ADHD, anxiety or depression, a general medical condition, or poor study habits). It can be argued that an LD is better characterized as a poor *aptitude* for an academic skill than as underachievement, and this change in emphasis may be reflected in new federal guidelines for schools.

What kind of a problem is an LD?

Two hundred years ago, a mother would never have thought to take her child to the doctor to evaluate a learning problem because, at that time, most children attended school for only a few years (if at all) and because academic ability was irrelevant to most peoples' livelihood. A member of a hunter-gatherer society would not care (or know) if his brain was not suited for reading or math, as long as his capacity for survival, reproduction, language, social interaction, and everyday activities was not affected.

An LD does not affect life span, cause pain or physical impairment, or affect a person's ability to have children. Most people with an LD, as adults, discover a career that suits them and find fulfillment in their job, family, social life, and leisure activities. (By the same token, *not* having an LD is no guarantee of success or happiness.) For all these reasons, an LD should not be considered a "disease," but rather a neurological variant. A perspective that every person's brain is better at some kinds of tasks than at other kinds of tasks is valid and may be shared with parents and patients.

Having said this, we recognize that people with an LD experience a great deal of frustration while in school and that it is the physician's roll to offer them insight and guidance.

How the problem comes to attention

Signs of an LD may be first recognized at any age. The preschool-age child at risk for an LD may have difficulty learning to identify numbers, letters, or shapes; may be unable to comprehend verbal directions; or may be said to have a "behavior problem" that is eventually recognized to result from confusion and frustration. Learning-disabled children in grade school are often slow to learn to read, have difficulty comprehending what they read or hear, may be unable to retain mathematical facts, and often struggle with mathematical word problems. Learning-disabled junior high school and high school students usually have difficulty in classes that stress reading comprehension, abstract thinking, and essay writing. Some people are not diagnosed with an LD until they are enrolled in college or embarked on a postgraduate career, at which point they come to realize that a particular type of cognitive task is much more difficult for them than their peers.

Neurological basis of learning disability and classification of learning disability

Our understanding of the neurological basis of LD has been enhanced by the results of research published during the last several decades. Studies using functional magnetic resonance imaging (MRI) show that people with dyslexia use different regions of the cerebral cortex to read than nondyslexic individuals (3). Other research suggests that the phonemic recognition speed of patients with a language-based LD may be slower than normal (4–6). Neuroanatomical correlates of LD, such as a less lateralized (more symmetrical) brain, have been reported for many years (7,8). *Left handedness* has also long been associated with LD.

Functional imaging studies are particularly intriguing, and emerging technologies such as functional MRI may, in the future, be widely used to characterize specific types of LD. Currently, however, there are no widely available neurological diagnostic tests to confirm the presence of an LD or aid in the classification of LD. The *diagnosis and classification of LD is still based entirely on the results of cognitive and psychoeducational testing.*

An important consequence of the nonneurological basis of LD classification is a theoretical and descriptive nomenclature. Thus, a child with an LD may be said by the educational psychologist to have a *processing problem* (poor listening comprehension or reading comprehension), a *decoding problem* (trouble recognizing or pronouncing the syllables he reads), a *sequencing problem* (trouble performing tasks requiring multiple steps or remembering sequences), or a *visuomotor integration problem* (difficulty recognizing shapes and drawing). Another popular term is *executive function*, which refers to the ability to make decisions, prioritize, and organize. All of these terms are ultimately models for what is happening in the child's brain but may sound like medical diagnoses and confuse parents who are trying to grasp the cause of their child's problem. It is important to explain that we do not really know the underlying neurological cause of most kinds of LD, no matter how specific the nomenclature may sound.

The system of classification determining eligibility for special accommodations used by Child Study Teams may not be helpful in this regard, although it has recently been improved. Unfortunately, a child with an LD was, for many years, classified under the heading of "perceptual impairment," whereas the child with ADHD was classified as "neurologically impaired," erroneously suggesting that while ADHD is a neurologically based condition, an LD is not. Fortunately, children with an LD are now straightforwardly classified as *specific learning disabled.*

The diagnosis of an LD ultimately has political and legal implications since the government's (public school's) obligation to pay for supportive services depends on whether and how the Child Study Team classifies a child. Since interventions for an LD are expensive to provide, financial limitations and federal guidelines may allow Child Study Teams to classify a student as learning disabled only when his or her LD is relatively severe, making children with a milder but still significant LD ineligible for many kinds of assistance. Federal guidelines state that a parent who disagrees with Child Study Team findings has a right to a second-opinion evaluation paid for by the school. In some cases, however, litigation has resulted when parents persistently disagree with the evaluation or the interventions proposed to remedy the problem.

Heritable Factors

A history of relatives who have had learning problems is often reported. A parent may remember that he had difficulty learning to read or mention that he did not finish high school. Many parents of learning-disabled children say that they *do not read for pleasure.* In other cases, a parent will say that mathematical calculation (balancing the checkbook or doing a tax return) or visual-spatial thinking (map reading) is difficult for him or her. One or more siblings often have been diagnosed with an LD. This kind of family history is common and suggests that an LD is, in all likelihood, a genetically inherited trait, although a specific genetic basis for LD has not been described.

Developmental and medical factors

Children with a history of *delayed language acquisition* or a *speech disorder* often have trouble comprehending what they hear (receptive language deficit) and may have difficulty reading because of poor phonemic awareness. These children should, of course, have an audiological evaluation, but their peripheral hearing usually is found to be normal. Children with a history of premature birth or low birth weight are at risk for developing an LD (9). Children with fetal alcohol syndrome, fragile X syndrome, neurofibromatosis type I, and many other syndromes of congenital malformation often have an LD, if not a more severe cognitive impairment.

Physical examination and laboratory testing

The physical examination of the patient with a suspected LD may be concise if there are no other medical complaints; the cognitive/behavioral part of the examination is more important. Stigmata suggesting a congenital syndrome should be noted. The child's behavior may suggest ADHD. The child's speech may reveal poor articulation. "Soft signs" and a preference for using the left hand to write should be noted.

The child's venous lead level should be checked. Other laboratory tests are not necessary unless a specific underlying disorder (fragile X syndrome, for example) is suspected. MRI is almost never necessary, and an electroencephalogram (EEG) should not be ordered.

LEARNING EVALUATION

Primary care physicians and neurologists are not trained to administer psychoeducational tests. These tests are also not practical to give in a physician's office since they require many hours. However, the following *screening evaluation* for LD can be administered in about 15 minutes. On the basis of this evaluation, it should be possible to get a sense of the child's strengths and weaknesses, assess the severity of her learning problem, and suggest whether or not formal testing by an educational psychologist will be necessary.

Testing children ages 5 and younger

The *Draw-a-Person Test* (10) is easily administered to preschool children and provides a rough initial estimate of cognitive development. Children in the preschool age group also may be asked to identify pictures of common objects, match and copy geometric shapes, and follow multistep directions. Five-year-old children should be able to recognize upper-case letters and numbers.

The child's comprehension and speech should always be assessed. Children 3 to 4 years of age should be able to follow a two-step verbal direction and engage in a simple conversation. Five-year-old children should be able to answer questions about more complex sentences (e.g., "A man saw a girl who was holding a balloon. Who was holding the balloon?"), and follow three-step commands ("Give me the pen, then the block, and then the scissors."), and spatial directions ("Put the paper under the book and then put the block on top of the book.").

The *Pediatric Examination of Educational Readiness* (11) is a concise screening test for the preschool child containing many of these items. The *Clinical Evaluation of Language Fundamentals* (12) is a more comprehensive test of language skills.

Testing school-age children and adolescents

If the patient is in grade school, junior high school, or high school, his or her reading level may be broadly evaluated with the single word reading section of the *Wide Range Achievement Test* (WRAT) (13). The examiner should also ask the patient to *define* some of the words he or she has read. If the child is in the second or a higher grade, he or she should read a paragraph of age-appropriate difficulty and be able to answer questions about the content. *The Gray Oral Reading Test* (14) is often given to evaluate fluency and comprehension.

The *Pediatric Early Elementary Examination* for grade-school children and the *Pediatric Evaluation of Educational Readiness at Middle Childhood* (11) for students in middle school and high school are very useful screening tests. Some of the skills tested are ability to recall a series of digits, rhyme words and substitute phonemes, recall and interpret complex sentences, and match and copy geometric figures. Older children (>9 years) and adolescents are also asked to deduce answers from verbally presented paragraphs, interpret sentences with double meanings, and answer questions requiring sequential reasoning.

The patient should also be asked to solve a few age-appropriate computation and mathematical word problems. Alternatively, the mathematics portion of the WRAT (11) may be administered. The following are some suggested math questions:

First grade: If you have two cookies and I give you three more, how many cookies do you have now? If you give me one cookie back, how many do you have left?

Second grade: Use questions like those stated for first-grade students, but use a number of objects that will sum to two digits and subtract to one digit, such as $8 + 5 = 13$ and $12 - 3 = 9$. How much is each coin worth (show a dime, nickel, or penny)?

Third grade: How much money is this? (Show the patient some mixed change.) If I give you 5 dollars to go to the store, and you buy three things for a dollar each, how much money will you have left over?

Third and fourth grade: Administer a quiz on a few multiplication facts (e.g., 3×4, 5×8, etc.). Use word problems like the one stated for third-grade patients but with larger numbers. Time questions can also be used: What time does my watch say? How many minutes after 11 o'clock is 11:30?

Fourth and fifth grade: Use questions like those stated for third- and fourth-grade patients but with still larger numbers, and use division problems ($12 \div 3$).

Middle school into high school: Depending on age, test understanding of fractions (What is larger, one half or one third? How much does one half *plus* one third equal?) and percentages (What is 10% of 200?).

If you drive at 60 miles per hour for one-half hour, how far have you gone? If your car used 10 gallons of gasoline to travel 300 miles, how many miles per gallon did your car get?

Formal Psychoeducational Testing

If the screening evaluation suggests that the patient may have an LD, a formal evaluation should be scheduled. Only an educational psychologist or neuropsychologist can formally diagnose an LD. In most cases, the school's Child Study Team will arrange for a psychologist to test the child at no cost to the family. Alternatively, testing can be privately arranged, although it will be costly and currently is usually not covered by medical insurance. Some parents still opt for private testing to avoid the usual lengthy wait for a Child Study Team evaluation, and so the results can be kept confidential. It should be pointed out, however, that if the child turns out to have an LD and requires extra help, the school will need to know the results of testing. Table 3.1 is a list of some tests often given by educational psychologists.

TABLE 3.1

Commonly administered formal tests of learning and cognition

Test	Purpose
Stanford-Binet (15)	IQ, ages 2–23
Wechsler Preschool and Primary Scale of Intelligence (WPPSI) (16)	IQ, ages 4–6 1/2
Wechsler Intelligence Scale for Children (WISC) (17)	IQ, ages 6–16 years, 11 months
Wechsler Adult Intelligence Scale (WAIS) (18)	IQ, age >17 years
Gray Oral Reading Test (14)	Reading fluency; can be used to assess comprehension
Woodcock-Johnson Test (19)	Comprehensive reading and language assessment; may be used as an intelligence test
Raven's Progressive Matrices (20)	Visual perceptual ability, reasoning
Bender Gestalt Test (21)	Visual perceptual ability, hand-eye coordination
Test of Visual-Motor Integration (22)	Visual perceptual ability, hand-eye coordination
Rey Complex Figure (23)	Visual perceptual ability

CLASSIFICATION OF LEARNING DISABILITIES

Many parts of the brain are functionally interconnected, and many similar cognitive functions share a common neuroanatomical substrate. Thus it is more common for a person to have an LD that impacts two or more related academic skills (i.e., both reading and auditory comprehension) than only a single skill. *Therefore, the following common types of LD should not be considered mutually exclusive categories. Learning disabilities also can be mild and perhaps better characterized as relative weaknesses.* Many people have some difficulty reading, for example, but would not be considered dyslexic.

Reading disorder

Reading disorder, or *dyslexia*, is diagnosed on the basis of a patient's below-average aptitude for reading despite his normal (or above average) intelligence. The problem, in many cases, stems from a difficulty *sounding out read syllables*. This is often called *decoding ability*. Children with reading disorder usually can read the letters of the alphabet but do not pronounce the letters and syllables as they are meant to sound in words. Therefore, during the first grade, words are read slowly or incorrectly, or similar appearing words are substituted. Once these children finally master the ability to sound out simple words (e.g., "cat," "see," "job"), words with blended syllables (e.g., "first," "twist," and "struck") present an even greater challenge, and as a result, the children fall further behind.

Other children with reading disorder pronounce basic syllables well enough but struggle with *polysyllabic* words. This group of students also tends to have difficulty with tasks involving the memorization of *sequences*, such as recalling a series of digits or days of the week in order or solving mathematical problems with multiple steps. These patients are sometimes said to have a *sequencing problem*.

In still other cases, a child masters phonemes and polysyllabic words but has trouble sight reading small words that are not easily dissected (e.g., "who," "ask," "know"). These children often seem to have trouble with visual-perceptual tasks (shape recognition), suggesting a right-hemisphere (visual spatial) deficit.

The child with reading disorder usually hates to read. Homework is a nightly battle that intensifies as the child advances from one grade to the next and required reading material becomes more demanding. Many academic subjects are affected. Grades are low from the start or fall off over time, and the child's confidence and self-esteem almost always suffer.

When they are given the WRAT (13) or Gray Oral Reading Test (14) children with reading disorder read slowly, mispronounce words, or substitute similar looking words. Their ability to perform tests of rhyming, phonemic substitution, and digit span tests (contained in the Pediatric Evaluation of Educational Readiness series) (11) often is below average for age.

A reading level *two or more grades below the norm for age* was once a primary criterion by which dyslexia was diagnosed, but this criterion is no longer used. Reading disorder is now recognized to represent a broad spectrum; many children struggle to read without lagging two grades behind their peers. Additionally, since children are not expected to learn to read until the latter half of kindergarten or the first grade, it is impossible to test two grades below level in reading ability until the latter half of second grade at the earliest.

Letter reversals and dyslexia

The concept of dyslexia as a syndrome of letter and word reversals is erroneous. Although some people who have difficulty reading reverse the letters or words they read or spell, most do not; conversely, many children who have no trouble reading "flip" their letters. *The presence or absence of reversals is not relevant to the diagnosis of reading disorder.* If a young child is reading well and is keeping up in other academic areas but occasionally reverses letters, there is no problem, and his reversals are best ignored.

Auditory comprehension

Many individuals with a history of poor academic performance have *difficulty comprehending what they hear.* A parent or teacher may have noted that the child has trouble following multistep verbal directions, understanding conversations, or, when he or she is older, taking notes during lecture. In many cases, the teacher complains that the student is "not focusing" and suspects ADHD. Prekindergarten children with this kind of LD often are initially said to have a "behavior problem" that is eventually recognized to result from a combination of poor comprehension and frustration.

Many of these individuals have a history of delayed language milestones. Testing in the office often reveals below-average performance on tasks requiring multistep verbal direction following, sentence repetition, complex sentence interpretation, and digit span.

A standard hearing test is almost always within normal limits. The *central auditory processing test,* administered by many audiologists, has become a popular tool for evaluating these patients. Despite its name, this test is not a physiological assessment of brain function (such as an EEG) but, instead, a performance test assessing the child's ability to interpret complex aurally presented material. The test does not yield a positive result in all cases of auditory comprehension difficulty. Many audiologists also feel that this test is not useful for children under the age of 7 years.

Reading comprehension

In many cases, the student with an LD affecting *reading comprehension* can read fluently and did well academically until junior high school, when the content of assigned reading material became more challenging. Individuals with this LD usually must read a passage multiple times before they comprehend the meaning. They often receive poor grades in *social studies* and *science*.

When given the single-word WRAT (11), the student with this kind of LD often reads fluently and at grade level but may be *unable to define the meaning* of many words. After reading through an age-appropriate paragraph once, the child will have trouble answering questions about the content. The Pediatric Evaluation of Educational Readiness at Middle Childhood (11), Gray Oral Reading Test (14), and the Woodcock-Johnson Test (19) are useful tests for evaluating these patients.

Dysgraphia and poor handwriting

Most people with *dysgraphia*, an LD affecting writing ability, also exhibit deficiencies in other language-based academic skills. Many patients who are thought to have dysgraphia really have trouble concentrating or are discouraged or oppositional. Writing is arguably the most concentration-demanding academic skill. If concentration ability is suspected to be the main problem, a trial of a stimulant medication may be worth considering. In many other cases, the problem is poor motivation, oppositional behavior, low self-esteem, perfectionism, or anxiety and can be managed with behavioral modification, assistance from a learning consultant, or psychotherapy.

The patient with *messy handwriting* may be asked to write a few sentences about a subject of his/her or the examiner's choice. If the result is illegible or the letters are poorly constructed or spaced and the neurological examination reveals immature fine motor abilities or "soft signs," the problem is neurodevelopmental, and the patient may be referred for occupational therapy. Although their handwriting usually gets better as they mature, children with fine motor problems can also be taught to do their written assignments on a computer keyboard. If the child's handwriting is easily legible in the office, there is probably no neuromotor basis for the messy handwriting, and the problem is most likely behavioral or caused by a lack of focus.

Learning disability in mathematics

Mathematics disorder is an LD specifically affecting mathematical ability (22). The patient with mathematics disorder typically has difficulty with tasks requiring computation. However, if the patient has trouble with mathematical *word problems* but *not* computation, the problem is more likely *reading comprehension* or *listening comprehension*.

Visual-perceptual learning disability

Some individuals have a great deal of trouble performing *visual-spatial* tasks. Not surprisingly, these people find *geometry* a particularly challenging subject. Children with this kind of LD also often have difficulty (or dislike) drawing, putting together puzzles, and playing with building toys. As adults, they may have trouble reading maps and following place directions.

Some of these patients also have a history of behavioral and social problems. This complex is sometimes referred to as the *syndrome of nonverbal learning disabilities (NLD)* (24,25). Since the right cerebral hemisphere mediates many visual-perceptual tasks and may also be responsible for cognitive functions in social interactions (reading facial expressions, etc.), this syndrome is sometimes called *right-hemisphere learning disability*. It should be noted that NLD is a relatively recent diagnostic category. Some psychologists believe that visual-perceptual learning disability and NLD are not synonymous.

Young patients with NLD are often hyperactive, and many are initially diagnosed with ADHD, but a trial of a stimulant medication does not result in behavioral improvement. NLD also resembles Asperger syndrome (an autistic spectrum disorder; see Chapter 9) in some respects, but ritualistic behaviors and stereotyped interests, poor eye contact, and failure to develop age-appropriate fantasy play (all features of Asperger syndrome) are not typical of NLD.

The diagnosis of an NLD usually requires the finding of a *significantly lower* (>15 point difference) *nonverbal than verbal IQ score*. Interventions are discussed in the following sections.

ASSISTANCE FOR PATIENTS WITH AN LD

Discussing the problem with the family

The patient with an LD and his or her parents should be informed that, although he or she has many strengths and talents, certain kinds of academic tasks are nevertheless very difficult for the patient. It is best to be straightforward and practical: *this is the problem area* (e.g., "testing shows that reading comprehension is a weakness"); *these interventions may help; and here are some things to think about when you are planning your child's future*. Theoretical terms (e.g., "processing," "decoding," and "executive function") should be avoided if possible. The family already has enough to digest.

Interventions for the student with an LD

If the patient has a mild LD, assistance from a tutor or a qualified learning specialist may address his or her academic needs. However, in most cases of an LD, the child's school must become involved. Children who have trouble learning to read or struggle in mathematics are usually initially offered remedial or *basic skills instruction classes* that review elementary material more intensively. The patient who fails to make progress in this setting is usually referred to his school's Child Study Team for evaluation. If this evaluation results in a formal *classification* on the basis of a specific LD, *resource room* placement in appropriate subjects, a *classroom aide*, referral to a *self-contained classroom*, or even placement in a *specialized school* may be recommended, depending on the severity of the problem and the resources available. Instruction in these settings is more individualized, moves at a slower pace, and may incorporate one or more of the following specific interventions.

The *Orton-Gillingham* and the *Wilson methods* are designed to help children diagnosed with *reading disorder* (dyslexia). These methods primarily rely on *intensive and repetitive phonetic drilling*. A multisensory approach using visualization and other associative techniques is often incorporated. Children with a severe reading disability usually require many years of instruction. A recently published review of current approaches to treating dyslexia (26) is recommended for the doctor who wishes to learn more about these methods. Patients who have trouble *comprehending what they hear* (auditory comprehension disorder) may benefit from *presentation of material in a written format* (in handouts or on the blackboard). A *frequency modulated (FM) radio system* raises the volume of the teacher's voice above background noise level and is often recommended. Individuals for whom *reading comprehension* is difficult can be taught to more efficiently glean information from the material they read, use word visualization techniques, and enlarge their vocabulary.

Waiver of the foreign language requirement is recommended for patients with any language-based LD.

Assistance with *organizational skills* and *occupational therapy* may be useful for patients with a visual-perceptual LD. The behavioral problems associated with NLD are addressed via *individual and group psychotherapy* focused on improving social skills. Some patients with an NLD take a medication such as clonidine or risperidone to help control impulsive behavior.

High school students with an LD may be allowed extra time when taking the Standardized Achievement Test (SAT). Formal testing by an educational psychologist is *required* by the SAT board in order for the student to be allowed this modification. The SAT board does not accept a doctor's note stating that the patient has an LD.

Many high school students with an LD who continue to struggle in school despite receiving appropriate supplemental services eventually choose a *technical education program*. Technical classes (in mechanics, carpentry, or culinary arts, for example) offer these students a welcome respite from difficult academic subjects and provide an opportunity to learn a trade that they may wish to pursue after graduation.

Nontraditional therapies

Eye movement exercises to enhance reading ability and auditory training sessions to improve listening comprehension ability are nontraditional interventions, claimed to enhance learning and improve academic performance, that are offered by some centers. These methods were evaluated by the

American Academy of Pediatrics and were not found to produce objective improvement (27,28).

Long-term issues

Hard work and appropriate accommodation in school will often result in steady, measurable academic progress for the child with an LD. Magical, overnight improvement is not to be expected. An LD is almost never "cured." Therefore, the patient should not spend his entire childhood being ferried from one learning consultant, psychologist, tutor, or learning center to the next in the hope that someone will "unlock the key."

The patient's self-esteem is the most important priority. The patient should be encouraged to do his or her best in all academic subjects, especially subjects that call upon the patient's strengths (e.g., mathematics in the case of a patient who mostly has difficulty reading, or history in the case of a patient who struggles in math but is a good reader). People with an LD should also be encouraged to develop an interest in sports, music, theatre, or art and to work during the summer vacation. Success in one of these activities will help the patient maintain confidence and a positive outlook and might even point the way to a future career. Good friendships and a happy family life are also very important.

Individuals with an LD should carefully plan their post–high school future. Some people with an LD choose to enroll in one of many available college programs or junior colleges offering modifications for learning-disabled students. Other people with an LD attend a post–high school program providing training in a nonacademic field, such as graphic design, culinary arts, computer programming, cosmetology, or audio engineering. A patient with an LD primarily affecting a particular academic subject may attend a 4-year college and select appropriate courses. The patient for whom mathematics has always been a struggle, for example, may major in English rather than physics, which the patient will find easier and also enjoy more. Other individuals work after high school rather than attend college or become apprentices at a trade. It is recommended that the student and family meet regularly and early with the high school guidance counselor to help plan an appropriate program. Many people with an LD do well once they have found the right occupation, and patients and parents should be encouraged to remain optimistic about the long-term outlook.

That having been said, it is not easy for a child or teenager to live with an LD, and the student may struggle to maintain a positive outlook. Other students may cruelly tease the child. Tantrums, outbursts, episodes of disruptive behavior in the classroom, and bouts of depression, especially during adolescence, are often reported and are distressing to the family. The physician can help by being knowledgeable about available educational and therapeutic options and by maintaining a sympathetic and constructive perspective. In many cases, the child with LD is also found to have ADHD, and significant improvement results from treatment with a stimulant medication. Psychotherapy is helpful for some patients. Finally, patients may be reminded that most people with an LD feel much happier after they complete high school, whatever future they choose.

Case 3.1

A 7-year-old boy is brought to the office because of school-related problems. Ever since kindergarten, his teachers have complained that he is easily distracted and does not complete his work in class, is restless, and often gets out of his seat. He has had trouble getting along with other children as a result of being overly "physical." At home, he is occasionally able to sit quietly and play with Lego and jigsaw puzzles but rarely for more than 15 minutes. Homework has been a nightly battle.

About 3 months ago, the child was prescribed a stimulant medication for ADHD by another doctor. The medication has helped him to settle down in class and to focus on his work more easily. However, he still is struggling in school, and he often becomes frustrated and angry when he tries to do his homework.

The child was born following a normal pregnancy and attained motor milestones on schedule but did not start to talk until 2 years of age.

His father had difficulty in school and does not like to read. A cousin was diagnosed with ADHD.

The general physical examination is unremarkable. The child is friendly, not hyperactive or restless, and not distractible. His mother states that he took his medication 2 hours earlier. He does have trouble articulating some words. Reading ability tests below grade level. He has trouble comprehending complex sentences and following multistep directions.

Diagnosis: *Probable language-based learning disability; previously diagnosed ADHD, Combined Type.*

Outcome: The boy was referred to his school's Child Study Team for a formal evaluation. He was diagnosed with a learning disability and placed in a resource room. His parents arranged for FM system (see page 83) in the classroom. He is making steady progress and is happier.

ATTENTION-DEFICIT HYPERACTIVITY DISORDER

During the last decade, ADHD has virtually become a household word and also, for some people, a diagnosis that provokes strong feelings. Many people suspect that ADHD is overdiagnosed or are concerned about the potential adverse effects of the medications for ADHD that are prescribed to millions of children. Other people, often parents whose children have benefited from treatment for ADHD, feel equally strongly and may attribute *any* school-related or behavioral problem to ADHD. For the physician, the main consequence of all this attention is that the possibility of ADHD is almost always raised when a patient is referred for a school-related problem. In many cases, the patient's parents and school specifically request that ADHD either be "ruled out" or diagnosed and treated.

Many people equate ADHD with hyperactivity and are unaware that it is possible for a nonhyperactive child to have ADHD. In fact, many children with ADHD are not hyperactive, and even for patients who are, *the most disabling manifestation of ADHD is usually a high level of distractibility.* Distractibility is also the manifestation of ADHD that usually persists into adult life, whereas hyperactivity typically diminishes by adolescence (29).

It has been estimated that 5% of the population of the United States, including 8% of American boys and 2% of American girls, has ADHD (30,31). Prevalence rates (not segregated by gender) in other countries are generally in the range of 5% to 10% (32).

It is often helpful to review the criteria for ADHD (Table 3.2) with parents; the *Diagnostic and Statistical Manual of Mental Disorders, 4th Edition* (DSM-IV) criteria are the "gold standard" and the most straightforward means of diagnosing ADHD. A child's behavior may fulfill the criteria for the *hyperactive-impulsive type,* the *inattentive type,* or the *combined type* of ADHD. The diagnostic term *attention-deficit disorder* or "ADD" has not been in formal usage since the publication of the DSM-IV in 1993.

In addition, the following general criteria listed in Table 3.2 for ADHD must be met:

1. Many of the behaviors were noted prior to 7 years of age.
2. Impairment both at home and in school.
3. Clear evidence of clinically significant impairment in social, academic, or occupational functioning.
4. Signs and symptoms do not reflect another cause or disorder (e.g., learning disability, anxiety, mood disorder, oppositional behavior, autism, psychosis, etc.).

The third general criterion for ADHD, which states that the condition must cause *clinically significant impairment,* is important. It implies that a patient may be somewhat hyperactive or distractible but still not meet the criteria for ADHD if he or she is doing well academically, is socially well-adjusted, and his or her behavior is not a serious problem. Treatment for these patients, who are sometimes said to have "ADHD–Not Otherwise Specified" (33), tends to be conservative and often does not include medication.

TABLE 3.2

Diagnostic criteria for attention-deficit hyperactivity disorder (33)

A	B
Makes frequent careless mistakes in schoolwork	Often fidgety or restless
Difficulty maintaining attention during concentration-requiring activities (usually avoids these activities)	Often gets out of seat in class, walks around classroom, goes to bathroom or nurse, etc.
Often doesn't appear to be listening when spoken to (not due to oppositional behavior)	Often runs or climbs excessively
Usually very slow to complete class work and homework	Has trouble playing by himself
Disorganized	Constantly on the go; "driven by a motor"
Highly resistant to doing homework	Constantly talking
Always losing things	Frequently blurts out answers
Easily distracted	Butts into line/can't take turns
Very forgetful	Frequently interrupts

Classification: *Inattentive Type*: ≥6 items from column A and all general criteria; *Hyperactive-Impulsive Type*: ≥6 items column B and all general criteria; and *Combined Type*: ≥6 items from both column A and column B and all general criteria (see text).

Clinical features

Signs of ADHD–Inattentive Type are often first noticed in school. The child's teacher typically complains to a parent that the child lacks the ability to remain on task, is unfocused and easily distracted, and cannot complete class work in a reasonable amount of time. Initially these tendencies are often attributed to immaturity. As the child advances from grade to grade and the required work becomes more difficult, distractibility, forgetfulness, disorganization, and procrastination begin to take a toll on the child's performance in school. Homework is not brought home or is not handed in to the teacher. The child may become unwilling to do homework when the assignments become more demanding, and the child's grades start to decline. The parents typically become frustrated or angry, and the situation at home deteriorates. In many cases, the child with ADHD also has an LD, and the child's lack of attentiveness makes it more difficult for him or her to concentrate on schoolwork that is already difficult for the child, leading to tantrums and refusal to do any work at all.

Children with ADHD–Combined Type are often brought for evaluation at a younger age, in many cases before the start of kindergarten. Hyperactive preschool-age children constantly run, climb, and move from one activity to the next. Inappropriate touching, pushing, and hitting are often reported by a teacher. In grade school, these children are restless, often out of their seat, make frequent trips to the bathroom or water fountain, blurt out inappropriate comments, or try attention-getting stunts (play the class clown). Relationships with other children are strained as a result of the child's tendency to be excessively physical and difficulty adjusting to other children's priorities. Hyperactive children often enjoy risky or dangerous activities (e.g., reckless play, jumping from high places) and are frequently evaluated by doctors for lacerations, fractures, and concussions. Life at home is chaotic, with constant fighting between siblings; tantrums and behavioral outbursts; battles over homework; and relentless, exhausting hyperactivity.

Teenagers with ADHD–Combined Type are usually not as hyperactive as they were when they were young children but are often impulsive. They are more likely than their peers to engage in risky behaviors or prefer "extreme" sports, use alcohol and drugs, have an automobile accident (34,35), and get into trouble with the law (36).

A relatively small percentage of children exhibit signs of hyperactivity/impulsivity but not distractibility/disorganization (i.e., have *ADHD–Hyperactive Type*). These patients tend to do better academically than children with ADHD–Combined Type and ADHD–Inattentive Type, but their impulsive behavior often gets them into trouble and makes it difficult for them to fit in socially.

Many people with ADHD are *easily frustrated* when attempting a task requiring planning and patience. Although there are exceptions, children with ADHD generally do not enjoy playing with building toys, reading, drawing, crafts, putting together puzzles or models, and other activities requiring concentration and an ability to delay gratification. However, video games are magnets for these children, and an ability to focus while playing video games or watching television in no way precludes the diagnosis of ADHD. Some children with ADHD are good athletes but find it difficult to sustain attention during the "waiting" periods in baseball games ("he counts the daisies when he is in the outfield") or during soccer and basketball games when they do not have control of the ball themselves.

Myths and misconceptions about ADHD

Many books have been published about ADHD in the lay press, and an even larger number of Internet Web sites provide information for parents. The quality of these sources varies, and many are strongly ideological or primarily rely on anecdotal information. Many of these sources make partly accurate or even false statements about ADHD, for example:

1. *No one had this when I was growing up.* In all likelihood, people did. They struggled in school and have had more than their share of problems in life as adults.
2. *ADHD is a made-up diagnosis; by current criteria, everyone has ADHD.* It is true that many peoples' behavior suggests a few *features* of ADHD, such as occasional forgetfulness, impulsiveness, or trouble concentrating. It is far from true that everyone's behavior fully meets the DSM-IV criteria for ADHD, especially with respect to the criterion of clinically significant impairment.

3. *People with ADHD can focus on things that interest them.* Many children with ADHD can "hyperfocus"; in other words, they can become entranced during passive or high-stimulation activities such as watching television or playing computer or video games. Other children with ADHD who have a particular talent, for example, playing the piano well, are, not surprisingly, able to maintain focus during that activity for a reasonable length of time. These examples are often cited as evidence that children with ADHD can focus on *any* activity that interests them. Although we recognize that many people subscribe to this theory, we do not.

   The neuroanatomical structures that mediate concentration, alertness, and impulse control are located in the brainstem, basal ganglia, and prefrontal lobes. These parts of the brain are not task specific. If someone has a neurologically based problem paying attention, that person's ability to concentrate on a range of cognitive tasks should be affected. There is no such thing as "ADHD for reading"; *if someone can focus well while doing math problems or playing chess but not while reading, it is likely that they have more of a problem reading than a problem paying attention.* In our experience, most people with ADHD *avoid activities that require concentration and patience* such as reading, crafts, puzzles, board games, practicing a musical instrument, and school work. A patient with ADHD may be able to focus well while engaged in an activity that is easy for him or her. However, if a person can focus for a prolonged period of time while engaged in a variety of attention-requiring tasks, the person probably does not have ADHD.

4. *Children with ADHD are bright.* In fact, children with ADHD often are found to also have a specific learning disability.

5. *Children with ADHD do best in "one-on-one" situations rather than large groups.* Many children with learning and behavioral problems as well as many children with no problem like to do their work with a grown-up.

6. *ADHD is often misdiagnosed.* That is doubtless true. Some children who have trouble focusing or appear restless are anxious, unhappy, excessively introverted, or have an LD and are mistakenly diagnosed with and prescribed medication for ADHD. The converse is also true. Many patients with ADHD–Inattentive Type are well behaved in school and are thus labeled underachievers and never receive appropriate treatment.

7. *Drugs for ADHD are addictive.* Stimulant medications are discussed later in this chapter. Addiction means different things to different people. By accepted criteria, stimulant drugs are not addictive.

Comorbidity

Many adults and some children with ADHD are also diagnosed with an *anxiety disorder* or *depression* (37,38). *Conduct disorder* and *oppositional-defiant disorder* are often associated with ADHD (37,38; see Chapter 5). Experts in the field disagree about the relationship of ADHD to *bipolar disorder* (36).

Family history

In most cases, a sibling, parent, or another relative of the patient either has been diagnosed with ADHD or offers a history of ADHD-like symptoms or behaviors. A father may remember that, as a child, he was hyperactive and often got into trouble in school, or he may say that he has never been able to concentrate well. A history of family members who are disorganized, procrastinate, have difficulty completing tasks, frequently change jobs, engage in risky behaviors, or have had many automobile accidents is frequently elicited. Indeed, if the diagnosis of ADHD is not clear-cut, a lack of a family history suggesting ADHD may be another reason to consider alternative diagnoses.

Other causes of hyperactivity and distractibility

Premature birth, fetal cocaine exposure, and perinatal asphyxia often result in childhood hyperactivity and distractibility. Children with fragile X syndrome, fetal alcohol syndrome, neurofibromatosis type I, and many other syndromes of congenital malformation are often hyperactive or distractible (39). The frequency of hyperkinetic behavior and inattentiveness in children with a history of a congenital syndrome or injury affecting neurological development gives meaning to *minimal brain dysfunction*, an early term for what is now called ADHD.

Anxiety often makes a child seem restless and distracted (see Chapter 5). Children who are anxious about their school work and especially children who also have an LD often withdraw or throw a tantrum ("shut down") when confronted with a challenging task, which is sometimes misinterpreted as an inability to focus. An *emotionally upsetting circumstance at home* may also be the cause of restlessness. Children with an *autistic spectrum disorder* (see Chapter 9) may be hyperactive or seem distracted. A history of "ADHD and delayed speech" or "ADHD and obsessive/compulsive disorder" suggests that autism may be the underlying diagnosis. If there is a history of *a poor response to multiple stimulant medications* ("Ritalin and Adderall didn't work" or "only made him more hyper"), an alternative diagnosis such as a *learning disability with secondary inattentiveness* should be considered.

Sleep apnea often leads to classroom inattentiveness caused by fatigue. Rarely, a *medical condition*, such as diabetes mellitus, hyperthyroidism, rheumatic fever, or a *degenerative disorder of the nervous system* (classically, adrenoleukodystrophy), presents with signs of hyperactivity. A careful history and examination should reveal other symptoms or signs more characteristic of the underlying disease. In most cases, the child was not hyperactive in the past.

Physical examination

Observation of the child's behavior is an important part of the examination. The child with ADHD–Hyperactive Type or ADHD–Combined Type may be obviously hyperactive, impulsive, fidgety, restless, and excessively silly or theatrical. The only sign of ADHD–Inattentive Type may be easy distractibility, which is most apparent during cognitive testing. The child also may appear anxious, sad, or angry, suggesting the possibility of comorbid anxiety or depression. The evaluation of patients with suspected ADHD should include a *learning assessment*. Other than nonspecific "soft signs," the rest of the neurological examination usually reveals no significant abnormalities. Occasionally, stigmata of a congenital disorder, such as neurofibromatosis type I, are recognized.

Laboratory and diagnostic tests

Many physicians order thyroid function tests and a venous lead level in cases of possible ADHD, although the yield is low. Laboratory tests to screen for metabolic disorders and MRI should not be ordered. The EEG may demonstrate a slow background rhythm, a nonspecific finding.

Quantitative and functional imaging studies (volumetric MRI, functional MRI, positron emission tomography, and single-photon emission computerized tomography) have revealed possible neuroanatomical and metabolic correlates of ADHD (40,41). These studies suggest that ADHD is associated with underdevelopment of some basal ganglia nuclei (involved in motor activity) and hypometabolism in the prefrontal lobes (planning, inhibition, and executive function) and cingulate gyrus. The findings are important but are based on small samples. Functional imaging currently plays no role in the diagnosis of ADHD and is either not available or prohibitively expensive for almost all patients.

Behavioral rating scales and computerized and formal tests of attention

Behavioral rating scales attempt to quantify a child's hyperactivity and inattentiveness and suggest whether these behaviors result from ADHD, an LD, or another cause (anxiety, oppositional behavior, etc.). Rating scales are also sometimes used to evaluate a patient's response to medication. The *Connors Rating Scale* (42), the most commonly used assessment tool, is completed by both parents and the child's teachers and scored using a key. The *Child Behavior Checklists* (43) are teacher- and parent-completed scales that are scored by computer. Many other rating scales are available, and several manufacturers of medication for ADHD provide a rating scale.

Unfortunately, each person who fills out a rating scale will have a different view of the child, often resulting in multiple diagnoses suggested by the observers' assessments. Furthermore, even when all the observers are in agreement, each scale may generate several elevated scores (e.g., for hyperactivity, anxiety, learning problems, and oppositional behavior), a result that does not indicate what the primary diagnosis is or point to a treatment approach likely to be effective.

The Connors' Continuous Performance Test (MHS Windows Compatible Software, North Tonawanda, NY) and Test of Variables of Attention (TOVA; Universal Attention Disorders, Los Alamitos, CA) are *computerized tests* that can be given in the office to assess the patient's ability to concentrate. The *Stroop Color and Word Test* (44), usually administered by an educational psychologist, is among the more commonly administered formal tests of attention.

Formal cognitive and computerized tests of attention are more reliable than behavioral rating scales. However, it is best to use scales and these tests to provide supportive rather than primary evidence for ADHD. *ADHD remains a clinical diagnosis.* The DSM-IV criteria, strictly interpreted, are still the most reliable standard.

TREATMENT

School and behavioral interventions

A *504 plan*, a provision of the Rehabilitation Act of 1973, can be implemented by the school. The 504 modifications for ADHD usually include extra time to complete tests, preferential seating, and organizational assistance. A 504 plan usually requires approval from the student's Child Study Team. Some 504 modifications (i.e., extra time and special seating) may also be available for students with ADHD who are taking the SAT or attending college but only if the diagnosis of ADHD is supported by the results of formal cognitive testing (by an educational psychologist or neuropsychologist).

During homework time, the child with ADHD should be given a quiet place to work, and competing stimuli should be minimized. A timer can be used to encourage the child to work steadily and efficiently. *Curtailment of television, online, and video game privileges during school nights* is suggested, despite the child's objections. Electronic entertainment distracts the child, makes the child rush, and is not conducive to quiet concentration.

A child diagnosed with ADHD should still be held responsible for his or her actions. The child should learn to make a list of his daily school assignments, initially with parental help and later on his own. The child should be taught to *avoid saying that she "forgot her homework"*; rather, *she should simply say that she did not bring the homework home.* When the homework is not brought home, the child's parents should give the child an assignment to do.

To the extent possible, the child with ADHD should be treated like any other child. Standards for behavior in and outside of the home, respect for others, and requirements for doing household chores should not be influenced by the fact that the child has been diagnosed with ADHD.

Cognitive behavior therapy may encourage good organizational and work habits. *Biofeedback* has been helpful for some patients. *Psychotherapy* is recommended if there is a history of chronically oppositional behavior, family problems, or difficulty getting along with other children.

The parents may contact the national support group *Children and Adults with Attention-Deficit Disorder* (CHADD, Landover, MD) for other recommendations. Suggestions for managing common childhood behavioral problems are included in Chapter 5.

STIMULANT MEDICATIONS FOR ADHD

Indications for treatment with a stimulant medication

ADHD often responds dramatically to treatment with a *stimulant medication*. In many cases, a distractible or hyperactive child becomes noticeably calmer, more settled, and more organized and can concentrate more easily after taking a stimulant drug. The child's grades typically improve, and there is often a marked improvement in the child's social life and overall behavior. Parents, usually initially wary of medication, are generally pleased by the improvement in their child's performance in school and note that life at home is generally happier.

The following are common reasons for prescribing a stimulant medication for ADHD:

1. To help with poor academic performance, even though support in school and structure at home has been provided
2. To help address a learning disability
3. To help with significant behavioral problems (hyperactivity, impulsiveness, or disruptive behavior)
4. To help a child who is experiencing great frustration or whose self-esteem is declining

The decision to start a stimulant medication may be more difficult to make when a child is less substantially impaired. Some physicians hardly ever use medication in mild cases of ADHD, whereas other doctors believe in aggressive treatment for almost every patient with ADHD-like symptoms. Acknowledging this diversity of opinion and practice style, the authors believe that the known short-term adverse effects of stimulant medications and the possibility of unknown long-term consequences are legitimate reasons to proceed conservatively. There is little to lose by trying nonpharmacological methods first in mild cases.

Which medicine to use

All stimulant drugs for ADHD are either a *methylphenidate*-based drug or an *amphetamine*-based drug. Most physicians no longer prescribe *pemoline*, once a mainstay of treatment, due to reports of hepatotoxicity. Commonly prescribed methylphenidate brands include Ritalin, Metadate, Concerta, and Focalin. The amphetamine class includes two drugs: *dexedrine* and a

TABLE 3.3
Medications for attention-deficit hyperactivity disorder

First line: sustained release stimulant medication: methylphenidate, D-threo-methylphenidate, mixed amphetamine salt, dexedrine. A few patients may prefer or have a better response to a short- or medium-duration drug.

Second line or for atypical cases: atomoxetine, clonidine, guanfacine.

Occasionally used, or for a comorbid condition such as depression or oppositional behavior: buproprion, risperidone, serotonin-selective reuptake inhibitor, mood-stabilizing drug, tricyclic antidepressant

mixture of amphetamine salts (Adderall and generic products) (Table 3.3). Methylphenidate- and amphetamine-containing medications are available as brands that vary in rate of release and duration of action. These products are all effective, but a given patient may respond better to one drug or brand than another or experience fewer adverse effects with a particular brand. Unfortunately, there is no way to predict in advance which product will be most effective and least side effect–producing for any particular patient. A trial-and-error approach is unavoidable.

Long-acting stimulant medications

Until a few years ago, a short-acting methylphenidate brand (Ritalin) was frequently prescribed to children with ADHD. Because the drug was effective for only 4 hours, children were required to go the school nurse to take their noon and sometimes late afternoon dose. Parents had to deliver the medication to the school nurse once a month. If the dosage was changed, the nurse had to be notified, and a new bottle of pills and doctor's note had to be provided. Many children felt that having to go to the school nurse to take medication stigmatized them, and some refused to take medication.

These problems were eliminated for most patients a few years ago when long-acting stimulant brands first became available. Three long-acting standard methylphenidate-based products (Concerta, McNeil; Ritalin LA, Novartis; and Metadate CD, Celltech) are currently marketed in the United States. Recently, an extended-release isomeric form of methylphenidate (D-threo-methylphenidate; Focalin XR, Novartis) was approved and is now available. Among amphetamine-based drugs, Adderall XR (Shire) is the only long-acting product.

Concerta, Focalin XR, and Adderall XR are effective for about 10 hours, and Ritalin LA and Metadate CD are effective for about 8 hours, albeit with considerable variability from patient to patient. Dexedrine Spansules (GlaxoSmithKline) are intermediate- to long-duration capsules that can be taken as a single daily dose medication by some patients.

Intermediate- and short-duration stimulant medications

Intermediate-duration stimulant drugs, effective for about 5 to 6 hours, include amphetamine salt tablets (Adderall, Shire; and generic brands); Dexedrine tablets (GlaxoSmithKline); and intermediate-duration methylphenidate (e.g., Ritalin SR, Novartis; Methylin ER, Mallinckrodt). These medications are less frequently prescribed now that the long-acting formulations have become the first-line treatment for ADHD. However, college students and adult patients sometimes prefer an intermediate-duration medication since it may be effective only during a particular time of day, such as for morning or afternoon classes, without committing to a full day on medication.

A few patients seem to respond better to a short-acting stimulant drug taken once, twice, or three times a day than to a long-duration drug. A short-duration drug is also sometimes administered prior to homework time (after the long-acting stimulant has worn off) or before weekend events such as church, weddings, and parties and sports activities, assuming the child does not require medication for the rest of the day. All of the short-duration brands are methylphenidate products (Ritalin, Novartis; Metadate, Celltech; Methylin, Mallinckrodt). D-threo-methylphenidate (Focalin, Novartis) is also effective.

Starting the medication

A stimulant medication is always started at a low dosage, for example 18 to 27 mg of Concerta or 10 to 20 mg of Ritalin LA and Metadate CD. Adderall XR, Dexedrine spansules, generic amphetamine products, and Focalin XR are more potent, milligram for milligram, than methylphenidate and often started at a dose of 5 to 10 mg. Short- and intermediate-duration stimulant drugs for ADHD are started at a dose of 5 to 10 mg. D-threo-methylphenidate (Focalin, Novartis) is available as a 2.5-mg tablet since it is twice as potent as standard methylphenidate.

Swallowing the pill

Young children often have trouble swallowing a pill. With the exception of one short-acting methylphenidate product (Methylin, Mallinckrodt), liquid and chewable forms of stimulant drugs are not available due to problems with intestinal absorption. Most long-acting stimulant drugs come in capsules that may be opened and the contents sprinkled on food. The Concerta capsule must be swallowed whole due to a unique drug delivery system. Short-acting stimulant drugs are produced as tablets that can be crushed and mixed with food. Children can often learn to swallow a pill by practicing with small, hard candies (M&Ms) or breath mints.

Judging effectiveness and titration

Once a stimulant medication has been started, the parents and teacher should notice an improvement in the child's attentiveness, academic performance, and behavior *almost immediately*. It is *not* necessary to "get the medicine into the child's system" over a period of weeks, as with antidepressant drugs. If there is no improvement or only a slight improvement after a few days, the dose may be increased. If there is little improvement after two increases in dose, the drug should be discontinued, and another drug should be tried. A different *drug* (e.g., a trial of amphetamine salts following a lack of response to methylphenidate) as opposed to a different *brand* of the same drug should be prescribed if the first drug was not effective. However, if a drug *appears to work*, but *causes adverse effects*, a *different brand* of the same drug may be substituted.

Drug holidays

Unlike many drugs prescribed for behavioral disorders, a stimulant drug for ADHD may be discontinued during weekends and vacations without rebound or withdrawal symptoms resulting. Whether discontinuation on nonschool days is best for the child is controversial. Many physicians believe that, if a child's behavior and performance improve when he is taking a stimulant medication, he should take it every day. Medication allows many children and adults with ADHD to function better at home and in social situations as well as in school. For teenagers and adults, driving an automobile is also a reason to consider taking a stimulant drug on weekends and holidays.

Some patients with ADHD, however, function reasonably well outside of school even when they have not taken their medication. There is less justification for daily use in these cases, and many physicians do not suggest that children who are primarily symptomatic in the school setting take their medication on the weekend. Adverse effects, especially suppression of appetite and insomnia, can be avoided when the child does not take his medication. Furthermore, if experience with other drugs is a guide, tolerance may result from long-term use of a stimulant medication and might be less likely to develop if drug holidays are given. Everyday use of a stimulant medication may lead to decreased reliance on behavioral strategies for managing ADHD by the parents and may also remove a stimulus for the patient to develop appropriate coping skills. However, a special circumstance (writing a term paper or studying for an exam over the weekend, going to church, or competitive sports) may be a valid reason even for these patients to take medication occasionally during nonschool hours. A short-acting brand may be useful in these situations.

Follow-up visits

The child's progress should be assessed after about one month and then every 3 to 6 months, depending on the effectiveness of the medication and any other issue that may arise. Positive feedback from the family and good grades are the best indication that the medication is working. Rating scales are sometimes used to track the child's progress, although they may involve a burdensome amount of work; a conversation with the child's teacher is often more helpful than interpreting a rating scale. The physician should ask the patient and family about adverse effects such as decreased appetite and insomnia, any undesirable changes in behavior, and tics (see the following section). Interval medical problems and any new medications taken for other reasons should be noted. Blood pressure and heart rate should always be checked (Table 3.4).

TABLE 3.4

Common adverse effects of stimulant medications for attention-deficit hyperactivity disorder (ADHD)

Adverse effect	Suggested management
Decreased appetite	Encourage a good breakfast. If appetite is suppressed for both lunch and dinner, consider a shorter duration product. If possible, discontinue the drug on weekends and vacation.
Headache	If persistent (and not due to another cause), try changing brand.
Stomachache	Take the medication after breakfast. If stomachache is persistent, try a different brand or drug.
Late afternoon hyperactivity or mood swings	Symptoms often improve over the course of a few weeks. If not, try a different brand or drug, or add a short-duration drug in the afternoon at a low dose (e.g., Focalin, 2.5 mg).
Insomnia	Change to a shorter duration product.
Undesirable change in child's affect or behavior while on the medication (flat affect, sedation, jitteriness, or drugged appearance)	Try reducing the dose. If no improvement, change drug or brand.
Tics	Discontinue the drug for a few days to see if tics disappear. If no change, restart the drug (tics were probably not related to the drug). If tics stop occurring when medication is discontinued and a stimulant drug for ADHD is required, try a different drug. If tics are worsened by all stimulants, a drug for tic control may need to be added (see Chapter 4)
Tachycardia	Lower the dose or change the drug. Consider cardiology evaluation.

Adverse effects

All stimulant drug brands for ADHD can cause the same side effects, which, however, will vary greatly from patient to patient. In many cases, the problem can be addressed by reducing the dose, changing *brand* (e.g., from one methylphenidate product to another) or changing *drug* (e.g., amphetamine to methylphenidate).

The following is a summary of common side effects:

1. *Decreased appetite* is common during the middle of the day. The child's appetite should *return to normal by the evening*. A good breakfast should be encouraged. Some patients have a poor appetite for dinner as well as lunch. When this occurs, a *shorter duration brand* may be prescribed. Some *weight loss* may occur if a stimulant drug is taken 7 days a week.
2. *Stomachaches*. Taking the medication on a full stomach may help. If not, a different brand or drug may be substituted.
3. *Mood swings* or *rebound hyperactivity may be noted in the afternoon* when the medication wears off. In most cases, the patient's behavior returns to normal after about a half hour. Additionally, these fluctuations in behavior tend to disappear during the first few months of treatment. If the rebound symptoms are severe, a different brand or drug should be tried.
4. *Headaches* occasionally are bothersome and may respond to a change of brand or drug.
5. *Insomnia* is a common side effect of long-acting stimulant drugs. Changing to a slightly shorter acting product (e.g., from Concerta to either Ritalin LA or Metadate CD) is recommended.

More problematic adverse effects include:

1. In some cases, medication results in an *undesirable change in affect or behavior*, such as sedation, exaggerated hyperactivity, or a flat (zombie-like) affect. Parents generally *hate* to see these kinds of personality changes in their child. In some cases, however, parents who are used to their child's extremely hyperactive behavior and are suddenly confronted with a well-behaved, nonhyperactive child will not notice the negative changes in affect. Therefore, the parents, and the child if he or she is old enough, should be specifically asked about changes in personality and mood. The loss of a child's personality and spirit is not an acceptable price to pay for improved behavior and attention. The dose should be reduced, or the brand or drug should be changed.
2. *Motor and vocal tics* may first be noted or may occur or worsen during the course of treatment with a stimulant medication. Other tic-like behaviors, such as picking at the nails, may be exacerbated. However, many children (and up to 50% of children with ADHD and other neurobehavioral disorders) have tics, even when they are not taking medication (Chapter 4). Any

stimulant, including caffeine and over-the-counter cold medications *can* precipitate tics in those prone, exacerbate any underlying tics or movement disorder, or even cause them, whereas other patients' tics are very often unaffected by or unrelated to the same substances. A recent study (45) found that methylphenidate did not exacerbate tics in a majority of patients with ADHD who had tics prior to treatment. Moreover, in the experience of the authors, some patients' tics *improve* during the course of treatment with a stimulant. Atomoxetine has also not been shown to increase, and may even improve the frequency of tics (see following section). If the patient develops a tic while taking a stimulant drug and the tic is bothersome and persistent, the drug should be stopped for a few days to see if it disappears. If the tic goes away, a different stimulant drug may then be tried. If tics worsen during treatment with several medications, the patient may either be taken off stimulant drugs altogether, or, if that is not possible, a medication for tic suppression such as clonidine, pimozide, or risperidone (see Chapter 4) can be added. Discussing the natural waxing and waning history of tics with the parents as well as their spontaneous resolution in the great majority of cases may encourage the family to agree to a wait-and-watch approach, particularly if the medication is helping the patient and the tics are not that bothersome.

3. *Sudden death* of a small number of children in Canada who were taking a mixed amphetamine product (Adderall) has been reported. Most of these children had underlying heart disease, however, and for this reason and because of the small number of these cases, the United States FDA did not further restrict the use of this drug in the United States. The sale of Adderall XR and Adderall has been discontinued in Canada, however. More recently, an FDA advisory panel, following rare reports of cardiac arrest and stroke among patients taking a stimulant drug, recommended that a "black box" warning be included in the package insert of all stimulant drugs for ADHD. At this time, it is not known whether this recommendation will be followed. **If the patient has a history of heart disease or if young people in the child's family have a history of heart disease or stroke, consultation with a cardiologist must be requested prior to initiating treatment with a stimulant drug.**

4. *Tachycardia and chest pain.* If these symptoms are severe or recurrent, the stimulant medication should be discontinued. The child should by seen by a cardiologist. A serious cause is unusual. Lowering the dose or changing to a different stimulant drug often prevents recurrence.

5. *Abuse.* Stimulant medications for ADHD can induce euphoria if crushed and "snorted." Adolescents requiring an unusually large dose of a stimulant or frequently requesting a new prescription may be abusing or selling their drug. Stimulants are Class II substances; refills cannot be prescribed, which tends to limit abuse. Long-acting stimulant products are difficult to abuse because they cannot easily be crushed into a powder and are therefore preferable.

Growth suppression was thought to be a long-term consequence of treatment with a stimulant medication (46–48). More recent studies do not support the theory that stimulant drugs impact children's growth (49,50).

Drug interactions

Stimulant drugs for ADHD interact with few prescription drugs. If there is any question about the compatibility of a stimulant drug and another medication, a neurologist or psychiatrist should be consulted.

On those days when the patient is taking a stimulant drug, the patient should *avoid nasal decongestants* containing drugs ending in *"-ephrine" or "-ephedrine"* (e.g., pseudoephedrine), which might cause an additive sympathomimetic effect.

Drugs frequently prescribed to pediatric patients, such as antibiotics, corticosteroids, antihistamines, and drugs for asthma, do not generally interact with methylphenidate or amphetamine-based drugs, although occasional patients taking a beta-agonist medication for asthma and a stimulant drug report feeling jittery. Antiepileptic medications, serotonin-selective reuptake inhibitors (SSRIs), buproprion, and tricyclic antidepressants are generally safe in combination with a stimulant drug for ADHD. Many patients taking a stimulant drug also take clonidine (see following section). Periodic monitoring with EKG is recommended given rare reports of cardiac arrhythmia associated with this drug combination. Neuroleptic medications (e.g., risperidone, haloperidol) do not interact with stimulant drugs, and the combination of a neuroleptic and a stimulant is often effective in cases of severe hyperactivity, autism, or bipolar disorder. Monoamine oxidase inhibitors may, in some cases, be given in combination with a stimulant drug, but they are intrinsically high-risk drugs that should never be prescribed by any physician other than a psychiatrist.

The parents of adolescent and college-age patients often ask about the interaction between drugs of abuse and stimulant medications. All drugs of abuse should be counseled against, and the physician should specifically mention that the *combination of cocaine and a stimulant is exceptionally dangerous and could be life threatening* due to the additive sympathomimetic effect of these substances.

Duration of treatment: "Will my child take this for the rest of his life?"

There is no single answer to this question. Hyperactivity usually has become less noticeable by the onset of adolescence, but previously hyperactive patients often are still impulsive and continue to get into trouble in and out of school. These patients will still require treatment.

Most patients with ADHD remain inattentive and distractible, but the degree of clinical impairment caused by these symptoms is variable. Most patients with ADHD continue to take their medication throughout high school, but occasional patients who have good study habits find that they are able to function well without medication. Patients who do not have an LD are more likely to be able to discontinue their medication.

Many individuals attending college find that they continue to need medication but only take it when their workload is heavy (for example, when studying for final examinations). Adults with ADHD also may take a stimulant drug on a pragmatic basis, such as when the demands of their job are overwhelming. However, patients with ADHD should consider taking a stimulant medication before driving an automobile, given evidence that people with untreated ADHD are more likely to have an accident (34,35). We often suggest that they consider driving a car with a manual transmission to keep them focused on their driving.

If the patient has been doing well academically and behaviorally for several years, a brief trial period off medication once a year may be suggested. Cognitive behavior therapy or biofeedback may be helpful for patients with mild symptoms who wish to discontinue medication.

Addiction: "Is this medicine addictive?"

Many parents ask this question. "Addiction" means different things to different people, so it is best to review the following with the family:

1. The accepted psychiatric definition of addiction is *continued use of a substance despite negative consequences*. For example, an alcoholic continues to drink despite developing cirrhosis of the liver, and a cocaine addict continues to use cocaine even if his drug use leads to the loss of a job, family problems, or trouble with the law. *Use of a stimulant drug for ADHD as prescribed never leads to this kind of compulsive, self-destructive behavior.*
2. *Use to achieve euphoria.* Short-acting methylphenidate and amphetamine tablets can be crushed and "snorted" to induce a state of euphoria. However, when a stimulant is taken orally, even at a high therapeutic dose, euphoria does not result. Long-acting stimulant drugs for ADHD are difficult or impossible to crush and abuse.
3. *Withdrawal symptoms.* Some patients who have been taking a stimulant drug at a high dose every day and then stop taking the drug report feeling a little "flat." No other symptoms typically follow the abrupt discontinuation of a stimulant drug.
4. *Tolerance.* Many drugs induce tolerance. Little research has examined this issue with respect to stimulant medications. Clinical experience suggests that some patients do become tolerant to a stimulant medication and requires a somewhat higher dose, but this usually occurs only after many months to years of regular use.
5. *Future substance abuse.* Parents also may worry that taking a stimulant medication during childhood or adolescence increases the chance that

a person will become an illegal drug abuser. In fact, research suggests the opposite: patients treated for ADHD with medication during childhood are less likely than untreated ADHD patients to abuse drugs later in life (51).

Routine laboratory tests

Because methylphenidate and another stimulant drugs may occasionally cause a slight elevation of hepatic enzymes and mildly increased or decreased platelet and leukocyte counts, patients are sometimes sent for routine blood tests. Clinical signs of hepatotoxicity or cytopenia do not accompany these laboratory findings, suggesting that routine blood work is probably unnecessary.

What to do if a stimulant drug is not working

Sometimes a child who appears to have ADHD does not respond to any stimulant drug, or the drug prescribed only makes the child appear agitated ("even more hyper"). In other cases, a stimulant drug causes a transient improvement lasting only a few days. The dose is then usually increased, again resulting in only a temporary improvement. A trial of a second stimulant drug also does not yield sustained improvement. The child is then brought back to the office for reevaluation.

Three questions should be asked when a child is not responding to a stimulant drug:

1. Is the problem a lack of improvement or adverse effects?
2. Has an appropriate dose been prescribed (i.e., at least two titrations)?
3. Has the child had a trial of both a methylphenidate- and an amphetamine-based drug?

Adverse effects and their management were discussed earlier. If the child has been given both methylphenidate and an amphetamine at an adequate dose and has not responded, a trial of atomoxetine (Strattera; see following section on atomoxetine) may be considered.

If trials of methylphenidate, an amphetamine, and atomoxetine do not lead to a sustained improvement, the diagnosis of ADHD should be rethought. Other possible causes for the child's problem include an LD with secondary inattentiveness, an *autistic spectrum disorder*, an *anxiety or mood disorder*, and *oppositional-defiant disorder*. A neuropsychological or psychiatric evaluation is recommended if the diagnosis remains elusive.

Finally, if the problem is a noticeable but still incomplete response to medication despite an adequate dose, it is likely that child also has a comorbid condition such as a learning disability, depression, or anxiety.

OTHER MEDICATIONS USED TO TREAT ADHD

Alpha-2 agonist drugs

The alpha-2 agonist drug *clonidine* (Catapres, Boehringer Ingelheim) is often prescribed to children who are impulsive or hyperactive. Clonidine is also taken at bedtime to treat *insomnia*, a problem for many children with ADHD. The usual starting dose of clonidine is 0.025 mg (a quarter of a 0.1-mg tablet) in the morning or before bedtime. The dose may be cautiously increased by 0.025-mg (quarter tablet) increments. Some patients also are given clonidine in the afternoon. Clonidine is also available as a patch (Catapres patch, Boehringer Ingelheim) that is placed on the child's skin. *Guanfacine* is a pharmacologically similar drug that is preferred by some physicians.

Treatment with an alpha-2 agonist often produces an improvement in the child's behavior and ability to get to sleep. However, alpha-2 agonists do not generally treat the symptoms of inattention and distractibility.

The most common adverse effect of both clonidine and guanfacine is *somnolence*. Many children are very sensitive to these drugs and become tired or sleepy even when given a very low dose; when this occurs, the drug should be discontinued. Hypotension, syncope, and paradoxical agitation are much less common adverse effects.

Atomoxetine

Atomoxetine (Strattera, Lilly) was approved in 2002 for the treatment of ADHD in children and adults. Unlike the stimulant medications, which increase the synaptic reuptake of norepinephrine and dopamine, atomoxetine is a *selective norepinephrine reuptake inhibitor*. Atomoxetine is not a Class II substance and can be prescribed with refills and samples. The recommended daily dose of atomoxetine is 0.5 mg/kg taken once daily, but lower doses are equally or more effective for many children. Unlike a stimulant drug, atomoxetine must be taken *7 days a week* and usually must be taken for *several weeks before a clinical improvement is noted*. Clinical trials were promising (52). Clinical experience has been mixed, however. To date, no controlled study has directly compared the efficacy of atomoxetine and a stimulant drug for the treatment of ADHD symptoms. Our experience has been that atomoxetine is most effective for children who are inattentive as a result of excessive *anxiety*. Adverse effects of atomoxetine and stimulant medications are quite similar. A recent study (53) demonstrated that atomoxetine did not exacerbate and, indeed, may have even improved the frequency of tics in children and adolescents with ADHD.

Atypical neuroleptics

Children who are exceptionally *hyperactive, impulsive, or aggressive* and have not responded adequately to treatment with a stimulant drug, an alpha-2 agonist, or atomoxetine may be prescribed *risperidone* (Risperdal, Janssen).

Risperidone is classified as an atypical antipsychotic drug. The usual starting dose is 0.25 to 0.5 mg once to twice daily; the maximum daily dose prescribed to children rarely exceeds 3 mg. Risperidone is a very effective drug, but it frequently causes adverse effects. The most frequent is a marked *increase in appetite* that often causes significant weight gain. Fatigue and somnolence are also common. Rare but serious adverse effects of risperidone include fatty liver, type II diabetes mellitus, neuroleptic malignant syndrome, and irreversible movement disorders (see Chapter 4).

The atypical antipsychotic drugs quetiapine (Seroquel, AstraZeneca) and aripiprazole (Abilify, Otsuka America) are sometimes prescribed for other childhood neurobehavioral disorders (e.g., autism, bipolar disorder) and occasionally to children with ADHD. Aripiprazole is less likely to cause weight gain than the other "atypicals" and, at this point, has not been found to cause irreversible motor dyskinesias. The FDA has not approved any atypical antipsychotic medication for use in children and adolescents, although they are often prescribed in practice. The physician is referred to Finding's extensive discussion of the role of these medications for the treatment of a number of adult and pediatric disorders (54).

Buproprion and other antidepressants

Buproprion (Wellbutrin, GlaxoSmithKline) is sometimes prescribed in cases of *ADHD associated with signs and symptoms of depression or dysthymia.* A dose of 100 to 300 mg divided in two daily doses is often prescribed. A single daily dose form of buproprion (Wellbutrin XL, GlaxoSmithKline) has been recently introduced. Common adverse effects of buproprion include fatigue and nausea. Buproprion also *lowers the seizure threshold*, most significantly at doses above 300 mg per day, and is, therefore, *contraindicated for patients with epilepsy.* Serotonin-selective reuptake inhibitors (see Chapter 5) generally are not effective for treating the symptoms of ADHD.

Dietary modification and alternative medications

Alternative medicine advocates as well as many other people believe that certain foods and food additives cause or worsen the symptoms of ADHD and thus that dietary modification may help treat the symptoms. A large number of parents are convinced that the right diet will improve their child's behavior and performance in school. They are usually unaware that the *blood–brain barrier* prevents many substances from entering the brain, limiting the effect of most diets on behavior.

Dietary modifications claimed to be beneficial for children with ADHD are reviewed by Wolraich (55). The most popular ADHD diet is the *Feingold diet*, the basis of which is removal of artificial ingredients such as food coloring. Studies varying in design, criteria, and quality have demonstrated marked, mild, and no improvement in the behavior of children with ADHD placed on the Feingold diet (55–59). Since parents generally know what their child eats, it is difficult to assure placebo control in studies measuring the effect of diet on behavior. A diet that restricts sugar-containing foods, which are widely believed to cause hyperactivity, has not been shown to improve children's behavior (60). (Did you ever act or feel "hyper" after eating a candy bar or an ice cream cone?)

The FDA currently is not authorized to test or regulate nontraditional drugs, and therefore, it is probably best not to recommend these drugs to patients. The High Commission E, the German equivalent of the FDA, has carried out a number of studies of alternative drugs. The reader may consult the *Physician's Desk Reference for Herbal Medicines* (61), which summarizes available information.

REFERENCES

1. Pastor PN, Reuben CA. Attention-deficit disorder and learning disability: United States, 1997–98. *Vital Health Stat.* 2002;10:1–12.
2. National Institutes of Health. Learning disabilities. NIH Publication No. 93-3611. Bethesda, MD: National Institutes of Health, 1993.
3. Shaywitz S. The working brain reads. In: *Overcoming Dyslexia.* New York: Random House; 2003:71–89.
4. Tallal P, Stark R. Speech discrimination abilities of normally developing and language-impaired children: acoustic analysis. *J Acoust Soc Am.* 1981;69:568.
5. Lieberman Am, Cooper FS, Shankweiler DP, et al. Perception of the speech code. *Psychol Rev.* 1967;74:431.
6. Renvall H, Hari R. Diminished auditory mismatch fields in dyslexic adults. *Ann Neurol.* 2003;53:551–557.
7. Geschwind N, Levitsky W. Human brain: right-left asymmetries in the temporal speech region. *Science.* 1968;161:186.
8. Galaburda A. The pathogenesis of childhood dyslexia. In: Plum F, ed. *Language, Communication, and the Brain.* New York: Raven Press; 1987:127–138.
9. O'Keefe MJ, O'Callaghan M, Williams GM, et al. Learning, cognitive, and attentional problems in adolescents born small for gestational age. *Pediatrics.* 2003;112:301–307.
10. Goodenough FL, Harris DB. *Goodenough-Harris Drawing Test.* San Antonio, TX: Psychological Corp; 1963.
11. Levine MD. *Pediatric Examination of Educational Readiness, Pediatric Early Elementary Examination, Pediatric Examination of Educational Readiness at Middle Childhood.* Cambridge, MA: Educator's Publishing Service; 2002.
12. Semel E, Wiig ET, Secord WA. *Clinical Evaluation of Language Fundamentals.* 4th ed. San Antonio, TX: Psychological Corp; 2003.
13. Jastak JF, Jastak S. *Wide Range Achievement Test.* Wilmington, DE: Jastak Assoc; 1992.
14. Robinson H, ed. *Gray Oral Reading Test.* Indianapolis, IN: Bobbs-Merrill; 1963.
15. Roid GH. *Stanford Binet Intelligence Scales.* 5th ed. Itasca, IL: Riverside Publishing Corp; 2003.
16. Wechsler D. *Wechsler Preschool and Primary Scale of Intelligence – III.* San Antonio, TX: Psychological Corp; 2002.

17. Wechsler D. *Wechsler Intelligence Scale for Children – IV*. San Antonio, TX: Psychological Corp; 2003.
18. Wechsler D. *Wechsler Adult Intelligence Scale – Revised*. San Antonio, TX: Psychological Corp; 1997.
19. Woodcock RW, Johnson MB. *Woodcock-Johnson Psychoeducational Battery III*. Itasca, IL: Riverside Publishing Corp; 2003.
20. Raven JC. *Raven's Progressive Matrices*. San Antonio, TX: Psychological Corp; 1998.
21. Bender L. *Bender Visual Motor Gestalt Test*. San Antonio, TX: Psychological Corp; 1946.
22. Beery KE, Buktenica NA. *Beery Buktenica Development Test of Visual-Motor Integration*. 4th ed. Eagan, MN: Pearson; 2003.
23. Meyers JE, Meyers KR. *Rey Complex Figure Test and Recognition Trial*. San Antonio, TX: Psychological Corp; 1995.
24. Gross-Tur V, Shalev RS, Manor O, et al. Developmental right-hemisphere syndrome: clinical spectrum of the nonverbal learning disability. *J Learn Disabil*. 1995;28:80–86.
25. Tranel D, Hall LE, Olson S, et al. Evidence for a right-hemisphere developmental learning disability. *Dev Neuropsychol*. 1987;3:113–127.
26. Alexander AW, Slinger-Constant AM. Current status of treatments for dyslexia: critical review. *J Child Neurol*. 2004;19:744–758.
27. American Academy of Pediatrics Committee on Children with Disabilities. Auditory integration training and facilitated communication for autism. *Pediatrics*. 1998;102:431–433.
28. Metzger RL, Werner DB. Use of visual training for reading disabilities. *Pediatrics*. 1984;73:824–829.
29. Wolraich ML, Wibbelsman MD, Brown TE, et al. Attention-deficit/hyperactivity disorder among adolescents: a review of the diagnosis, treatment, and clinical implications. *Pediatrics*. 2005;115:1734–1746.
30. American Academy of Pediatrics. Clinical practice guidelines: diagnosis and evaluation of children with attention-deficit/hyperactivity disorder. *Pediatrics*. 2000;105:1158–1170.
31. Rowland AS, Lesesne CA, Abramowitz AJ. The epidemiology of attention-deficit/hyperactivity disorder (ADHD): a public health view. *Ment Retard Dev Disabil Res Rev*. 2002;8:162–170.
32. Prince JB. ADHD in children and adolescents. Data presented in postgraduate course in child neurology. Harvard Medical School, Cambridge, MA, October 5–8, 2005.
33. American Psychiatric Association. *Diagnostic and Statistical Manual of Mental Disorders, Text Revision*. 4th ed. Washington, DC: American Psychiatric Association; 2000:92–93.
34. Barkley RA, Guevremont DC, Anastopoulos AD, et al. Driving-related risks and outcomes of attention-deficit hyperactivity disorder in adolescents and young adults: a 3- to 5-year follow-up survey. *Pediatrics*. 1993;92:212–218.
35. Cox DJ, Merkel RL, Kovatchev B, et al. Effect of stimulant medication on driving performance of young adults with attention-deficit hyperactivity disorder: a preliminary double-blind placebo controlled trial. *J Nerv Ment Dis*. 2000;188:230–234.
36. Weiss M, Weiss G. Attention-deficit hyperactivity disorder. In: Lewes M, ed. *Child and Adolescent Psychiatry*. Philadelphia: Lippincott; 2002:645–670.

37. Biederman H, Newcorn J, Sprich S. Comorbidity of attention-deficit hyperactivity disorder with conduct, depressive, anxiety, and other disorders. *Am J Psychiatry.* 1991;148:564–577.
38. Semrud-Clikeman M, Biederman J, Sprich-Buckminster S, et al. Comorbidity between ADHD and learning disability: A review and report in a clinically referred sample. *J Am Acad Child Adolesc Psychiatry.* 1992;31:439–448.
39. Johnson H, Wiggs L, Stores G, et al. Psychological disturbance and sleep disorders in children with neurofibromatosis type 1. *Dev Med Child Neurol.* 2005;47:237–242.
40. Bush G, Frazier JA, Rouch SL, et al. Anterior cingulate cortex dysfunction in attention-deficit/hyperactivity disorder revealed by fMRI and the Counting Stroop. *Biol Psychiatry.* 1999;45:1542–1552.
41. Castellanos FX, Lee PP, Sharp W, et al. Developmental trajectories of brain volume abnormalities in children and adolescents with attention-deficit/hyperactivity disorder. *JAMA.* 2002;288:1740–1748.
42. Connors CK. *Connors Rating Scales.* San Antonio, TX: Psychological Corp; 1996.
43. Achenbach T. *Child Behavior Checklists.* Burlington, VT: University Medical Education; 1997.
44. Golden C. *Stroop Color and Word Test.* Lutz, FL: Psychological Assessment Resources; 2002.
45. Kurlan R, Goetz CG, McDermott MP, et al. Treatment of ADHD in children with tics: a randomized controlled trial. *Neurology.* 2002;58:527–536.
46. Safer DJ, Allen RP, Barr E. Depression of growth in hyperactive children on stimulant drugs. *N Engl J Med.* 1972;287:217–220.
47. Mattes JA, Gittelman R. Growth of hyperactive children on maintenance regimen of methylphenidate. *Arch Gen Psychiatry.* 1988;45:1131–1134.
48. Loney J, Whaley KMA, Pinto LB, et al. Predictors of adolescent height and weight in hyperkinetic boys treated with methylphenidate [proceedings]. *Psychopharm Bull.* 1981;17:132–134.
49. Satterfield JH, Cantwell DP, Schell A, et al. Growth of hyperactive children treated with methylphenidate. *Arch Gen Psychiatry.* 1988;45:1131–1134.
50. Biederman J, Faraone SV, Monuteaux MC, et al. Growth deficits and attention-deficit/hyperactivity disorder revisited: impact of gender, development, and treatment. *Pediatrics.* 2003;111:1010–1016.
51. Wilens TE, Faraone SV, Biederman J, et al. Does stimulant therapy of attention-deficit/hyperactivity disorder beget later substance abuse? A meta-analytic review of the literature. *Pediatrics.* 2003;111:179–185.
52. Michellson D, Faries D, Wernicke J, et al. Atomoxetine in the treatment of children and adolescents with attention-deficit hyperactivity disorder a randomized, placebo-controlled, dose-response study. *Pediatrics.* 2001;108:E83.
53. Allen AJ, Kurlan RM, Gilbert DL, et al. Atomoxetine in children and adolescents with ADHD and comorbid tic disorders. *Neurology.* 2005;65:1941–1949.
54. Finding RL. Pediatric use of atypical antipsychotic medications: emerging psychopharmacologic options for the developing child. Monograph, Case Western University School of Medicine, Cleveland, OH, 2003.
55. Wolraich ML. Diet and behavior: what the research shows. *Contemp Pediatr.* 1996;13:39.
56. Gross MD, Tofanelli RA, Butzirus SM, et al. The effect of diets rich in and free from additives on the behavior of children with hyperkinetic and learning disorders. *J Am Acad Child Adolesc Psychiatry.* 1987;26:53–55.

57. Carter CM, Urbanowicz M, Hemsley R, et al. Effects of a few food diet in attention-deficit disorder. *Arch Dis Child.* 1993;69:564–568.

58. National Institutes of Health. Defined diets and childhood hyperactivity. National Institutes of Health Consensus Development Conference Statement. 1982. http://odp.od.nih.gov/consensus/1982/1982DietHyperactivity032html.htm.

59. Edelkind SS. Food-induced attention-deficit hyperactivity disorder: The research. 1998. http://www.diet-studies.com/lit_review.html.

60. Wolraich ML, Wilson DB, White JW. The effect of sugar on behavior or cognition in children. A meta-analysis. *JAMA.* 1995;274:1617–1621.

61. LaGow B, ed. *Physician's Desk Reference for Herbal Medicines.* Montvale, NJ: Thomson PDR; 2004.

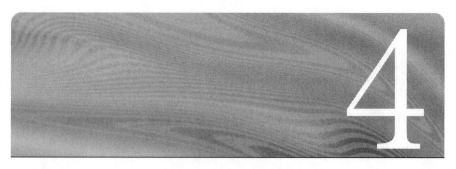

ABNORMAL MOVEMENTS

Table 4.1 summarizes important features of movement disorders and syndromes resembling movement disorders. Tic, tremor, and self-stimulating behaviors are often evaluated in the office or clinic. Partial motor seizures and myoclonus, both of which might be confused with a movement disorder, are less common but still regularly seen. Chorea and dystonia are rarer; a child neurologist in general practice may not see a single patient with either disorder during the course of a typical year.

COMMON MOVEMENT DISORDERS

Tic and Tourette syndrome

A *tic* is a habitual, stereotypic movement, vocalization, or behavior that can be temporarily suppressed by the patient. Many people develop a tic at some point during childhood. The number of patients considered to have tics increases when "nervous habits," such as biting the fingernails, twirling the hair, or chewing the shirt collar, are included. The distinction between a tic and a habit is not based on any medical criterion.

Simple motor tics, such as *blinking, grimacing, eye rolling, and neck stretching*, often cause parents to bring their child to the doctor. Children, and especially young children, are often unaware of or unconcerned by their tics. Simple vocal tics, such as throat clearing, humming, and sniffing, also are frequently evaluated. Vocal tics are not physiologically different from motor tics in as much as muscle contraction produces both movements and vocalizations.

Tics can be *temporarily inhibited* by the patient, a feature unique among the movement disorders. Adult patients often suppress their tics during social occasions or may deliberately "tic" repetitively before social occasions so that their tics are then less frequent. Tics also are affected by a patient's mental state. Stress, agitation, and fatigue often cause an increase in tic frequency.

TABLE 4.1

Movement disorders and similar conditions

Movement	Affected body part	Vocal manifestations	Occurrence during sleep	Character of movement	Frequency of movement	Can be temporarily suppressed
Tic	Any body part; facial and neck movements are most common; will often change over weeks or months	Common: often throat-clearing, sniffing; coprolalia is rare	No	Discrete, stereotypic	Highly variable	Yes
Chorea	Any	No	Rarely may persist	Fluid, continuous; movements migrate rapidly from one part of the body to another	Near constant	No, but patients may try to incorporate into normal movements
Focal Motor Seizure	Unilateral; face/arm most common; same body part often involved in every event	During a secondarily generalized seizure, occasionally	Common	Very stereotypic; clonic or tonic	Variable; in most cases, seizures occur less often than once a week	No

Movement	Affected body part	Vocal manifestations	Occurrence during sleep	Character of movement	Frequency of movement	Can be temporarily suppressed
Myoclonus	Shoulders or extremities; often bilateral	No	Yes (if only during sleep, a normal phenomenon; otherwise, always abnormal)	Lightning fast	Variable; may occur on awakening	No
Tremor	Usually hands	May affect voice	No	Continuous	Constant but variable in intensity	Somewhat
Dystonia	Any; may be focal or generalized	No	No	Torsional	Variable	Patient may learn tricks to suppress or mask movements
Self-Stimulating Behaviors of infancy	Usually head, neck, upper extremities	No	No	Stereotypic, repetitive	Sporadic; often during times of excitement	N/A (occur in infants)
Opisthotonos in infancy	Neck and back	No	Yes	Single or multiple episodes of arching	Variable	N/A (noted in infants)

111

The onset is usually between 5 and 10 years of age. Facial tics and minor vocal tics are often the first tics that parents notice. Other children's tics may be more idiosyncratic, such as an odd or complex movement of the trunk or limbs (complex motor tic), a quirky gait, or a habit of making an unusual sound. It is normal for a child's tic to wax and wane over a few weeks or months and for one tic to disappear and a different tic to evolve over the course of time.

The most "famous" tic, the compulsive blurting out of obscenities (*coprolalia*), which for many lay persons defines *Tourette syndrome* (TS), is rare.

Children presenting with a history of eye blinking, facial grimacing, and throat clearing may attribute their tics to a feeling of irritation in the eyes, nose, or throat (sensory tic). The family may offer a history of allergies or recent upper respiratory infection, although the physical examination reveals no sign of allergy or inflammation.

Some complex motor tics, such as the compulsive touching of objects, are indistinguishable from obsessive-compulsive behaviors, and, conversely, many people with obsessive-compulsive disorder manifest a variety of tics. Patients with a history of tic often have a mood disorder, anxiety disorder, attention-deficit hyperactivity disorder (ADHD), conduct disorder, or LD (1,2). Autistic children also are tic prone. There is also often a family history of individuals with one or more of these disorders and, in many cases, a family history of tic. A tendency to develop tics appears to be an autosomal dominant trait with variable penetrance (3–5). Boys are affected more often than girls.

Some patients' tics first occur or worsen following a streptococcal infection. This association has been called pediatric autoimmune neuropsychiatric disorders associated with streptococcal infection (PANDAS) (6–8). If the tics or obsessive behaviors clearly become increasingly worse with each episode of streptococcal infection, then PANDAS should be suspected. Whether management is affected in a practical sense is not clear. Issues relating to diagnosis and treatment of PANDAS are discussed later in this chapter.

Does my child have Tourette syndrome?

By formal criteria, (TS) is diagnosed by the presence of multiple motor tics and at least one vocal tic, persisting more or less uninterrupted for 1 year (9). A history of coprolalia is quite unusual and *not* necessary.

It is important to remember that *the tics of patients with TS can be the same as the tics of patients who do not meet the criteria for TS*. The distinction is based purely on the number of tics and their persistence. Previous versions of the *Diagnostic and Statistical Manual of Mental Disorders* required that *the patient experience significant distress* because of the tics in order to fulfill the criteria for TS. In the authors' view, it is unfortunate that this criterion was omitted, since the diagnosis of TS now applies to many patients whose tics are not debilitating. It is also worth remembering that a patient can have a disabling tic disorder but not meet the criteria for TS, for example, a patient with a loud vocal tic but no motor tics.

The essential point here is that TS, much like epilepsy and cerebral palsy, is a nonspecific but fear-provoking term. We suggest that this be explained to patients and parents, who often imagine a worst-case scenario.

Differential diagnosis, physical examination, and diagnostic testing

The first task is to make certain that the patient does not have a different movement disorder. A history of *discrete, stereotypic* movements or vocalizations that can be *inhibited by the patient* and of *disappearance of the movements during sleep* supports the diagnosis of tic/TS.

The patient's tics are often evident in the office. In many cases, the patient is also noticeably hyperactive, impulsive, or anxious. Some patients with tics also have a learning disability (LD) that is suggested by a history of poor grades and further suggested by a learning evaluation. The remainder of the examination should be unremarkable.

Tics do not normally result from a brain tumor, any other intracranial lesion, or a degenerative disorder and are usually readily differentiated on clinical grounds from other abnormal movements. Therefore, magnetic resonance imaging (MRI) and electroencephalogram (EEG) normally play no role in the diagnosis of a tic disorder. One exception is a "tic" that *always involves the same part and side of the body*. In that case, the abnormal movement may be a *focal motor seizure*, and EEG and MRI should be ordered.

If the history suggests a recent streptococcal infection or many infections, the antistreptolysin (ASO) antibody or anti-DNAase B titer can be checked to look into the possibility of PANDAS. The finding of an elevated titer would not prove that the tics are related to the streptococcal infection, however, nor suggest a specific form of treatment. In cases of suspected PANDAS, some physicians initiate penicillin prophylaxis, as in cases of Sydenham chorea. A recent study (8) does not support this practice. Immunological tests do not appear to distinguish between patients with PANDAS, patients whose tics are not related to streptococcal infection, and control patients (10).

When to consider medication

Since anxiety and stress often cause tics to increase in frequency, some patients may benefit from biofeedback and the learning and practice of relaxation techniques such as meditation, deep breathing technique, etc. Avoidance of caffeinated beverages is also advised. Particularly in mild cases, these modifications frequently suffice. In other cases, when behavioral therapies are of little benefit, the most important decision is whether or not to start medication to control the tics. The decision should be based on the *patient's* feelings about the tics, not his parents' feelings. If the patient is not embarrassed by his tics and is not being teased by other people and repetitive motor tics are not causing him physical discomfort, medication should not be prescribed. Parents, who may be horrified by the sight of their child's tics, may initially have difficulty accepting the idea that the best thing to do is nothing. Parents usually become more willing to defer pharmacological treatment when they learn that drugs to control tics are not always that effective, often become less effective over time, and may cause significant side effects. The fact that tics often spontaneously subside as the patient gets older should, of course, be mentioned. It also often helps to explain that the tics do not result from a serious underlying cause such as a brain tumor or a degenerative disease.

If a medication is not started, the family may be told to return for a follow-up visit if the tics begin to persistently bother their child. Physicians should make certain that parents are aware that a waxing and waning course is to be expected and that new tics often take the place of previously recognized tics. At all times, the paramount question should be, "How much do the tics bother the *child*?"

Case 4.1

The parents of a 7-year-old boy bring him for evaluation because he has developed a habit of blinking his eyes. This habit has been noted for 3 weeks. Sometimes, he will blink incessantly and, at other times, hardly at all. His habit can be suppressed for up to a minute but not longer. He remains alert and acts normally during the blinking episodes. He does not blink when he is asleep. Other children do not notice his habit of blinking, but his father is very worried and requests that the doctor order an MRI scan to make certain that nothing is wrong with his son's brain.

No other unusual behaviors are reported. However, in retrospect, the parents note that 6 months ago, the child developed a habit of clearing his throat that was attributed to allergy but persisted longer than expected. The child has no history of other significant medical problems. He had one episode of streptococcal pharyngitis 1 year ago that was treated with amoxicillin.

The child is a good student and gets along well with other children but is described as "a worrier." His maternal aunt was treated for obsessive-compulsive disorder.

Physical examination reveals a high-strung, alert boy in good general health. There are no signs of infection or inflammation in the pharynx, and no adenopathy is noted. The neurological examination reveals no focal deficits. The child frequently and forcefully blinks his eyes and also periodically stretches his neck.

Diagnosis: *Tic disorder.*

Outcome: The parents were counseled about the nature of tics. The fact that MRI does not yield information relevant to the cause of tics was emphasized.

The parents agreed with the physician that medication should not be started since the tics were not causing the child significant distress. The fact that anxiety often exacerbates tics was mentioned.

The family returned a year later. Although the child had stopped blinking, he had recently acquired a new habit of rolling his eyes. This habit was diagnosed as another tic. The fact that tics often evolve over time was discussed. Medication was again not prescribed. During the next several years, the patient exhibited a number of different tics. They never bothered him especially; his parents learned to ignore the tics and did not feel the need to take him to the doctor. The patient was last seen at age 14 because he was experiencing panic attacks, but he reported that his tics had become less frequent during the previous year.

Medications to control tics

Medication is usually started if a patient's tics are persistently distressing, physically painful, or socially disabling. Drugs from the *neuroleptic* class are usually the most effective. *Pimozide* (Orap, Gate) is a good choice for many patients. Treatment is usually initiated at 0.5 to 1 mg twice daily and titrated based on the patient's response. The total maximum daily dose of 8 mg is rarely necessary. High doses of pimozide may cause drowsiness, but other adverse effects are uncommon. Pretreatment EKG and yearly monitoring is recommended because pimozide may, in rare cases, prolong the Q-T interval and provoke cardiac arrhythmia (Table 4.2).

Haloperidol is among the most effective drugs used for tic suppression and is prescribed at a dose ranging from 0.25 mg twice daily to 2 mg three times daily. The use of haloperidol to treat tics has declined during the last decade as the result of concern about the possibility that the drug will cause an irreversible movement disorder (*tardive dyskinesia* or *tardive dystonia*) or a syndrome of high fever, rigidity, and altered mental status (*neuroleptic malignant syndrome*). These feared complications are uncommon, however, and haloperidol remains an important medication for the control of refractory tics. *Risperidone*, prescribed at a dose of 0.5 to 1.5 mg twice daily, is also effective. Common adverse effects include sedation and weight gain; rare complications include diabetes mellitus, tardive dyskinesia/dystonia, and neuroleptic malignant syndrome. Since haloperidol and risperidone also control hyperactivity, impulsivity, and aggressiveness, they are often prescribed to patients with tics who also have a behavioral disorder or ADHD.

Clonidine (0.25 to 1 mg twice or three times daily; see Chapter 3) and *guanfacine* are often prescribed to control tics. These medications also may be behaviorally beneficial for patients who are impulsive or hyperactive. Sedation is a common adverse effect of these drugs that prevents many patients from tolerating them.

Antidepressant medications from the *serotonin-selective reuptake inhibitor* (SSRI) class, such as fluoxetine (10 to 30 mg daily; see Chapter 5),

TABLE 4.2
Drugs used to control tics

Drug	Adverse effects
Alpha-2 agonists: clonidine, guanfacine	Fatigue, sedation, lightheadedness, agitation.
Neuroleptics: risperidone, haloperidol, pimozide	Fatigue, sedation, acute dystonic reaction; rarely, tardive dyskinesia/dystonia, neuroleptic malignant syndrome, seizures. *Risperidone*: often increases appetite, causing weight gain; rare reports of fatty liver and diabetes. *Pimozide*: less often associated with above adverse effects but, in rare cases, causes prolongation of Q-T interval with potentially serious consequences; EKG monitoring required.
SSRIs: Fluoxetine, sertraline, others. Usually prescribed for tics exacerbated by anxiety or comorbid with obsessive-compulsive symptoms.	Changes in appetite, sedation, sexual dysfunction; rare reports of suicidal ideation.
Less often used: antiepileptic drugs, benzodiazepines, other antidepressant drugs	See Chapters 5 and 6 for adverse effects of specific drugs

are sometimes effective in cases of tic comorbid with an *anxiety disorder* or *obsessive-compulsive disorder.*

Maintenance on medication

Regardless of the drug used, a low dose is always prescribed initially. The dose may be gradually increased after 2 weeks if there is little or no improvement. The physician should try to achieve a 75% reduction, approximately, in the frequency of the patient's tics. Complete control is generally unattainable or comes at the price of oversedation. If the medication does not appear to be working after the dose has been titrated upward twice, it should be tapered off, and another drug should be substituted.

Once control is achieved, the improvement usually lasts for several months or longer in some cases. Unfortunately, tolerance to the drug develops fairly quickly in many cases, and the tics again become frequent. If that occurs, the dose of the drug may be increased. If the increased dose does not lead to an improvement or results in sedation, the drug may be tapered off, and another drug can be substituted. For some patients, acceptable control is maintained by changing their drug every few months. In other cases, a combination of drugs (often a neuroleptic and either an SSRI or clonidine) is effective. An antiepileptic drug, such as carbamazepine, topiramate, or gabapentin (see Chapter 6) or a benzodiazepine, is sometimes added to help control refractory tics. It is worth remembering that, in many cases, a patient's tics spontaneously worsen or improve *regardless* of the medication or dose prescribed.

Prognosis

In the great majority of cases, the tics are either eventually outgrown or continue to occur in adult life but do not cause the patient significant distress; the patient's tics are assumed by others to be common nervous habits (11). In many cases, a marked improvement is noted during adolescence. This is fortunate because adolescents, unlike young children, are likely to cruelly tease the patient with tics.

In about 5% to 10% of cases, the patient's tics do not diminish over time and continue to be frequent and socially disabling. These patients carry the diagnosis of TS into adult life and most will continue to require medication.

Self-stimulating behaviors of infancy

Many infants are brought to the doctor to evaluate what are known as *self-stimulating behaviors*. Their parents usually have observed that the infant has developed a habit of shaking his head or making characteristic, repetitive movements of one or both hands. These behaviors may be noted a few or many times during the day, but they never occur during sleep.

Self-stimulating behaviors are common. They are not a precursor to tics. The possibility of an epileptic seizure should only be considered if an alteration of consciousness, cyanosis, tonic eye deviation, or nystagmus is also noted; if the movements are extremely stereotyped; or if the movements always involve the same side of the body. EEG and MRI should be ordered if a seizure is suspected. If there is uncertainty about the nature of the movements, the parent may be asked to *videotape the episodes*. In many cases, review of the videotape will clearly show the movements to be nonepileptiform habits. If the spells cannot be taped because they are too infrequent or if their nature remains elusive, an ambulatory EEG or video EEG can be ordered to capture these spells and help determine their nature.

Tremor

The parents of a child brought for evaluation of a tremor often worry that their son or daughter has Parkinson disease. They are reassured to hear that juvenile parkinsonism typically causes rigidity, not a tremor, and is extremely rare.

TABLE 4.3
Causes of tremor in children and adolescents

Common causes:

Medications and drugs of abuse

Essential/familial tremor

Mildly delayed neurological development (infants and young children)

Anxiety

Tonic spasms in cases of cerebral palsy and other disorders causing spasticity

Rare causes:

Disorders of calcium, phosphorus, and magnesium metabolism

Hyperthyroidism

Degenerative disorders (tremor is almost always accompanied by other abnormal neurological findings)

Brain tumor or other focal lesion (suspect if tremor is unilateral or an intention tremor)

Classification of tremor

A tremor most often involves the hands and is either classified as a *postural*, an *intention*, or a *resting* tremor. In the pediatric population, a *postural tremor* that is noticeable when the patient's *arms or hands are held in a fixed position* (outstretched or when writing) is the most common. An *intention tremor* caused by cerebellar disease is observed only during *gross purposeful movement* (reaching for an object). In cases of adult-onset Parkinson disease, a *resting tremor* is evident when the hands are *supported and at rest* (on the patient's lap). A resting tremor is virtually never observed in children.

Common causes of tremor

Currently taken medications and the possibility of *drug abuse* should always be considered (Table 4.3). Drugs that may cause or exaggerate a tremor include valproate, other antiepileptic drugs, lithium, methylphenidate, amphetamines, tricyclic antidepressants, cocaine, and caffeine. In fact, almost any substance affecting the central nervous system can cause a tremor. *Withdrawal* from chronic alcohol, barbiturate, opiate, or benzodiazepine use also often causes tremulousness.

Essential tremor is an *intrinsic* condition that often presents during the second or third decade. A postural tremor is usually noticeable when the patient's arms are outstretched. The tremor impacts fine motor tasks such as drawing or knitting. Handwriting is also affected, and handwriting samples may demonstrate the tremor. Sometimes the patient's voice has a quavering quality. Anxiety and stress exacerbate the tremor. There is often a family history of tremor, and in these cases, the condition is called *benign familial tremor*. If an adult relative accompanying the patient also has a history of tremor, the relative may be asked if the *tremor disappears after he or she has a glass of wine or an alcohol-containing drink*. If so, the relative and the patient probably can be diagnosed with a benign familial tremor. The tremor is thought to result from mildly abnormal midbrain and cerebellar activity (12).

Essential/familial tremor is treated with clonazepam, diazepam, topiramate, primidone, or propranolol (13). Many patients prefer to take no medication due to the mild impact of the disorder on most activities and the high frequency of adverse effects, especially sedation, caused by these drugs.

Tremulousness in young children often is a sign of mild neuromaturational delay. There is often a history of delayed fine or gross motor skills (see Chapter 8). The tremor usually is noticed during activities such as drawing or cutting with scissors. It should disappear as the child grows older.

Anxiety is a common cause of tremulousness and should be suspected if the patient with a tremor has a history of panic attacks, phobias, or generalized anxiety disorder. In cases of cerebral palsy, tremulousness is often the observable manifestation of a *tonic spasm* (see Chapter 10).

Less common causes of tremor in children and teenagers

Uncommon causes of tremor in children and adolescents include *hypoglycemia, hypocalcemia, phosphorus or magnesium deficiency,* and *hyperthyroidism*. These disorders usually cause symptoms and signs other than the tremor and can be excluded by routine laboratory tests. The plasma *ceruloplasmin level* is often added. In cases of Wilson disease, a very rare degenerative disorder usually associated with multiple clinical neurological abnormalities, ceruloplasmin is decreased, hepatic transaminases are almost always elevated, and Kayser-Fleischer rings are noted on ophthalmologic examination (14).

In the case of a *tremor that is unilateral*, MRI of the brain should be ordered to exclude a structural abnormality in the brain such as a tumor or an arteriovenous malformation (AVM). *Intention tremor* is also an indication for MRI.

Tremor in the neonate and infant

A *neonate* with a tremor may be experiencing *opiate, cocaine, or barbiturate withdrawal*. A urine specimen from the mother should be sent for drug screening. *Hypoglycemia, hypocalcemia, hypomagnesemia, and hypophosphatemia* are other possible causes that should be excluded by laboratory tests.

During *infancy*, tremulousness and jitteriness are often signs of *neurological immaturity* and should disappear during the first month or two of life.

OTHER MOVEMENT DISORDERS

Chorea

Clinical features

Chorea is a relatively uncommon disorder characterized by *continuous*, non-purposeful movements that move *rapidly and fluidly* from one part of the body to another. The fluid quality of choreiform movements is unique and distinguishes chorea from tics, myoclonus, tremor, and seizures. The patient *cannot suppress* choreiform movements, although some patients attempt to incorporate their choreiform movements into purposeful movements to disguise them.

Physical examination

Choreiform movements are usually obvious. The examination may also reveal mild hypotonia and diminished deep tendon reflexes. The patient may appear restless or excessively emotional. The *"milkmaid sign"* (repetitive squeezing when the patient grasps the examiner's fingers) and an *inability to hold the tongue in a protruded position* are classic but not invariable accompanying findings. Clinical signs of drug toxicity, hyperthyroidism, rheumatic fever, and systemic lupus erythematosus should be noted, as should any focal neurological abnormalities.

Causes of chorea

Sydenham chorea, which is associated with rheumatic fever, *is the most common etiology for chorea in the pediatric population.* Unless another cause is demonstrated, the patient with chorea should be assumed to have Sydenham chorea. In a majority of cases, no other signs of rheumatic fever are noted. An elevated ASO antibody titer is a nonspecific finding that cannot be relied upon to diagnose Sydenham chorea.

Prescription drugs (oral contraceptives, antipsychotics, antidepressants, and antiepileptic medications) and *drugs of abuse* (amphetamines and cocaine) can occasionally provoke choreiform movements. *Systemic lupus erythematosus, hyperthyroidism, and Wilson disease* are also potential causes of chorea. Chorea can be caused by *encephalitis, stroke or tumor affecting the basal ganglia, and degenerative diseases* of the nervous system and can follow *kernicterus* in the neonate (see Chapter 10). *Huntington disease* is a rare hereditary cause of chorea in children; more often, this disease causes parkinsonian rigidity. "Chorea gravidarum," or chorea associated with pregnancy, is probably caused by an occult autoimmune or thyroid disorder (Table 4.4).

TABLE 4.4
Causes of chorea
Sydenham chorea (rheumatic fever)
Medications and drugs of abuse
Hyperthyroidism
Systemic lupus erythematosus
Tumor, infarct, infection, or other lesion in basal ganglia
Wilson disease and other degenerative diseases

Diagnostic studies

Laboratory tests should include toxicology screening, antinuclear antibody titer, erythrocyte sedimentation rate, hepatic function panel, ceruloplasmin level, and thyroid stimulating hormone level. Contrast-enhanced MRI of the brain is ordered to search for an abnormality in the basal ganglia or signs of a degenerative disorder. Wilson disease causes a hyperintense appearance of the basal ganglia.

Treatment

Chorea usually responds to an antipsychotic drug. Risperidone, pimozide, and haloperidol are often prescribed at the dose used to control tics (see earlier section on tics). Antiepileptic drugs (gabapentin, carbamazepine, and others) and benzodiazepines are also used. Immune globulin has been used successfully to treat Sydenham chorea (15).

Chorea caused by a drug usually disappears after the drug is discontinued. Chorea associated with hyperthyroidism and autoimmune disorders improves with treatment of the underlying disorder.

In cases of Sydenham chorea, treatment with a medication to suppress choreiform movements is usually continued for at least 6 months. The patient should be *referred to a pediatric cardiologist* because of the possibility of associated rheumatic heart disease, and *prophylaxis against future streptococcal infection with penicillin* should be initiated. The chorea eventually remits in most cases, although relapses may occur.

Myoclonus

Myoclonus is a *very rapid* ("lightning-fast") involuntary movement, most often of the upper extremities. Myoclonus can be distinguished from tics and chorea on the basis of the quality of the movements and, in many cases, *occurrence during sleep*. Unlike tics, myoclonic jerks cannot be voluntarily suppressed.

Sleep myoclonus, which is common at all ages, even infancy (16), is a normal phenomenon. Myoclonic jerking of the legs is typical and occurs only during sleep.

In contrast, *during wakefulness, myoclonus is never normal*. Myoclonus during wakefulness is often a manifestation of an *epileptic seizure*, in which case the EEG often shows generalized spike-and-wave or polyspike discharges. *Juvenile myoclonic epilepsy* (JME) (see Chapter 6) responds well to several broad-spectrum antiepileptic drugs. Much less commonly, myoclonus is an early sign of a *neurodegenerative disease*. In such cases, the onset of myoclonus is accompanied or followed by ataxia, spasticity, and progressive dementia. This syndrome is called *progressive myoclonic epilepsy* and has many possible causes (see Chapter 14). Myoclonus also may be noted in the aftermath of a severe hypoxemic injury (as in cases of asphyxiation, near drowning, and cardiorespiratory arrest).

In rare cases, a *spinal cord lesion* gives rise to *nonepileptic* (segmental) myoclonus, usually affecting a single muscle group (often in the trunk).

Approach to diagnosis

An EEG should be ordered to evaluate myoclonic jerks noted during wakefulness. If the patient is an adolescent and the EEG suggests JME, further studies, including MRI, are not necessary, and the patient should simply be treated with an appropriate antiepileptic drug. If routine and prolonged EEG monitoring fails to show evidence of JME or if the patient is an infant or a young child, the physician should order MRI and consider testing the patient for a degenerative disease (see Chapter 14). A history of segmental (nonepileptic) myoclonus supported by a normal EEG suggests the need for MRI of the spinal cord.

Dystonia

Dystonia occurs as the result of the simultaneous action of agonist and antagonist muscles. The movements are *sustained and torsional*, may be restricted to a single limb or segment of the body (*focal dystonia*), or may affect the entire body (*generalized dystonia*). The affected part of the body typically appears *hyperextended or twisted*. In the most severe cases of dystonia, the patient's position and posture are grossly distorted, and the patient is in considerable and sometimes agonizing discomfort.

Dystonia is not usually difficult to distinguish clinically from other movement disorders. Dystonic movements *cannot be voluntarily suppressed*, although, as in cases of chorea, patients may attempt to disguise their dystonic movements as purposeful movements.

Dystonia is distinguished from other movement disorders clinically. *MRI, EEG, and electromyography do not help prove that the movements are dystonic*, except by excluding other possibilities. However, MRI and laboratory tests sometimes point to the *cause* of dystonia.

Possible causes of dystonia

Dystonia can be an acute, reversible reaction to a recently started neuroleptic medication (*acute dystonic reaction*). The causative medication must be discontinued. Benztropine or an antihistamine is effective for treating the symptoms, which are self-limited. In contrast, *tardive dystonia*, an uncommon and serious complication of *long-term* neuroleptic and (rarely) other psychiatric drug therapy, often does *not respond to discontinuation of the drug*. Treatment is difficult and often unsatisfactory. Benzodiazepines, trihexyphenidyl, antiepileptic drugs, and tetrabenazine (not available in the United States) may be somewhat effective.

Dopa-responsive dystonia is a genetically inherited movement disorder (17) that responds, sometimes dramatically, to treatment with levodopa. The child's gait is often affected, and consequently, this disorder is sometimes mistaken for the diplegic form of cerebral palsy (see Chapter 10). In many cases, the disorder worsens late in the day and with fatigue. Since this disorder is often dramatically responsive to levodopa, a trial of this drug is usually recommended in cases of unexplained childhood dystonia. *Wilson disease* (discussed earlier) should also be considered when looking for the cause of dystonia. Rarely, dystonia can result from a lesion in the brain such as infarction, bleeding, or tumor in the basal ganglia, which can be visualized by MRI.

In still other cases, dystonia is an autosomal recessive hereditary disorder (*idiopathic torsion dystonia*) that is caused by a gene on chromosome 9 (18,19). Idiopathic torsion dystonia in its severest form is severely disabling, but the disease can also present as an intermittent and mild focal dystonia. A commercially available laboratory test can confirm the presence of the gene.

Writer's cramp is a form of dystonia mostly affecting adults that causes tightening of the hand and wrist muscles when the patient attempts to write with a pen. In other cases, dystonia is a *psychogenic* disorder, often a conversion reaction (see Chapter 6).

Dystonia is usually difficult to treat. An anticholinergic medication, such as trihexyphenidyl, or a benzodiazepine is often used. A recent study (20) suggests that a surgically placed deep brain stimulator is beneficial in some cases. Referral to an expert in the field of movement disorders is recommended.

Opisthotonos

Opisthotonos means arching of the back and neck. An infant with *Sandifer syndrome* has episodes of opisthotonic posturing caused by *gastroesophogeal reflux disease*. Once the underlying condition is effectively treated, the episodes of arching stop occurring.

In other cases, opisthotonic posturing often has more ominous implications. A *malformation of the cervical spine or posterior fossa* or a *cervical or brainstem tumor* is a possible cause. In such cases of opisthotonos, generalized hypertonicity and exaggerated deep tendon reflexes are usually noted.

There is often a history of developmental delay. Cranial nerve palsies suggest a brainstem tumor. MRI of both the brain and cervical spine must be ordered.

Opisthotonic posturing can also be an *early sign of cerebral palsy* (see Chapter 10). *Infantile spasms* (see Chapter 6), a serious form of epilepsy, may present as episodes of intermittent opisthotonic posturing. EEG should be ordered if episodes of opisthotonic posturing occur in clusters or are associated with cyanosis, a change in mental status, or any other signs of a seizure.

REFERENCES

1. Kurlan R, McDermott MP, Deeley C, et al. Prevalence of tics in schoolchildren and association with placement in special education. *Neurology.* 2001;57:1383–1388.
2. Gadow KD, Nolan E. Tics and psychiatric comorbidity in children and adolescents. *Dev Med Child Neurol.* 2002;44:330–338.
3. Pauls DL, Leckman JF. The inheritance of Gilles de la Tourette's syndrome and associated behaviors: evidence for autosomal dominant transmission. *N Engl J Med.* 1986;315:993–997.
4. Kurlan R, Eapen V, Stern J, et al. Bilineal transmission in Tourette's syndrome families. *Neurology.* 1994;44:2336–2342.
5. Sadovnick D, Kurlan R. The increasingly complex genetics of Tourette's syndrome. *Neurology.* 1997;48:801–802.
6. Swedo SE, Leonard HL, Mittleman BB, et al. Identification of children with pediatric autoimmune neuropsychiatric disorders associated with streptococcal infections by a marker associated with rheumatic fever. *Am J Psychiatry.* 1997;143:110–112.
7. Kurlan R. Tourette's syndrome and 'PANDAS': will the relation bear out. *Neurology.* 1998;50:1530–1534.
8. Kurlan R, Kaplan EL. The pediatric autoimmune neuropsychiatric disorders associated with streptococcal infection (PANDAS) etiology for tics and obsessive-compulsive symptoms: hypothesis or entity? Practical considerations for the clinician. *Pediatrics.* 2004;113:883–886.
9. American Psychiatric Association. *Diagnostic and Statistical Manual of Mental Disorders, Text Revision.* 4th ed. Washington, DC: American Psychiatric Association; 2000.
10. Singer H, Hong JJ, Yoon DY, et al. Serum autoantibodies do not differentiate PANDAS and Tourette syndrome from controls. *Neurology.* 2005;65:1701–1707.
11. Leckman JF, Zhang H, Vitale A, et al. Course of tic severity in Tourette syndrome: the first two decades. *Pediatrics.* 1998;102:14–19.
12. Pinto AD, Lang AE, Chen R, et al. The cerebellothalamocortical pathway in essential tremor. *Neurology.* 2003;60:1985–1987.
13. Janovik J, Madisetty J, Dat Voung K. Essential tremor among children. *Pediatrics.* 2004;1114:1203–1205.
14. Prashanth LK, Taly AB, Sinha S, et al. Wilson's disease: diagnostic errors and clinical implications. *J Neurol Neurosurg Psychiatry.* 2004;75:907–909.
15. Garvey MA, Snider LA, Leitman SF, et al. Treatment of Sydenham's chorea with intravenous immunoglobulin, plasma exchange, or prednisone. *J Child Neurol.* 2005; 20: 424–429.

16. Volpe JJ. *Neurology of the Newborn*. Philadelphia: Saunders; 1995:189.
17. Tassin J, Durr A, Bonnet AM, et al. Levodopa-responsive dystonia: GTP cyclohydrolase or Parkin mutations? *Brain*. 2000;123:1112–1121.
18. Spinella GM, Sheridan PH. Research opportunities in dystonia. *Neurology*. 1994;44:1177–1179.
19. Bressman SB, Sabatti C, Raymond D, et al. The DTY1 phenotype and guidelines for diagnostic testing. *Neurology*. 2000;54:1746–1752.
20. Vidalihet M, Vercueil L, Houeto J, et al. Bilateral deep-brain stimulation of the globus pallidus in primary generalized dystonia. *N Engl J Med*. 2005;352:459–467.

5

BEHAVIORAL AND SLEEP PROBLEMS

Behavioral disorders and problems that may present during childhood or adolescence and bring the patient to medical attention include depression, anxiety, oppositional or antisocial behavior, bipolar disorder, and psychosis. A psychiatrist should manage the care of any patient who has a serious behavioral disorder. The general practitioner should be able to diagnose many of these conditions and treat less severely affected patients. The primary care provider should also be familiar with the medications used to treat psychiatric disorders and their adverse effects. In many other cases involving young children, a behavior problem can be effectively addressed by means of effective parenting skills and limit-setting strategies.

TOPICS TO EXPLORE WHILE TAKING THE HISTORY

1 The *age of onset* of the behavioral problem can be diagnostically helpful. A behavioral problem presenting during the first 5 years of life often is a manifestation of an *underlying neurological or neurodevelopmental condition.* *Autism* (see Chapter 9) is always a possibility. Prader-Willi, Williams, fragile X, and fetal alcohol syndromes as well as many other congenital disorders should be considered, especially if the child has *dysmorphic facial features or a history of a recognized congenital anomaly.* Children who do not have a definable genetic disorder but who have a history of *low birth weight* or *delayed language milestones* also are at risk for developing a behavior disorder (1,2).

School-age children may have a *learning disability* (LD) or *attention deficit/hyperactivity disorder* (ADHD). *Anxiety disorders and mood disorders* may present during middle childhood. The onset of a behavioral problem during middle childhood may result from a *stressor in the child's family.* A close relative with a serious illness, divorce, abuse, alcoholism, financial hardship, a traumatic event (e.g., a house fire), and frequent changes of residence are commonly reported stressors that may impact the child.

Depression, anxiety disorders, and *eating disorders* are often diagnosed during adolescence. The teenager with an *LD* may have outbursts. *Family problems* continue to be a potential source of concern. *Bipolar disorder* and *schizophrenia* often first present during adolescence.

Occasionally the first manifestation of a *medical disorder*, such as hyperthyroidism, diabetes mellitus, or systemic lupus erythematosus is a change in the patient's personality. A brain tumor or a degenerative neurological disease also sometimes initially causes a change in behavior.

2 *Where* the problematic behavior occurs is important. Behavior that is significantly *worse at home than in school* often reflects *inadequate parenting skills*. A behavioral problem that is *mostly evident in school* suggests the possibility of an *LD*. In particular, an auditory comprehension problem (see Chapter 3) should be suspected in the case of a preschool child who often "acts out." ADHD–Combined Type and ADHD–Hyperactive Type, mood and anxiety disorders, autism, and psychosis are *evident in multiple settings*.

3 The *family history* should be explored. Family members may have been diagnosed with depression, an anxiety disorder, bipolar disorder, schizophrenia, ADHD, or a personality disorder. Family members with a history of chronic unemployment, alcoholism or substance abuse disorder, or incarcerations may be recalled.

4 The examiner should inquire about the patient's *performance in school*. If the child's grades are poor, an LD or ADHD should be suspected, and a screening evaluation for LD should be included (see Chapter 3).

5 *Teenagers should be interviewed privately during part of the visit* and asked about their experiences in school and with family members and friends. The subjects of *alcohol* and *drug use, sexual activity*, and eating habits should be discussed. A withdrawn or odd-acting patient should be asked if he or she has had *hallucinations* (usually hearing voices), and questions should be asked to determine whether the patient has *delusional or paranoid thoughts*. The physician must specifically ask about *suicidal thoughts, plans, or acts. If there is a history of recurrent suicidal thoughts or a suicidal attempt, the patient should be referred to a psychiatrist or sent to the emergency room.*

PHYSICAL EXAMINATION

Obesity or an emaciated appearance suggests an eating disorder. Features that may suggest a syndrome of congenital malformation should be noted, especially in young children. The thyroid gland may be enlarged or contain a nodule. "Soft signs" (see Chapter 1) are sometimes noted when examining young children with behavioral and neurodevelopmental problems. A focal neurological deficit is rarely noted, but if discovered, it is an indication for magnetic resonance imaging (MRI).

The patient may appear agitated, anxious, depressed, angry, apathetic, or aloof. The physician should make note of the patient's speech, thought process, and style of interaction.

SUGGESTIONS FOR MANAGING COMMON BEHAVIORAL PROBLEMS

Many childhood behavioral problems are not serious but do need to be addressed by the family. Physicians should be able to suggest effective strategies. Parents may benefit by reading through the excellent handbook *Redirecting Children's Behavior* (3), from which many of the following suggestions are derived.

Structure in the home is important. Behavioral limits teach children to act considerately and responsibly. Most parents try to set limits but do so inconsistently and ineffectively. When limits to behavior are poorly defined or inconsistently enforced or when punishments are overly harsh or poorly conceived, the result is often oppositional behavior and, in many cases, problems in and outside of the home. The following are useful strategies.

Natural and logical consequences

An approach to limit setting that emphasizes *natural consequences* and *logical consequences* is generally effective.

Natural consequences

Many parents do not let their children learn from experience. A *natural consequence* is the spontaneous result of a child's behavior when an adult does not intervene. For example, if a 7-year-old child stubbornly insists that he can play in the snow wearing only a tee shirt and is permitted to do so, he will soon feel cold (the natural consequence). If a child takes an hour to get ready in the morning and is therefore late to school, the teacher will reprimand the child (the natural consequence). The lessons for the child are clear: wearing a coat in winter is a good idea if you want to stay warm, and teachers do not like tardiness. In addition to teaching children important lessons, a reliance on natural consequences may prevent parents from being drawn into power struggles with their child ("Put your coat on or you'll freeze to death!" or "If I told you once, I've told you a thousand times to get ready or you'll be late for school!").

Logical consequences

If some natural consequences are permitted to occur, the child may be harmed. A 5-year-old child who insists on running into the street cannot be allowed to learn that cars are dangerous from the experience of being hit by one. The natural consequence for a teenager who plays video games instead of doing homework is likely to be a poor report card, possibly damaging his or her chances of getting into college, which is a high price to pay for a poor sense of priorities. In other situations, the natural consequence of a child's behavior does not directly affect the child, for example, when he or she disrupts a birthday party by constantly demanding special favors.

In these situations, a *logical consequence* imposed by a parent should be substituted for the natural consequence. The general form of a logical consequence is as follows: *"I am not willing to (allow the natural consequence to occur), so if you cannot (stop a behavior that will lead to the natural consequence), I will (have to restrict a relevant privilege)."*

The following are examples of a logical consequence that might be imposed in the previously mentioned situations:

> "I am not willing to take the risk that you will be hit by a car, so if you keep trying to run into the street, you will not be allowed to play outside."
>
> "I am not willing to let you jeopardize your future because you are not doing your homework, so if you can't buckle down, I will limit your video game time to weekends."
>
> "I am not willing to let you act that way at a party, and if that happens again, you will not be allowed to go to parties for the next month."

In formulating a logical consequence, the word *logical* should always be kept in mind. *A logical consequence is not a randomly chosen punishment.* Here is a typical example of an arbitrary punishment: "After Johnny failed his math test because he didn't study, we grounded him for the weekend." Here, the "grounding" has no logical relationship to Johnny's failure to study, is probably considered a mean and pointless punishment by Johnny, and is likely not going to encourage him to study harder. (An adult may imagine what his or her reaction would be if the penalty for driving too fast was the loss of vacation time, as opposed to the driver's license.) A more logical consequence, in the case of Johnny and the poor test grade, might take the form of eliminating television privileges on school nights to encourage better study habits.

The pitfalls of rewarding

Many parents, teachers, and doctors suggest a reward system to encourage appropriate behavior. Typically, the child is either given a symbolic reward (point on a "star chart") or a tangible reward (e.g., video game time) in return for good behavior.

Rewarding often produces a short-term improvement in behavior but rapidly loses effectiveness. Children often "up the ante"; in other words, they ask for a continually bigger reward ("I want two stars" or "I want extra time") in return for continued "good" behavior. Furthermore, a reward system suggests that the only reason to behave appropriately is to "get something out of it," which is not the best philosophy to teach a child. A system of natural and logical consequences works better and teaches more appropriate lessons.

How to use time-outs

The "time-out" has become a popular and probably overused way of managing difficult behavior. A time-out is not a punishment. The purpose of a time-out is to *distract* a young child when he is behaving inappropriately (having a tantrum, fighting with a sibling, or being obstinate). A time-out should be a chance for the child to unwind and refocus. The child should be sent to a quiet place where she may color or play with a favorite toy. Children older than 4 or 5 years of age may be told to return when they feel ready.

Once a child is old enough to remember what he was given a "time-out" for, this strategy will no longer be effective. Children who have behavioral outbursts caused by ADHD, autism, and psychiatric disorders also often do not respond to time-outs.

Negative attention and positive attention

Children cannot tolerate feeling ignored. *Many childhood misbehaviors are attempts to get parental attention.* Parents should be aware that "positive attention" (praise, affection, or enjoyable activities shared with a parent) and "negative attention" (being scolded, punished, etc.) are *both* forms of attention, in a child's eyes, and are *both* viewed as are better than no attention at all. *A child deprived of positive attention will often misbehave*; a little positive attention from a parent (playing a board game or a sport together or going to the movies) will often go a long way toward preventing misbehavior. Parents should also try to keep a level head and not "blow up" at a child when he or she is acting badly, thus denying the child negative attention as a reward for misbehavior.

Lying

Many parents complain that their child lies. It is usually best to focus on *what it is that the child is lying about*. For example, if the child is dishonestly denying having any homework to do, she may be having trouble understanding the homework. If a teenager has denied smoking cigarettes when she, in fact, does smoke, the discussion should be about smoking rather than lying about smoking. By avoiding the subject of lying, the underlying issue can often be addressed more effectively, and the child or teenager may feel more comfortable talking other matters over in the future.

Sibling disputes

It is unrealistic to expect siblings to always get along with each other. Parents should *avoid taking sides* in sibling conflicts, even if one child appears to have been the instigator. (The other child might have done something 5 minutes earlier that the parent did not see.) The focus of parental intervention should be on stopping the fighting or bickering and not on assigning blame. *Consequences should be applied to both children.* In other words, if a child takes a toy from his brother, *both* children should lose the toy; children who are bickering should *both* be told to leave the room. This is known as *"putting them both in the same boat."*

Morning and dinner time

Many young children are oppositional about getting ready for school in the morning. A simple way of managing this kind of behavior is to give the child a choice: "You have 5 minutes to get yourself dressed, or I will have to do it for you." If the child does not get himself or herself dressed, the parent should return to the room in 5 minutes, get the child dressed without making a fuss, and leave the room.

Children who run away from the dinner table every 5 minutes should be told, "Dinner is on the table for 15 minutes." If the child persists in going away from the table, the table should be cleared after 15 minutes, and the child should not be given a late meal.

Many family conflicts revolve around food. A parent raised in a family with a small income, where food was not assumed to be available, may be offended when his child refuses to eat a lovingly prepared dish. A parent raised in a more wealthy family may feel guilty about wasting food. Children will not allow themselves to starve, but parents often force their child to eat, and reprimand the child if he or she refuses. The child *always* wins these battles. If battles continue, the child may figure out that he or she can manipulate the parents by not eating or by only eating certain kinds of food. The parent then may go to great lengths to prepare a meal that the child is willing to eat. In these situations, it can be tactfully suggested that indulging the child is not a good idea. A reasonable meal should be served to everyone in the family, and special meals should not be prepared.

In addition to being a source of unnecessary conflict, forcing food often leads to obesity, which has become a nationwide problem. In other cases, the result is an eating disorder.

Choosing battles

Finally, parents should *choose their battles.* They should identify a small number of behavioral problems that are most significant and stay focused on these problems. Less significant issues are best ignored. No child is perfect.

Case 5.1

A 12-year-old girl is brought to the office because she has been feeling removed from her surroundings. This sensation has been noted a few times a week, and she reports that it often lasts for as long as a half hour. She reports that objects look far away when she has these spells. She remains alert and is able to converse with other people. She denies any history of headaches, other disturbances of vision, weakness, or incoordination. She is not groggy or tired after these events.

Her general health has been good. Menarche occurred 3 months ago. Her mother states that her daughter has been happy and reports no change in her personality. Her performance in school has also been good, and her mother describes her as very perfectionistic.

The physical examination is unremarkable. Neurological examination reveals normal optic discs, visual acuity, and visual fields. Strength and reflexes are normal, and no cerebellar signs are noted. Throughout she is alert and pleasant.

Brain MRI and 48-hour EEG yield no evidence of a structural abnormality or epileptiform activity. During the EEG recording, the girl experienced two episodes of the visual disturbance, but no abnormal electrical activity was recorded.

When asked again about the episodes, she now remembers that they occur mostly when she is in large crowds or outdoors in open spaces.

Diagnosis: *Anxiety disorder.*

Outcome: The girl was given a prescription for sertraline 25 mg, which was increased to 50 mg after 2 weeks. At 50 mg, she reported that the episodes stopped occurring. She was also referred for psychological counseling. One year later, she was taken off sertraline and has remained asymptomatic.

BEHAVIORAL DISORDERS OF CHILDHOOD AND ADOLESCENCE

The following section covers specific behavioral disorders presenting during childhood and adolescence. The reader will note that two important conditions are discussed in other chapters: ADHD is discussed in Chapter 3 because of the relevance of ADHD to the school setting, and autism is discussed in Chapter 9.

Depression in children and adolescents

Depression is a common condition in the pediatric and, especially, adolescent age group. Complaints (from a parent or the patient) suggesting depression include *social withdrawal, irritability, outbursts of anger, a loss of interest*

in formerly enjoyable activities, frequent feelings of sadness, and distur-
bances of sleep or appetite (4). *Suicide is the greatest danger associated*
with depression and is a leading cause of death during adolescence (5).
Suicidal thoughts may be openly admitted or revealed only in a confidential
discussion with a doctor or psychologist. Although most suicidal remarks
made by young patients to family members are made primarily to get attention ("I'll kill myself if you make me go school today"), the physician should
never downplay the significance of a suicidal thought or remark. *If the physi-*
cian feels that the patient may be at risk for suicide, the patient should be
sent to the emergency room.

The interview may reveal a stressor in the depressed patient's life, such as
a seriously ill family member, a divorce in the family, abuse, a parent with a
drinking problem, or trouble fitting in with a peer group. The patient's family
often reports poor grades in school, which often are the result of lack of
effort but may suggest an undiagnosed LD contributing to low self-esteem.

The *family history* often reveals that relatives of the patient have been
diagnosed with depression, bipolar disorder, or anxiety disorder or have a
history of alcoholism or drug abuse.

Assessment of very young children

The behavior of preschool-age children with a history of *delayed language*
milestones may suggest depression, as these children are often quiet and
withdrawn. Their eye contact is often poor, suggesting an autistic spectrum
disorder (ASD). If there is no history of ritualistic or stereotyped behaviors,
the child is unlikely to be autistic. A series of sessions with an experienced
child psychologist often helps clarify the diagnosis.

Examination

A depressed patient may be sad and tearful or irritable. Sometimes signs of
self-mutilation are visible on the patient's forearms. Patients who are severely
depressed are usually withdrawn and have a flat affect (are *abulic*). An odd
affect or a history of delusional thinking, hallucinations, or bizarre thoughts
suggests psychosis, not depression. The physical examination should be otherwise unremarkable. Focal neurological signs or papilledema are rarely
noted but, if present, suggest an occult brain tumor.

Diagnostic testing

Depression is primarily a clinical diagnosis. Neuropsychological testing may
be helpful when the diagnosis of a mood disorder requires confirmation.
Thyroid function tests should be sent because laboratory evidence of
hypothyroidism is sometimes discovered. MRI should be ordered when there

is no family history of a mood disorder and no history of a recent psychological stressor or when the neurological examination reveals abnormal findings.

Can you test my child for a chemical imbalance?

A "chemical imbalance" is a tactful term for a mood disorder. As is the case when many such metaphorical terms are used with good intention to communicate with the family, many people take the term too literally; they assume that there is a specific blood test to detect a chemical abnormality, such as a lack of serotonin, in the brain and ask that their child be tested. Unfortunately, since the blood–brain barrier prevents many chemicals from entering and leaving the brain, levels of serotonin and other neurotransmitters in plasma cannot be assumed to reflect levels in the brain. There is no blood test that can diagnose a mood disorder.

Treatment

The initial treatment for children and teenagers with mild symptoms of depression should be psychotherapy. Either cognitive behavior therapy or psychodynamic psychotherapy may be helpful. The response to therapy, however, is highly dependent on the patient's attitude, the skill of the therapist, and the compatibility of the therapist and patient. Many children and adolescents, not to mention adults, are incapable of the introspection required to make psychotherapy a successful experience. Some patients refuse to go for counseling or will not talk to the therapist if they do go. Other patients simply do not benefit. However, psychotherapy can be very helpful for some patients and should be recommended.

The U.S. Food and Drug Administration (FDA) has recently approved fluoxetine (Prozac, Lilly), a *serotonin-selective reuptake inhibitor* (SSRI), for the treatment of pediatric patients diagnosed with depression. Sertraline (Zoloft, Pfizer), another SSRI, had previously been approved for children and adolescents diagnosed with obsessive-compulsive disorder (OCD). No other SSRI has been approved for use in children and adolescents, although in practice, many of these drugs are prescribed.

The FDA has recently required that a "black box" warning, citing an increased incidence of suicide among depressed patients taking SSRIs, must be included in the package insert accompanying these drugs. Previously, the FDA had discouraged the prescription of one SSRI (paroxetine) to children and adolescents based on similar concerns. Some physicians have, as a result, gone so far as to suggest that these drugs should never be prescribed to a child or adolescent; many other physicians equally strongly disagree. Currently, despite the suicide warning, the FDA does not contraindicate the prescription of SSRIs to children and teenagers. We feel that these drugs should, obviously, be used with caution, but note that they are effective for many patients and are usually well tolerated.

Frequently prescribed SSRIs include sertraline (Zoloft, Pfizer), fluoxetine (Prozac, Lilly), fluvoxamine, and citalopram. For older children and adolescents, a low initial dose (10 mg of fluoxetine or 12.5 to 25 mg of sertraline) given daily for 2 weeks, followed by an increase (to 20 mg of fluoxetine or 50 mg of sertraline) is usually prescribed. Some patients do not respond adequately until the dose is further increased, but if there has been no clinical improvement after two increases in dose and a 4- to 6-week trial period, the SSRI should be tapered off over the next 2 to 3 weeks. The SSRI should not be abruptly discontinued since severe mood swings may result. A trial of a second SSRI may then be attempted, although the chance of a response is relatively low if the first drug was not helpful; a drug from a different antidepressant class, such as buproprion, may be a more appropriate choice. SSRIs may cause nuisance side effects such as fatigue, nausea, diarrhea, and suppression of appetite. Adult patients taking an SSRI often report sexual dysfunction.

A *tricyclic antidepressant* (TCA) may be effective for treating the vegetative symptoms (lack of energy and appetite and insomnia) of depression. However, most primary care physicians avoid TCAs because these drugs often are sedating and, in rare cases, cause cardiac arrhythmia and provoke epileptic seizures.

Buproprion (Wellbutrin, GlaxoSmithKline) is an antidepressant that is neither in the SSRI nor TCA family. The effective dose ranges from 100 to 300 mg (occasionally 400 mg) divided once or twice daily. Buproprion is also sometimes used to treat ADHD (see Chapter 3). Most patients tolerate buproprion well. However, the drug may provoke a *seizure* (0.1% to 0.4% incidence, according to the manufacturer). The risk is highest when the dose exceeds 300 mg per day. Therefore, buproprion is contraindicated in cases of epilepsy. Buproprion may cause nuisance side effects (sedation, nausea, etc.) similar to those caused by the SSRIs.

Venlafaxine (Effexor, Wyeth-Ayerst) is an antidepressant and anxiolytic with a mode of action intermediate between the SSRI and TCA medications. Experience in the pediatric population has been limited, and a recent warning from the manufacturer advises against the use of venlafaxine for children and adolescents.

Duration of treatment and management of refractory depression

If the patient's signs and symptoms improve following the initiation of antidepressant treatment, the *antidepressant should be taken for at least 6 months.* A short treatment period is a common reason for relapse. Many patients diagnosed with depression are treated for 2 years or longer.

If a depressed patient does not improve during treatment with either of two medications, he or she should be referred to a psychiatrist. Patients with signs of major depression should be referred immediately. Bipolar disorder is a possibility in cases of refractory depression.

Bipolar disorder in children

Until fairly recently, children were not diagnosed with bipolar disorder; specific criteria for childhood bipolar disorder are still not included in the *Diagnostic and Statistical Manual of Mental Disorders*, 4th Edition, Text Revision (DSM-IV-TR). However, clinical experience shows that some children and adolescents have exaggerated mood swings and outbursts of anger and are hyperactive or intensely anxious. This complex of behaviors is now thought to represent the pediatric equivalent of bipolar disorder (6). In such cases, there is often a family history of mood disorders, ADHD, obsessive-compulsive disorder (OCD), or autism. Many of these children are initially thought to have ADHD but only partially respond to treatment with a stimulant medication. The intensity and variety of their behaviors soon makes it apparent that the diagnosis is not just ADHD.

A child psychiatrist should manage the care of any young patient exhibiting signs of bipolar disorder. Treatment is difficult, and more than one drug is invariably required. Medications often prescribed include mood-stabilizing drugs, antidepressants, antipsychotics, stimulant drugs, clonidine, and lithium.

Mood-stabilizing medications

Patients diagnosed with bipolar disorder or who have a history of frequent behavioral outbursts are often prescribed a *mood-stabilizing* medication. In most cases, the medication is an *antiepileptic drug* (AED). Valproate, carbamazepine, oxcarbazepine, gabapentin, lamotrigine, and topiramate are often prescribed as mood stabilizers. These drugs are reviewed in Chapter 6. *Lithium* has traditionally been used to treat bipolar disorder. Renal, hematological, and neurological adverse effects can be significant and require careful monitoring.

Panic and anxiety

Patients with a history of *panic attacks* report episodic symptoms of intense anxiety or fear of impending doom and simultaneously experience heart palpitations, chest tightness, flushing, shortness of breath, or light-headedness. Fainting spells (*psychogenic syncope*) may occur. These events often occur at random; no clear precipitating cause is usually identified. A medical and cardiological evaluation to exclude hypoglycemia, hyperthyroidism, anemia, and cardiac arrhythmia is usually ordered (see Chapter 7), although the evaluation rarely reveals an underlying disorder. MRI and electroencephalogram (EEG) are not necessary to evaluate stereotypic panic attacks but should be considered if there is a history of prolonged unresponsiveness after an attack suggesting a post-ictal state (see Chapter 6).

Common *specific phobias* include fears of airplane travel, bridges, elevators, storms, fires, insects, animals, enclosed or open spaces, high places, and crowds.

Young children with symptoms of *generalized anxiety* are usually shy, overly dependent on their mothers, and afraid of strangers and unfamiliar situations. Some patients' symptoms of anxiety are recognized to have first occurred or to have worsened following a traumatic event, such as the unexpected death of a family member or friend, an accident, a violent crime, a house fire, or a horrifying event in the news (such as the September 11, 2001, attacks). In these cases, the patient is said to have *posttraumatic stress disorder*.

Separation anxiety is common among children starting preschool or with a newborn sibling. *Performance (test) anxiety* is common and often exacerbated if the patient has a learning disability. Children with *autism* are often extremely anxious in novel situations.

A *family history* of individuals diagnosed with chronic anxiety, panic attacks, or a mood disorder is frequently reported in all these cases.

"Neurological" symptoms of anxiety

Some patients who are chronically anxious report intermittent symptoms of disorientation, seeing nearby objects that appear distant (*micropsia*), or a general sense of removal from their surroundings ("like a person looking in"). MRI and an EEG are often appropriately ordered to exclude a seizure or a temporal or frontal lobe tumor.

Obsessive-compulsive disorder

Patients with OCD typically report *persistent, intrusive thoughts* (*obsessions*), often about cleanliness, germs, disease, or death, or are preoccupied with *orderliness and symmetry*. *Compulsions* (hand washing, cleaning, counting numbers, or other rote mental tasks) are the *acts* committed by the patient as a result of his thoughts. OCD is classified as an anxiety disorder. Many patients with *Tourette syndrome* (see Chapter 4) are diagnosed with OCD.

Patients with autism may *appear* to exhibit obsessive-compulsive behaviors, but these behaviors are *not ego-dystonic*. In other words, patients with OCD are usually *troubled by their obsessions and compulsions and seek medical help*, whereas autistic patients appear unconcerned by or even may derive pleasure from their routines and rituals.

Treatment

Cognitive-behavior therapy plays an important role in the treatment of anxiety disorders; traditional psychodynamic psychotherapy tends to be less effective. In adults, for the pharmacological treatment of occasional panic attacks that occur in predictable situations (airplane travel), a *benzodi-azepine* such as alprazolam (0.25 to 0.5 mg per dose) or clonazepam (0.1 mg per dose) is often effective. However, chronic use of benzodiazepines may lead to the development of tolerance, and withdrawal symptoms including seizures can occur following abrupt discontinuation. For these reasons, it is unusual to prescribe a benzodiazepine to a patient in the pediatric age group for anxiety. A benzodiazepine should also not be prescribed to any patient with a history of substance abuse. *Propranolol* may be used, although it often causes sedation.

Pediatric patients with a history of frequent panic attacks or generalized anxiety often respond to an SSRI (7). A low dose (e.g., sertraline 12.5 to 25 mg or fluoxetine 5 to 10 mg daily) is often most effective; higher doses may worsen the patient's anxiety. For OCD, however, high doses (e.g., sertraline up to 200 mg daily) are often necessary.

Disruptive behavior disorders

Diagnostic criteria for *oppositional-defiant disorder* (ODD) and *conduct disorder* are summarized in Table 5.1.

ODD is characterized by chronically noncompliant, argumentative behavior. In many cases, there is a history of a disruption of family life such as a difficult divorce or a child who has been shuttled from one relative's home to another's. Excessively harsh punishments, poorly conceived limit-setting strategies, or inconsistently imposed consequences for misbehavior are often described. In addition, many patients diagnosed with ODD also have a history of LD or ADHD.

The child's oppositional tendencies should be addressed by means of effective limit setting, appropriate help in school when necessary, family counseling, and psychotherapy. An approach to limit setting that relies on natural and logical consequences (discussed earlier) is recommended. Treatment with a stimulant medication is often helpful if the patient has been diagnosed with ADHD. Risperidone is often effective if the patient is highly oppositional and disruptive and his or her behavior has not improved as a result of nonpharmacological interventions.

Conduct disorder is a precursor to adult *antisocial personality disorder*. Patients with conduct disorder lack a sense of remorse and respect for others' basic rights. They may steal from others, damage property, or cause physical harm to people or animals. As children and teenagers, these individuals are often suspended or expelled from school and may be arrested for vandalism, drug abuse, assault, or theft. The home environment is typically poorly structured; parental supervision is often limited, and abuse is frequently reported.

Patients with conduct disorder should be referred to a psychiatrist. Aggressive or impulsive behavior is managed with an antipsychotic drug,

TABLE 5.1
Disruptive behavior disorders

Oppositional-defiant disorder (*four or more required for diagnosis*)	Conduct disorder (*history of three or more required*)
Often loses temper	Often bullies/threatens others
Often argues with adults	Initiates physical fights
Often deliberately defiant/disobedient	Use of a weapon
Often deliberately annoying	Physical cruelty to people
Often blames others for own behavior	Physical cruelty to animals
Easily annoyed	Stealing associated with physical assault/aggression
Often angry/resentful	Forcing sexual activity on a person
Often spiteful/vindictive	Fire setting with intent to cause damage
	Deliberate property destruction
	Breaking into a car or home
	Lying to obtain goods/favors
	Shoplifting or forgery
	Staying out despite parental rules
	Running away from home
	Chronic truancy

Adapted from DSM-IV-TR (8).

a mood-stabilizing drug, or clonidine. A stimulant medication with a low potential for abuse (that does not come in the form of a tablet that can be crushed and "snorted") may be prescribed if the patient has a history of ADHD. A program for teenagers with a history of drug abuse, delinquency, or other behavioral problems may be helpful for some patients.

Psychosis

Psychosis is a state of disconnection from reality. Classic signs and symptoms of psychosis, most often noted in cases of schizophrenia, include: (a) delusional thinking; (b) hallucinations; (c) thought broadcasting (the concept that others are directly communicating with the patient via fantastic means, such as the television set); (d) ideas of reference (the patient believes that remote events over which he or she has no control are directly connected to his or her thoughts or actions); (e) bizarre behavior; and (f) marked social withdrawal.

Examination

The physical examination should first be directed toward excluding a medical cause for the patient's behavior. Psychosis may be a manifestation of medically caused delirium or a neurological disorder. *Signs of dehydration* suggest hyponatremia, which can cause psychotic behavior. The *thyroid* should be palpated for signs of enlargement or a nodule. *Fever or rash* suggests the possibility of encephalitis (see Chapter 13), an infection causing delirium, or an autoimmune disease such as systemic lupus erythematosus. *Dilated pupils* suggest intoxication with an amphetamine, cocaine, LSD, phencyclidine, or an anticholinergic medication. *Tremor* may result from withdrawal from chronic alcohol or other drug abuse. *Focal neurological signs* are rare but, if present, suggest a degenerative neurological disease or a localized abnormality in the brain.

The interviewer should make note of the patient's orientation, speech, social relatedness, and affect. The patient should be asked if he has used drugs or alcohol, has had suicidal thoughts, is hearing voices, or is having visual hallucinations. During the interview, an effort should be made to determine whether or not the patient has delusional or paranoid thoughts.

In cases of psychosis, a psychiatrist should be asked to conduct a formal interview and will usually assume responsibility for the case if no underlying medical cause is discovered.

Diagnostic testing

Urine toxicology should always be ordered. Other laboratory tests often include *complete blood count* with *erythrocyte sedimentation rate, electrolyte panel, thyroid studies, liver function tests, ceruloplasmin level, syphilis serology, antinuclear antibody*, and 24-hour *urine collection for porphyrins*. If the patient has a fever, a *lumbar puncture* should be performed. *MRI of the brain* should be ordered in the case of any patient with a history of unexplained psychotic behavior.

Schizophrenia

In practice, an underlying medical cause of psychosis is not often discovered, and the eventual diagnosis made is *schizophrenia*. The DSM-IV-TR criteria for schizophrenia are summarized in Table 5.2. Family members often report a prodromal phase during which the patient became socially withdrawn, disheveled, and uninterested in previously enjoyable activities; had strange thoughts; or became preoccupied with religion. A florid phase characterized by bizarre behavior and paranoid delusions or hallucinations typically follows. The patient may appear agitated, aloof, or withdrawn. The patient may spontaneously express delusional thoughts and report hallucinations, or

TABLE 5.2
Criteria for schizophrenia

At least two of the following: hallucinations, delusions, disorganized speech, grossly disorganized behavior, flat affect
Symptoms cause a significant disturbance in social, academic, or occupational functioning
Duration greater than 6 months
Symptoms not due to a mood disorder (agitated depression, bipolar disorder)
Symptoms not due to substance abuse or a general medical condition

Adapted from DSM-IV-TR (9).

these thoughts and experiences may be revealed only if the patient is questioned specifically about them. The interview may also suggest paranoid, tangential, or bizarre ideation.

Hospitalization is required in the great majority of cases. A psychiatrist should assume responsibility for the case.

Common adverse effects of psychiatric mediations and drugs of abuse

Patients taking a medication for a behavioral disorder may report side effects of the drug. In other cases, a parent or friend may notice a change in the patient's behavior. Table 5.3 lists the common and important adverse effects caused by these drugs. Substances of abuse are included.

Sleep disorders

Normal sleep occurs as five sequential stages: stages I, II, III, and IV followed by the rapid-eye movement (REM) phase. The first four stages of sleep coincide with progressively deeper somnolence and neurophysiologically are distinguished by the degree of *slowing of the EEG background rhythm* (10) (see Chapter 6), as well as by the presence, in some stages, of *sleep spindles and vertex sharp waves*. During REM sleep, the EEG demonstrates electrical activity of much lower amplitude and more irregular rhythm, characteristic *eye movements* occur, and *muscle tone decreases*. All *dreaming* occurs during REM sleep. The entire cycle, from stage I sleep through REM sleep, lasts up to 2 hours and is repeated several times during the night. *However, the percentage of time spent in stages III and IV decreases during the night, whereas the percentage of REM sleep increases. Therefore, most dreaming occurs during the predawn as opposed to near-midnight hours.*

TABLE 5.3

Adverse effects of psychiatric and abused drugs[a]

Drug class	Common effects	Uncommon to rare effects
Stimulant medications for ADHD (see Chapter 3)	Appetite suppression, afternoon mood swings, headache, abdominal pain, insomnia (*change brand or drug; see Chapter 2*)	Agitation, flat affect, zombie-like appearance, tachycardia, tics (*lower dose; consider changing or discontinuing drug; see below for symptoms of amphetamine abuse*)
Alpha-2 agonists (clonidine, guanfacine) (see Chapter 3)	Sedation, fatigue, paradoxical agitation (*lower dose or discontinue drug*)	Hypotension, syncope (*discontinue drug*)
Serotonin-selective reuptake inhibitors (SSRIs)	Nausea, change in appetite, fatigue (*change to different SSRI*); sexual side effects in older patients (*change to non-SSRI antidepressant*)	Serotonin syndrome (rare): agitation, myoclonus, shivering, and ataxia; suicidal ideation (in both cases, *discontinue drug; hospitalization*)
Tricyclic antidepressants	Sedation, paradoxical agitation, dry mouth, urinary retention in adults (*change to different antidepressant*)	Cardiac arrhythmia, seizures (*discontinue drug; appropriate consultations*)
Antipsychotics	Sedation, flat affect; increase in appetite (risperidone and other atypical antipsychotics; *try to reduce dosage*); acute dystonic reaction (*discontinue drug; treat with diphenhydramine or benztropine*)	Seizures (especially with thioridazine); neuroleptic malignant syndrome (NMS); tardive dyskinesia/dystonia. (*discontinue drug; see Chapter 4 for treatment of dystonia; NMS patient must be hospitalized in intensive care unit (ICU), treated with dantrolene*)
Mood stabilizers (antiepileptic drugs)	Fatigue, cognitive slowing (*reduce dose or change drug*); allergic rash (*promptly stop drug*)	See Chapter 6 for specific drugs

Drug class	Common effects	Uncommon to rare effects
Alcohol	Ataxia, slurred speech, loss of consciousness, withdrawal seizures (*observation only in mild cases; hospitalization in cases of withdrawal seizure*)	Tremulousness, delirium, hallucinations (in cases of withdrawal; rare in pediatric patients) (*hospitalize in ICU; close observation; benzodiazepine to help alleviate symptoms*); coma/death may occur in rare cases of alcohol overdose
Benzodiazepines	Oversedation, ataxia, sleep disturbance (*observe; reduce dose or discontinue drug*)	Withdrawal seizures; respiratory arrest at very high doses (*hospitalization*)
Marijuana	Mild euphoria, loss of motivation, increased appetite, dilated pupils (*observe only*)	Agitation, paranoid ideation (*may require admission and treatment with a sedative*)
Lysergic acid diethylamide (LSD)	Hallucinations, perceptual distortions, euphoria (*observe only; consider hospital admission*)	Agitation, frightening hallucinations or delusions, flashbacks, suicide attempts (*hospitalization; benzodiazepines may be helpful*)
Phencyclidine (PCP; "angel dust")	Mild hallucinogenic state, euphoria (*consider hospitalization*)	Marked disorientation, regression of behavior, impaired communication, agitation, suicide attempts; sympathomimetic effects (hypertension, tachycardia); procholinergic effects (sweating, drooling) (*hospitalize; treatment is controversial but may include haloperidol*)
Cocaine and amphetamine abuse (signs and symptoms almost identical)	Hyperactivity, euphoria, increased energy, insomnia (*observation; consider hospitalization*).	Chest pain, myocardial infarction, seizure, stroke, cerebral hemorrhage (*hospitalize for appropriate treatment*)

[a] Suggested treatment in italics.

Common non-REM sleep disorders

Night terrors occur only during *non-REM* sleep, during the *earlier part* (10 PM to 1 AM) of the night. They often first present between 2 and 4 years of age. The child abruptly awakens in the middle of the night, sits bolt upright in bed, appears terrified, and begins to scream uncontrollably. Some of these children get out of bed or run wildly through the house. There may be other signs of sympathetic nervous system involvement (dilated pupils, diaphoresis, or enuresis). The child does not respond to others and is inconsolable to attempts at comforting but, after 10 or 20 minutes, quiets down and goes back to sleep. The child looks perfectly well in the morning and does not recall the event. In most cases, the spells are eventually outgrown. Occasionally patients are treated with carbamazepine.

Sleepwalking is characterized by a trancelike state in which the patient gets out of bed and wanders about the house, sometimes performing complex tasks. Sleepwalking also occurs only during non-REM sleep. The onset is typically between 4 and 8 years of age. Since injuries sometimes occur, patients who sleepwalk are occasionally prescribed a benzodiazepine to be taken before bedtime. The condition may persist into adulthood.

A *family history of a non-REM sleep disorder* is common in cases of night terrors and sleepwalking.

Head banging and *body rocking* are common during late infancy. These behaviors occur during the early stages of sleep, and episodes usually continue to occur for more than a year but rarely beyond age 4. External injuries such as bruising and callous formation may occur; intracranial injuries are rare.

Other disorders of sleep

Nightmares only occur during *REM* sleep and, therefore, are experienced during the *later* hours of the night (2 to 5 AM). The time of occurrence and the fact that the child can be consoled after awakening and recalls the dream are helpful in distinguishing a nightmare from a night terror. No treatment is indicated, although frequent nightmares may suggest that the child is anxious or troubled about something.

Seizures often occur during sleep. Jerking (clonic) or stiffening (tonic) movements of the limbs or trunk, arrest of speech, cyanosis, tongue biting, and bowel or bladder incontinence suggest a seizure. *Benign Rolandic epilepsy* (see Chapter 6) is the most common cause of seizures during sleep. Screaming and agitation are not typical features of nocturnal seizures, although they may rarely be caused by frontal lobe seizures. Video EEG monitoring may be appropriate if "night terrors" occur late in the night or seem atypical.

The cause of *narcolepsy* is an abnormal sleep cycle in which the *REM* phase occurs at the *onset of sleep*. Clinically, narcolepsy is suggested by the following: (a) *excessive daytime somnolence*; (b) attacks of *cataplexy* (collapse, triggered by laughing or crying); (c) a history of *hypnogogic hallu-cinations* (vivid visual illusions while falling asleep); and (d) *sleep paralysis* (inability to move the body during presleep drowsiness) (11). The latter two symptoms can be understood as manifestations of an early-onset REM sleep phase, with dreaming while still awake causing hallucinations, and muscular hypotonia causing paralysis.

Narcolepsy usually develops during the second or third decade and is rare during childhood. It is sometimes a familial disorder.

The diagnosis of narcolepsy requires a positive *multiple sleep latency test*. The patient's EEG is monitored while he or she takes a series of daytime naps. A *REM pattern at the onset of sleep on at least two occasions* confirms the diagnosis of narcolepsy.

Narcolepsy is treated with a stimulant medication, such as methylphenidate or an amphetamine, to prevent daytime somnolence and a tricyclic antidepressant to prevent cataplexy, hypnogogic hallucination, and sleep paralysis.

Teenagers with a history of *insomnia* are often found to be habitual late sleepers who consequently stay up late at night. In these cases of *delayed sleep phase cycle*, the patient's sleep habits should be gradually adjusted towards a more normal schedule. In other cases, *anxiety* causes insomnia. *Melatonin*, which is sold without a prescription in pharmacies and health food stores, often helps patients fall asleep. Hydroxyzine is also useful. A benzodiazepine should not be prescribed for insomnia except in the most refractory cases.

Sleep disturbances associated with neurobehavioral disorders

Children with *ADHD* often have trouble falling asleep. Clonidine at bedtime (0.025 to 0.2 mg) is often helpful. *Autistic* patients often awaken during the middle of the night, get out of bed and play, make noise in their room, or walk around the house, disturbing other family members. Melatonin, clonidine, chloral hydrate, a benzodiazepine, or risperidone is given before bedtime to help prevent these nighttime disruptions.

REFERENCES

1. Gray RF, Indurkhya A, McCormick MD. Prevalence, stability, and predictors of clinically significant behavior problems in low birth weight children at 3, 5, and 8 years of age. *Pediatrics.* 2004;114:736–743.
2. Hack M, Youngstrom EA, Cartar L, et al. Behavioral outcomes and evidence of psychopathology among very low birth weight infants at age 20 years. *Pediatrics.* 2004;114:932–940.
3. Kvols K. *Redirecting Children's Behavior.* Gainesville, FL: INCAF Publications; 1993.
4. American Psychiatric Association. *Diagnostic and Statistical Manual of Mental Disorders, Text Revision.* 4th ed. Washington, DC: American Psychiatric Association; 2000:369–381.

5. Pfeffer CR. Suicidal behavior in children and adolescents: causes and management. In: Lewis M, ed. *Child and Adolescent Psychiatry*. Philadelphia: Lippincott; 2002:706–805.

6. Weller E, Weller RA, Sanchez L. Bipolar disorder in children and adolescents. In: Lewis M, ed. *Child and Adolescent Psychiatry*. Philadelphia: Lippincott; 2002:782–791.

7. Walsh KH. Welcome advances in treating youth anxiety disorders. *Contemp Pediatr*. 2002;19:66–82.

8. American Psychiatric Association. *Diagnostic and Statistical Manual of Mental Disorders, Text Revision*. 4th ed. Washington, DC: American Psychiatric Association; 2000:93–102.

9. American Psychiatric Association. *Diagnostic and Statistical Manual of Mental Disorders, Text Revision*. 4th ed. Washington, DC: American Psychiatric Association; 2000:312–313.

10. Fisch BJ. *Spehlmann's EEG Primer*. Amsterdam: Elsevier; 1991:229–241.

11. Aldrich MS. Narcolepsy. *Neurology*. 1992;42(suppl 6):34–43.

6

SEIZURES, EPILEPSY, AND RELATED DISORDERS

OVERVIEW OF SEIZURES AND EPILEPSY

A *seizure* is paroxysmal, caused by an involuntary, hypersynchronous discharge of neurons in the brain. Many studies have examined the prevalence of seizures, epilepsy, and specific forms of epilepsy. These data are summarized by Hauser (1). About 5% of the population has a seizure by 20 years of age, if febrile seizures are included.

Where in the brain do seizures originate and what causes them?

Most seizures originate from the *cerebral cortex*. Some seizures originate from the *hippocampus*. Myoclonic, atonic, and absence seizures are thought to originate from the *brainstem* or the *thalamus*. Seizures do not originate from the cerebral white matter, the cerebellum, or the basal ganglia.

Seizures often originate from a *structurally abnormal area in the brain*. A *severe metabolic disturbance, hypoxemia, and some drugs* also can provoke a seizure. *Fever* is the only cause of many childhood seizures. The cause of some *genetically inherited seizure disorders* may be a "channelopathy": a defect, in one of the sodium, potassium, or calcium channels or the ion pumps in the cell membrane that may cause cerebral neurons to discharge abnormally.

EPILEPSY

When a patient has had two or more seizures that were not the result of a general medical condition or fever, the patient is said to have epilepsy. Approximately five out of every 1,000 children are diagnosed with epilepsy (1).

Epilepsy is further classified as follows. When a structural abnormality in the brain causes seizures, a patient is said to have *symptomatic epilepsy*.

Causes of symptomatic epilepsy include tumor, congenital malformation, infarction, intracranial infection, hemorrhage, and traumatic brain injury.

Idiopathic epilepsy refers to seizures caused by a *genetically inherited trait*. The most common genetically inherited forms of epilepsy are absence epilepsy, juvenile myoclonic epilepsy, and benign Rolandic epilepsy. In all cases of genetic epilepsy, by definition, no structural abnormality exists in the brain that would account for seizures.

If there is no evidence that a patient's seizures were caused by a medical disorder, a structural abnormality in the brain, or an inherited disorder, the patient is said to have *cryptogenic epilepsy*. However, all seizures must have a cause. In some cases of unexplained epilepsy, a part of the brain from which intractable seizures originate is surgically resected, and pathological examination of the resected tissue demonstrates cortical dysplasia. Since the seizures stopped occurring following surgery, the cause is presumed to have been the subtle structural abnormality; in other words, the patient had symptomatic epilepsy.

Other possible causes of a seizure

As noted earlier, a seizure can be provoked by a *medical disorder* such as hyponatremia, hypoglycemia, or hypoxemia. Many young children have *febrile seizures*, which are seizures that are provoked only by fever. Withdrawal from alcohol and other drugs (especially benzodiazepines) and intoxication with cocaine or an amphetamine often causes a seizure. Prescription drugs, including tricyclic antidepressants, buproprion, and antiepileptic medications, occasionally provoke a seizure. **A patient who has a seizure provoked by one of these causes is not considered to have epilepsy, assuming the patient does not have a history of prior epileptic seizures**.

Case 6.1

A 16-year-old adolescent female is brought to the office for evaluation of a seizure. One week earlier, she had been in a shopping mall with her friends when she abruptly lost consciousness, fell to the ground, and "shook all over" for at least a minute. She regained consciousness gradually. She was found to have bitten her tongue and urinated. In the emergency room, she was awake and alert. No Todd's paralysis or other focal neurological deficit was noted. Laboratory tests, including electrolyte panel, glucose, and urine drug screen, were normal. She was discharged home, told that she cannot drive an automobile, and told to see her doctor as soon as possible.

Her mother states that her daughter has been clumsy lately, especially in the morning when her arms sometimes inexplicably jerk upward, once causing her to break a bathroom glass. Her general health, performance in school, and athletic ability has otherwise been good. She has no prior history of any significant medical problem. She takes no medication.

A cousin is said to have epilepsy.

On examination, she is pleasant and cheerful. She does not recall the seizure in the mall. Her general physical and neurological examination is entirely unremarkable.

The EEG reveals generalized 6-Hz spike-wave discharges.

Diagnosis: *Juvenile myoclonic epilepsy.*

Outcome: MRI was not ordered since the patient was diagnosed with a form of idiopathic primary generalized epilepsy. She was informed that she has a treatable disorder but that she will need to take medication for the rest of her life to prevent seizures. The patient was prescribed lamotrigine, but a week later, she developed a rash; the drug was discontinued. She was then prescribed valproate, which she has tolerated well. She has remained seizure free. Six months later, she was medically cleared to enroll in a driver's education class.

TYPES OF SEIZURES

To understand the treatment of epilepsy, the physician must know the difference between *partial (focal)* seizures and *primary generalized* seizures. The difference is important both for the purpose of understanding the nature of the seizures and because *several medications indicated for partial seizures do not control or may even worsen primary generalized seizures.*

PARTIAL SEIZURES

Partial seizures **originate from only** *one cerebral hemisphere.* **They are sometimes caused by a structural abnormality.**

A partial seizure usually *causes signs and symptoms reflecting the function of the neuroanatomical region from which the seizure arises.* Signs and symptoms of the seizure may include arrest of speech (seizure originating in the language cortex); stereotypic movements of a part of the body (motor area seizure); a stereotyped thought, emotion, or behavior (prefrontal cortex seizure); the perception of odd noises (auditory cortex seizure); unilateral paresthesias or numbness (sensory cortex seizure); or a disturbance of vision (visual cortex seizure). The physician should be aware that this list only begins to suggest the experiential and observable phenomena that may be caused by a partial seizure; many other examples are described (2–4).

After a *partial motor seizure* causing movements of one side of the body, *transient paralysis of the affected limb* is often noted that lasts for minutes to hours. This phenomenon is called *Todd's paralysis.*

A distinction is made between *simple* and *complex* partial seizures. Partial seizures that *do not impair the patient's responsiveness during the seizure or the patient's memory of the seizure* are called *simple* partial seizures. Partial seizures that *interfere with the patient's responsiveness and ability to recall the events of the seizure* are called *complex* partial seizures.

Complex partial seizures

Complex partial seizures are sometimes called temporal lobe seizures, but in fact, they may also originate from the frontal lobe. Complex partial seizures are classically preceded by a prodromal stage (*aura*) that is actually a part of the seizure. Typical symptoms during the aura include unpleasant olfactory sensations, a rising sensation in the abdomen as if coming down a roller coaster, a stereotypic thought, and a "deja-vu" spell or a feeling of impending doom or dread; in all such cases, the aura is the only part of the seizure that can later be recalled by the patient. A state of diminished responsiveness lasting for several minutes or longer typically follows, during which time the patient does not respond and appears to be in a trance. Associated *behaviors* may include staring, forced eye deviation or head turning to one side, nystagmus, blinking, lip smacking, and semi-purposeful movements of the hands. These are known as *automatisms.*

Following a complex partial seizure there is *often* a state of *sleepiness or grogginess* lasting several minutes to hours. This *postictal state* is an important clinical sign useful in differentiating complex partial seizures from absence seizures and also from syncopal episodes and other nonepileptic events.

Secondary generalization

Partial seizures that *spread* within one cerebral hemisphere and then, via the corpus callosum, spread to the opposite hemisphere are called *secondarily generalized partial seizures.* Once this occurs, a *generalized tonic-clonic ("grand mal") seizure* is often observed, manifesting as complete loss of consciousness and whole-body stiffening, followed by rhythmic jerking of the torso and extremities, clenching of the jaw, eye rolling, tongue biting, cyanosis, and loss of bowel or bladder control. A secondarily generalized seizure usually lasts 1 to 2 minutes; the postictal state that follows is often prolonged, sometimes lasting for hours or even days. The patient cannot recall any of this, other than the aura.

PRIMARY GENERALIZED SEIZURES

Primary generalized seizures affect *both cerebral hemispheres from the moment of onset.* Idiopathic primary generalized seizures by definition *never result from a structural abnormality in the brain.* It has been suggested, but not proven, that the thalamus or brainstem is the source of these seizures, although lesions in these areas do not cause seizures. A possible cause is a "channelopathy" (see earlier section, Where in the Brain Do Seizures Originate and What Causes Them?). These seizures are presumed to occur as the result of a genetically inherited trait.

Some types of seizure, in particular infantile spasms and atonic seizures, are considered primarily generalized despite the fact that they sometimes indirectly result from a structural abnormality. In these cases, there are often widespread abnormalities in the patient's brain.

Recognizable types of primary generalized seizure are *absence seizures, myoclonic seizures, tonic seizures, clonic seizures, tonic-clonic seizures,* and *atonic seizures.*

Differentiating primary generalized seizures from secondarily generalized seizures

After reading the previous sections, the physician may realize that a generalized tonic-clonic seizure could be either a primary generalized or a secondarily generalized seizure.

Features suggestive of a *primary generalized* tonic-clonic seizure are:

1. No aura preceding the event.
2. Involvement of both sides of the body from the moment of onset.
3. No deviation of the eyes to one side or Todd's paralysis after the seizure.
4. A generalized spike-wave electroencephalogram (EEG) tracing (Figs. 6.1 and 6.2).
5. A family history of epilepsy.

Features suggestive of a *secondarily generalized* tonic-clonic seizure include:

1. History of an aura that preceded the seizure.
2. Eye deviation to one side during or after the seizure.
3. Tonic or clonic movements mostly of one side of the body during the seizure.
4. Todd's paralysis after the seizure.
5. EEG showing epileptiform discharges from only one cerebral hemisphere (Fig. 6.3).
6. A family history of epilepsy is less often reported.

Grand mal and petit mal

Patients often use grand mal and petit mal to describe their seizures. A grand mal seizure means a generalized tonic-clonic seizure. A petit mal seizure, to neurologists of previous generations, meant an *absence seizure. However, laypersons tend to refer to any epileptic event that is not a generalized*

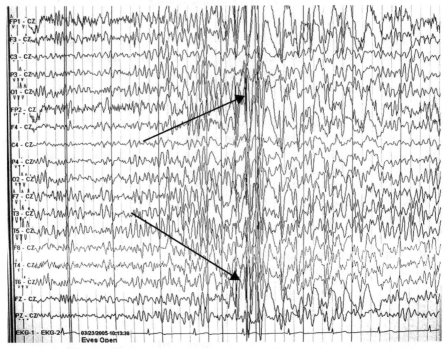

Figure 6.1 EEG showing burst of **generalized polyspike activity** in a 17-year-old male with a history of generalized tonic-clonic seizures.

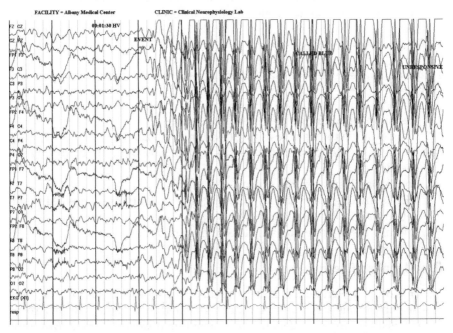

Figure 6.2 EEG of **absence epilepsy** showing 3-Hz, spike-wave complexes.

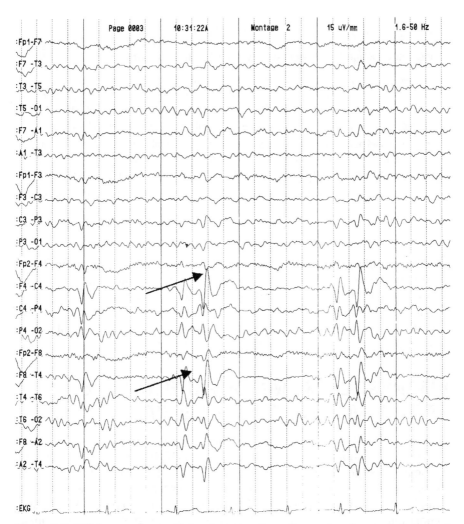

Figure 6.3 EEG from patient with benign rolandic epilepsy showing **centrotemporal spikes** (*arrows*).

tonic-clonic seizure as a "petit mal" seizure. Therefore, reports from patients that they have petit mal seizures should not be taken at face value. The patient may be describing almost any kind of seizure or even a nonepileptic event such as a panic attack or fainting spell.

PHYSICAL EXAMINATION

The general physical examination always must include *the skin.* Stigmata of a neurocutaneous disorder should be recognized (see Figs. 1.1–1.3). Dysmorphic facial features may suggest a syndrome of congenital malformation (Angelman

TABLE 6.1

Diagnostic testing for patients with a first nonfebrile seizure

In emergency room: serum glucose, electrolytes, urine drug screen (adolescents and adults), complete blood count, liver function panel. Noncontrast head CT is usually ordered, although not necessary if MRI can be promptly obtained. Consider LP if the clinical picture suggests meningitis or encephalitis (fever, altered mental status).

For hospitalized patients or outpatients: routine EEG; if normal, consider 24- to 72-hour ambulatory or video EEG. MRI should be ordered unless EEG suggests primary generalized epilepsy or a medical cause for seizures, such as hypoglycemia.

CT, cat scan; MRI, magnetic resonance imaging; LP, lumbar puncture; EEG, electroencephalogram.

syndrome, Williams syndrome) associated with epilepsy. A cranial bruit may signify an arteriovenous malformation. Odd behavior may suggest *autism*, which is associated with seizures in a significant percentage of cases. The physician must carefully examine the patient for *focal findings* and *signs of raised intracranial pressure* (papilledema), especially in the case of a new-onset, partial or poorly characterized seizure (Table 6.1).

DIAGNOSTIC TESTING FOR PATIENTS SEEN AFTER A FIRST NONFEBRILE SEIZURE

Plasma sodium, glucose, calcium, and magnesium levels should be drawn in the emergency room. The yield of these tests is highest in cases of a general medical illness that might cause dehydration, such as gastroenteritis, or in cases of endocrine dysfunction. Other laboratory tests often ordered include complete blood count, urine toxicology, and liver function panel. A computed tomography (CT) scan should not be performed if magnetic resonance imaging (MRI) can be done within the next few days assuming the neurological examination reveals no abnormal findings. If the patient has a fever or exhibits signs of nuchal rigidity or if there is a history of a change in his or her mental status *preceding* the seizure (not limited to the postictal period), a lumbar puncture is indicated. Recommendations for the evaluation of *febrile* seizures are suggested later in this chapter.

Brain imaging studies

MRI should be ordered to evaluate partial, secondarily generalized, and poorly characterized seizures. It is not necessary to order MRI to evaluate absence seizures or when *the EEG shows generalized spike-wave complexes*, since a structural lesion in the brain does not cause idiopathic primary generalized seizures. The yield of MRI (and EEG) in the evaluation of seizures resulting from a general medical disorder, such as hypoglycemia or hypocalcemia, is low, and these tests need not be ordered if the cause was obviously a metabolic disturbance. These tests are also not routinely indicated for children with febrile seizures (see section febrile seizures).

CT should not be ordered unless MRI is unavailable to prevent unnecessary radiation exposure.

MRI findings that account for a focal or secondarily generalized seizure include tumor, abscess, arteriovenous malformation (Fig. 2.9), cortical malformation (Fig. 6.4), recent or remote infarct (Fig. 10.2), and hemorrhage. *Mesial temporal sclerosis* refers to scarring or atrophy within the hippocampus that often causes complex partial seizures. *Agenesis of the corpus callosum* (Fig. 6.5) is associated with difficult to control seizures, developmental delay, and other structural abnormalities of the central nervous system. Uncommon congenital brain malformations that often cause focal seizures include lissencephaly, hemi-megalencephaly, polymicrogyria (Fig. 6.6) and schizencephaly.

In most cases, MRI reveals no abnormality. Although a normal MRI study is reassuring, patients and parents must be informed that this is no guarantee that more seizures will not occur.

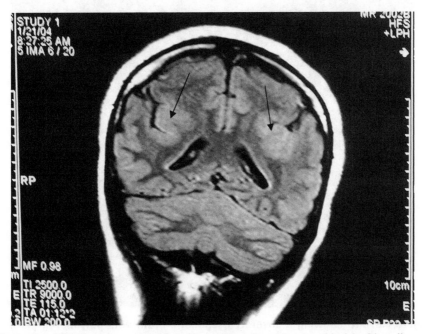

Figure 6.4 MRI showing **cortical malformations** in a 12-year-old girl with epilepsy. (Courtesy of Howard Seigerman, MD, and Eliot Lerner, MD, The Valley Hospital.)

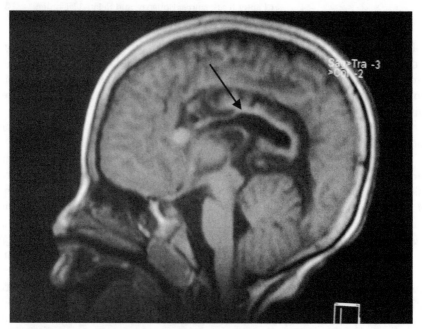

Figure 6.5 MRI showing **agenesis of the corpus callosum** in a 6-year-old girl. (Courtesy of Ajax George, MD, New York University School of Medicine.)

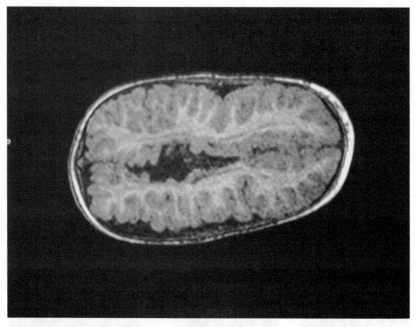

Figure 6.6 MRI showing a **severely dysgenetic brain with polymicrogryia** in a 3-year-old boy with a history of epilepsy. (Courtesy of Ajax George, MD, New York University School of Medicine.)

ELECTROENCEPHALOGRAM

How to think about the electroencephalogram

The following points address common misconceptions about the EEG:

1 The primary purpose of the EEG is to detect *epileptiform discharges* suggesting that part of a patient's brain is electrophysiologically abnormal and that a seizure may occur as a result. **A person does NOT have to have a seizure during the EEG recording for the EEG to reveal epileptiform activity.**

2 A single, 30-minute EEG demonstrates epileptiform activity in about 50% of all patients with a history of epilepsy. The sensitivity of the EEG varies markedly from patient to patient. The EEG of some patients with epilepsy is always abnormal, while the EEG of other patients with epilepsy is never abnormal. In the latter group of patients, epileptiform discharges are thought to originate from an area of the brain too distant from the recording electrodes to cause a recordable abnormality.

3 The sensitivity of the EEG can be increased to more than 80% if the EEG is repeated, if the patient is sleep deprived before the EEG, or if the patient is monitored for 24 to 72 hours.

4 If the history strongly suggests that a patient has had epileptic seizures but the EEG is persistently normal, *the patient is treated with an antiepileptic medication.*

5 The EEG of some patients who never have had a seizure reveals epileptiform discharges. The EEG of asymptomatic relatives of patients with a history of benign Rolandic epilepsy or absence seizures, for example, is sometimes epileptiform. *Patients with no history of seizure are rarely treated with an antiepileptic medication, regardless of what their EEG shows.* This is a good reason to think twice before ordering an EEG in the case of a patient who has never had a seizure.

6 The EEG may or may not normalize following initiation of antiepileptic drug (AED) therapy. In most cases, if the patient's seizures are controlled by the AED, it does not matter that the EEG remains abnormal. The treatment of certain conditions, such as infantile spasms, is expected to normalize the EEG.

7 The EEG is very helpful in distinguishing primary generalized seizures from secondarily generalized seizures.

8 The diagnosis of some forms of epilepsy requires specific EEG findings. These conditions include benign Rolandic epilepsy, absence epilepsy, juvenile myoclonic epilepsy, infantile spasms, and Lennox-Gastaut syndrome (Figs. 6.2, 6.3, and 6.7).

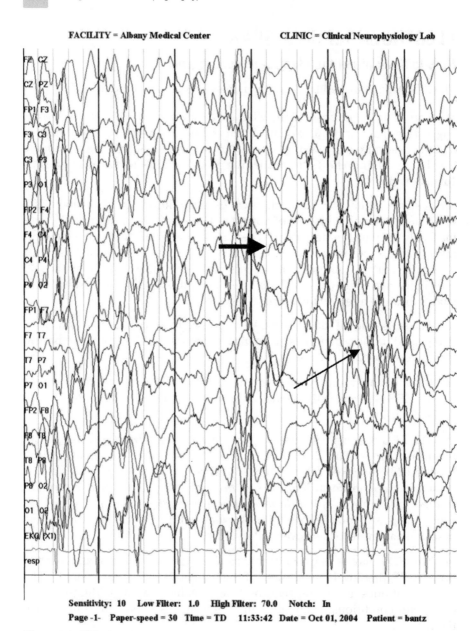

Sensitivity: 10   Low Filter: 1.0   High Filter: 70.0   Notch: In
Page -1-   Paper-speed = 30   Time = TD   11:33:42   Date = Oct 01, 2004   Patient = bantz

Figure 6.7 EEG showing **hypsarrythmia** in a patient with infantile spasms.
Note General Disorganization and High-Voltage Slow Waves (*large arrow*) Intermixed with
Multiple Spikes (*small arrow*).

9 A normal EEG helps to distinguish syncopal episodes, panic attacks, pseudoseizures, and tremors from epileptic seizures, particularly if the suspected spell is captured during the EEG recording.

10 An EEG is occasionally ordered to assess patients with a persistently abnormal mental status, such as coma. The EEG in these cases is often used to support the diagnosis of a specific cause, such as hepatic encephalopathy.

11 The EEG of patients with attention-deficit hyperactivity disorder (ADHD) and other disorders of behavior may be mildly abnormal (for example, showing a slow background rhythm in many cases of ADHD), but these results are nonspecific and should never be used to diagnose any behavioral disorder.

Recording the EEG

A routine EEG is recorded using electrodes, usually 20 in number, affixed in a standard pattern to the patient's scalp by a conductive gel. The duration of a standard EEG recording is 30 minutes for adults, but it may be less for young children. The patient is instructed to lie quietly on his back with his eyes closed except when instructed. Young children may be restless; they may lie on their parent's lap. If the child is old enough, he at one point is asked to hyperventilate for 3 minutes. A period of photic stimulation with a strobe light flashing at different frequencies is usually part of the study. (In some cases, hyperventilation or photic stimulation will trigger a burst of generalized spike-wave activity suggesting primary generalized epilepsy.) The patient is also permitted to become drowsy or fall asleep during the EEG.

Infants and young children often are uncooperative during the EEG recording, and their movements may cause excessive artifact, making the EEG difficult to read. These patients are often prescribed a sedative, but the drugs used (e.g., chloral hydrate, benzodiazepines) often cause excessive high-frequency beta activity that obscures many EEG features. Benzodiazepines are effective antiseizure medications and, if used for sedation, may mask epileptiform abnormalities. An EEG recorded while the child is asleep without sedation (e.g., after bottle feeding or after sleep deprivation) is preferable.

Common normal and abnormal features of the EEG

The primary care physician may not have an opportunity to learn to read an EEG, but she should understand the significance of common normal and abnormal findings described in EEG reports.

1 While the patient is *awake* (Fig. 6.8), a well-organized, medium- to high-amplitude background or *alpha rhythm* of 8 to 13 Hz is recorded over the posterior head regions. The background rhythm is of a lower frequency in young children, with 8 Hz being attained by about 3 years of age. The alpha rhythm is interrupted when the patient opens his or her eyes. In older children and adolescents, the frontal regions give rise to lower amplitude, >13 Hz *beta*

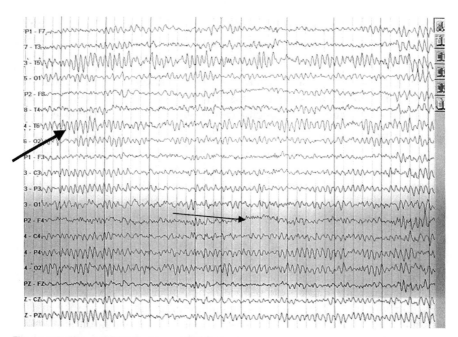

Figure 6.8 Normal EEG during wakefulness.
Note Posterior Alpha Rhythm (*large arrow*) and Faster Frontal Beta Activity (*small arrow*).

activity that generally is less consistently rhythmic and less influenced by eye opening than the alpha rhythm.

2 As the patient becomes drowsy, the alpha rhythm becomes fragmented, and slower *theta* (5 to 7 Hz) activity becomes more prominent. During sleep (and often during hyperventilation) the background rhythm slows further, and high-amplitude *delta* (2 to 4 Hz) waves appear. In the *earlier stages of sleep, vertex sharp waves* and clusters of beta-range waves, known as *sleep spindles*, are typical features (Fig. 6.9). During the *deeper stages of sleep*, delta waves are the dominant feature of the EEG.

3 *Artifacts* caused by movement, muscle contraction, eye blinking and eye movements, overflow from the electrocardiogram, medication, and loose electrodes are common in EEG tracings.

4 Commonly reported *EEG abnormalities* include: an *abnormally slow background rhythm*, due to *encephalopathy* of almost any cause (e.g., concussion, overmedication, sepsis, postictal state, coma, etc.); *focal slow waves* from one hemisphere due to a *structural lesion* (e.g., tumor, infarct, etc.); *focal sharp waves or spike discharges from one hemisphere*, typical in cases of *partial seizure* (see Fig. 6.3); and *generalized spike-wave or generalized polyspike discharges*, which are seen in cases of *primary generalized epilepsy* (see Figs. 6.1 and 6.2), including absence epilepsy and juvenile myoclonic epilepsy.

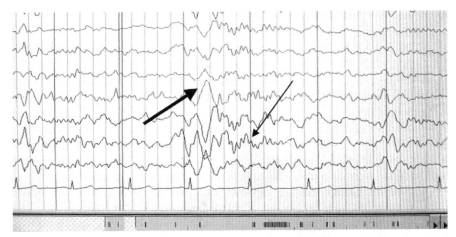

Figure 6.9 EEG detail showing **vertex sharp wave** (*large arrow*) and **sleep spindles** (*small arrow*) during sleep.

Hypsarrhythmia is associated with *infantile spasms*. This term refers to a grossly disorganized, high-amplitude EEG comprised of unsynchronized delta waves and spike discharges. *Burst-suppression* is a very abnormal EEG finding characterized by a flat tracing alternating with high-amplitude discharges. This pattern, which carries a very poor prognosis, is often noted in cases of severe generalized encephalopathy caused by a hypoxemic injury (as in cases of cardiac arrest or near drowning).

Many other normal and abnormal findings are noted in EEG reports. A neurologist should be consulted if there is uncertainty about the significance of reported EEG findings.

WHEN TO TREAT A PATIENT WHO HAS HAD A SEIZURE

Many pediatric neurologists *do not* initiate treatment with an AED if only one nonfebrile seizure has occurred, since at least 50% of these patients never experience a recurrence (5). We are more likely to prescribe an AED if MRI demonstrates a *structural abnormality*, if the EEG shows *epileptiform discharges*, or if the patient has a history of *neurodevelopmental delay*. The chance of recurrence is higher in all such cases (6). The risk of recurrence is also generally high if the patient is diagnosed with a form of idiopathic (genetically inherited) epilepsy characterized by recurrent seizures.

If the patient is old enough to *drive an automobile*, there are additional concerns. The great majority of states impose a time frame (6 months or longer) during which the patient must be documented to be seizure free in order to maintain driving privileges. For this reason, an AED is prescribed to many adolescent and adult patients even after a first seizure so that they will remain seizure free and can safely drive.

If the patient has had *two or more unprovoked seizures*, the risk of recurrence is greater than 70% (6), and most neurologists will initiate treatment. (Guidelines for initiating AED therapy are presented in the following sections.) However, many parents do not want their child treated with an AED even if there have been two or more seizures. They may be especially reluctant to initiate treatment if the child's seizures were brief or widely spaced. Parents are understandably concerned about the potential adverse effects of AEDs. They may argue that the possibility of an occasional, brief seizure is no reason to take a drug that might cause unpleasant short-term or even dangerous long-term side effects. Such parents need to be made aware of the danger of a very prolonged seizure (status epilepticus) that can damage the brain or even cause death; for most patients with epilepsy, the chance of this occurring is small, although never zero (6). The "kindling" model, based on animal studies, implies that ongoing epileptiform activity in the brain makes future seizures more likely to occur and also provides some justification for treating a patient with a history of multiple seizures. There is also evidence that multiple complex partial seizures might cause progressive memory impairment (7). The social implications, particularly for an older child, also need to be considered.

ANTIEPILEPTIC DRUGS

Indications, dosages, and adverse effects of AEDs are summarized in Table 6.2. The U.S. Food and Drug Administration (FDA) has approved all of these drugs for use in the pediatric population. However, some drugs are not approved for the treatment of a particular form of epilepsy or for monotherapy. Therefore, the table is partly based on current accepted practice.

AEDs for partial seizures

The AEDs traditionally prescribed to patients with partial epilepsy are phenytoin, carbamazepine, and phenobarbital. AEDs more recently approved include valproate, gabapentin, levetiracetam, topiramate, zonisamide, and oxcarbazepine. Overall, these drugs are about equally effective, but efficacy and tolerability vary considerably from patient to patient.

Patients taking one of the newer AEDs (gabapentin, levetiracetam, topiramate, zonisamide, and oxcarbazepine) do not require routine blood work (complete blood counts and liver function monitoring). Levetiracetam and gabapentin do not undergo significant hepatic metabolism and do not bind to plasma proteins, making these two AEDs preferable for patients with a history of a liver disease or who are taking a drug that is plasma protein bound.

TABLE 6.2

Antiepileptic drugs (AEDs)

Drug	Indication	Dose	Important adverse reactions
Phenytoin (Dilantin, Parke-Davis)	PS, SGS	Maintenance: 5 to 10 mg/kg divided bid. Loading for status epilepticus: 15 to 20 mg/kg intravenously (**not intramuscular**, as route can cause tissue necrosis).	AR, CBS, gum hyperplasia, coarse facial features, HLA. Zero-order kinetics at higher doses. Cardiac arrhythmia when given intravenously.
Fos-phenytoin (injection only) (Cerebyx, Eisai)	Status epilepticus	As above; may also be administered by intramuscular injection.	Generally well-tolerated; fewer adverse reactions than phenytoin.
Phenobarbital	PS, SGS	Maintenance: 3 to 6 mg/kg divided daily-bid. Loading for status epilepticus: 15 to 20 mg/kg intravenously.	AR, CBS (especially in young patients), HLA. **AVOID GIVING WITH VALPROATE**.
Carbamazepine (Tegretol, Novartis; Carbatrol, Shire)	PS, SGS	Maintenance: 10 to 15 mg/kg divided bid or tid. Adolescents: initial dose, 200 mg bid; increase as clinically indicated.	AR, HLA, SIADH (usually mild), CBS, aplastic anemia (R).
Oxcarbazepine (Trileptal, Novartis)	PS, SGS	150 to 300 mg bid; may increase to maximum of 1800 mg daily.	Lowered plasma sodium, CBS.
Valproate compounds (divalproex sodium, valproic acid) (Depakote, Depakene, Depakone; Abbott)	PS, SGS, PGS	Maintenance: 15 to 60 mg/kg divided bid or tid. Adolescents: initial dose, 250 mg bid; increase as clinically indicated. Depakore can be loaded intravenously.	AR, HLA, CBS, weight gain, tremor, hair loss, hepatic failure (R), pancreatitis (R). **USUALLY NOT GIVEN TO PATIENTS UNDER 2 YEARS OF AGE**.

(continued)

TABLE 6.2
(continued)

Drug	Indication	Dose	Important adverse reactions
Gabapentin (Neurontin, Parke-Davis)	PS, SGS	100 to 300 mg bid or tid; may increase to maximum of 900 mg tid.	CBS
Levetiracetam (Keppra, UCB)	PS, SGS, PGS	250 mg bid; may increase to maximum of 1500 mg bid.	CBS, behavioral disturbances.
Zonisamide (Zonegran, Elan)	PGS, PS, SGS	100 to 400 mg once daily.	CBS, hematological abnormalities, renal stones, oligohidrosis (R).
Topiramate (Topamax, Ortho-McNeil)	PS, SGS, PGS	Initial dose, 15 to 25 mg daily; gradually increase to 50 to 100 mg bid.	CBS (can be marked), appetite loss, renal stones (R), glaucoma (R), oligohidrosis (R).
Lamotrigine (Lamictal, GlaxoSmithKline)	PS, SGS, PGS	0.6 to 1.2 mg/kg divided bid; increase gradually to maximum of 5 to 15 mg/kg divided bid. **IF USED WITH VALPROIC ACID, CONSULT MANUFACTURER'S RECOMMENDED DOSAGE**.	AR, Stevens-Johnson syndrome (uncommon), CBS.
Ethosuximide (Zarontin, Parke-Davis)	Absence seizures (only)	250 mg tid; maximum dose, 500 mg tid.	AR, stomach pain, HLA, lupus-like reaction (R).
Benzodiazepines (diazepam, clonazepam, lorazepam, midazolam)	Status epilepticus; occasionally a maintenance AED; rectal diazepam used for febrile seizures	See Physician's Desk Reference for dosing.	High likelihood of developing medication tolerance, somnolence, respiratory depression (R); rebound seizures when drug tapered off.

AR, allergic rash; CBS, cognitive/behavioral symptoms; HLA, hematological and liver abnormalities; PGS, primary generalized seizures; PS, partial seizures; R, rare; SGS, secondarily generalized seizures; SIADH, syndrome of inappropriate antidiuretic hormone secretion.

AEDs for primary generalized seizures

Valproate (Depakote, Depakene, Abbott; and generic forms) for many years was the only AED that controlled primary generalized seizures. Newer medications that are effective for primary generalized epilepsy include topiramate, lamotrigine, levetiracetam, and zonisamide. Ethosuximide controls absence seizures but not other primary generalized seizures.

Phenytoin, phenobarbital, and gabapentin generally are not effective for the long-term control of primary generalized seizures. Carbamazepine and oxcarbazepine may cause *an increase in the frequency of primary generalized seizure, especially absence and myoclonic seizure* (8), and should never be prescribed to patients with primary generalized epilepsy.

Titration, maintenance, and duration of treatment

To minimize adverse effects, treatment with an AED is usually initiated at about one quarter to one half of the normal maintenance dose (see Table 6.2), and the dose is then gradually increased. If seizures still occur after the target dose has been attained, it is reasonable to further increase the dose as long as the patient does not complain of adverse effects. If good control without significant adverse effects cannot be achieved, the AED should be quickly tapered off while another AED is introduced.

After the seizures have been brought under control, the AED dose is not changed. However, if breakthrough seizures start to occur after a few months of good control, the dose should again be increased, assuming that the seizures did not occur as a result of noncompliance. Recurrent seizures also may occur in infants and children as a result of normal growth, which affects the volume of distribution of the AED. Therefore, many pediatric neurologists increase the dose every 6 months to a year on the basis of the patient's weight or the plasma AED level.

If the patient has remained seizure free for at least 1 year, the possibility of discontinuing the AED is often discussed. A repeat EEG is often ordered in this situation. It is more likely that seizures will recur if the frequency of seizures before the AED was started was high, if the EEG continues to be abnormal, or if a structural abnormality caused the seizures.

Plasma AED level

The plasma AED level should be drawn just before the morning dose (trough level). Levels obtained at other times vary greatly and are not reliable. All hospitals and clinical laboratories routinely measure plasma phenytoin, phenobarbital, carbamazepine, valproate, and ethosuximide levels. Plasma levels of the newer AEDs are often not readily available, and a blood sample usually must be sent to a specific laboratory or the manufacturer.

Some patients' seizures are well controlled by a plasma AED level below the normal range listed in laboratory reports. Therefore, an AED level that is somewhat below the normal range should *not* lead the doctor to increase the patient's dose as long as the seizures are well controlled. Conversely, if a patient requires a high dose for seizure control, a level even well above the listed normal range does *not* necessitate a decrease in dose, as long as the patient does not report significant adverse effects. The axiom "treat the patient, not the level" should always be heeded. The AED level may, however, be useful for documenting the therapeutic level (i.e., that provides good control) for a particular patient and may guide the doctor as he or she increases the dose of an AED prescribed to a growing infant or child.

Another reason to check the AED level is to make certain that the patient is taking the medication. Noncompliance, which is mostly a problem for adult and adolescent patients, often occurs after the patient has been seizure free for several months, lulling the patient into a sense of complacency. Noncompliance is a common cause of recurrent seizure. Patients and parents should be reminded that they *must* continue to take their AED as prescribed.

AED toxicity

When a patient who is taking an AED presents with lethargy, vomiting, or ataxia, *AED toxicity* should be suspected. If the patient's symptoms are severe, the patient may need to be sent to the emergency room or hospitalized. Liver function tests and a plasma ammonia level should be ordered if the patient is taking an AED (especially *valproate*) that undergoes hepatic metabolism. The AED level should be measured. The drug should be withheld until the patient becomes asymptomatic. Once the symptoms of toxicity abate, the AED may be restarted at a lower dose than the patient originally took.

If the symptoms of toxicity are mild, an AED level should be drawn, the next scheduled dose withheld, and the patient's daily dose reduced by 10%. The patient should be seen in the office the following day, with a repeat AED level to be checked in about 1 week.

Surgery and procedures requiring sedation

A patient taking an AED to control seizures who is scheduled for surgery or dental work (or the doctor who will perform the procedure) often asks if a history of epilepsy or the AED is a contraindication to anesthesia, conscious sedation, or surgery. Since general anesthesia and most sedatives are effective in *aborting* a prolonged seizure (see later section, Status Epilepticus), the patient will not have a breakthrough seizure in the operating room or the dentist's chair. The AED should be taken at the normal dose up to the time of the procedure. If the patient cannot be given medication by mouth after the operation, the AED may be administered intravenously (if the drug comes in that form), or an acceptable substitute may be given until the patient can take medication by mouth.

Pregnancy

Most AEDs have been found to cause congenital malformations. *Fetal hydantoin syndrome* is a craniofacial and digital malformation resulting from prenatal exposure to phenytoin. *Valproate* compounds increase the risk of fetal *neural tube defects*. Many other specific AED-linked syndromes are described (9). However, serious injury to the fetus or fetal demise can result if the mother has a *generalized tonic-clonic* seizure during pregnancy. If a woman with a history of *generalized tonic-clonic* seizures wishes to become pregnant, her AED *should not be discontinued*. Valproate-based drugs should be avoided. Myoclonic, absence, and nongeneralized partial seizures are *not* likely to be injurious to the fetus, and a woman with a history of only one of these types of seizure may reasonably elect to discontinue her AED before becoming pregnant. If she does so, she must not drive an automobile. These issues should be raised and discussed at length with her obstetrician and neurologist.

Hepatic and renal insufficiency

The plasma level of AEDs that are metabolized by the liver will tend to be higher if the patient has a history of hepatic insufficiency, and the AED level should be carefully monitored. The ammonia level should also be checked. The doses of AEDs that are primarily metabolized by the *kidney* (e.g., levetiracetam, gabapentin) may require adjustment in cases of renal insufficiency.

Important adverse effects of AEDs

Cognitive impairment

The most common adverse effect reported by patients taking an AED is *mild cognitive impairment*, including drowsiness, mental fatigue, lightheadedness, and difficulty concentrating. Treatment with an AED should be started at a low dose to help minimize these symptoms. Many patients report that their symptoms become less noticeable after a few weeks, but in some cases, the drug must be discontinued and another AED substituted.

Allergic rash

Phenytoin, carbamazepine, lamotrigine, phenobarbital, and occasionally other AEDs may cause an *allergic rash*, which is often accompanied by fever. The *AED must be immediately discontinued* to avoid progression to Stevens-Johnson syndrome.

Hematological abnormalities

Patients taking *carbamazepine* or *valproate* often are found to have mild *hematological abnormalities* such as anemia, neutropenia, or thrombocytopenia. Adjustment of the AED dose is not usually necessary since there are no clinical manifestations.

Aplastic anemia is an extremely rare but life-threatening complication of treatment with several AEDs, in particular *carbamazepine*. Although the complete blood cell count is usually monitored every 3 to 6 months when a patient is taking carbamazepine, it is not clear that routine monitoring prevents this complication. *Felbamate* (Felbatol, Wallace), an AED prescribed almost exclusively to patients with Lennox-Gastaut syndrome, causes aplastic anemia in a larger percentage of cases.

Hepatic effects

Valproate-based AEDs can cause *liver failure*. An aberrant metabolite of valproate that acts as a mitochondrial poison is thought to be the cause. The incidence of liver failure has been estimated at 1 per 600 in children under the age of 2 years who are taking valproate, but the incidence is only 1 per 100,000 among adults (10,11). Valproate is prescribed to patients under 2 years of age only to treat infantile spasms or Lennox-Gastaut syndrome and only when other AEDs have not been effective. Levocarnitine (Carnitor, Sigma-Tau), 50 to 100 mg per day, is sometimes prescribed with valproate to help prevent hepatotoxicity. *Pancreatitis* and *polycystic ovarian syndrome* also occasionally result from treatment with valproate.

Liver function tests are periodically monitored while a patient is taking a valproate-containing AED. Mild elevations of the hepatic transaminases are commonly noted but do not signify hepatic failure. Sometimes mild hyperammonemia, causing somnolence, also is noted. If the dose of valproate is reduced slightly, the ammonia level will usually decrease, and the patient will become more alert.

Other adverse effects of valproate-based AEDs

Valproate also may cause weight gain, hair loss, tremor, and mood swings. However, valproate is well tolerated by most patients and continues to be a very useful drug, especially in cases of primary generalized epilepsy. Multivitamins with zinc and selenium often help prevent hair loss and tremors from valproate.

Allergic hepatitis

Other AEDs that are metabolized by the liver (e.g., phenytoin, carbamazepine, and phenobarbital) occasionally cause *allergic hepatitis*. The AED is usually discontinued, and another AED, preferably a drug that does not undergo hepatic metabolism, is substituted.

Phenytoin

Patients who take *phenytoin* (Dilantin, Parke-Davis) often develop *gingival hyperplasia* and *coarse facial features*. As a result, this drug is not usually prescribed to pediatric patients, except (often in the form of its isomer *fosphenytoin*) for status epilepticus.

When phenytoin is taken as a maintenance AED, physicians must remember that *phenytoin is protein bound in plasma*. When the plasma protein-binding capacity of phenytoin is exceeded, the remaining free drug increases by *zero-order pharmacokinetics*. Therefore, a relatively small increase in the dose of phenytoin can sometimes cause clinical toxicity.

Phenobarbital

Phenobarbital, the AED most often prescribed to neonates and infants, often causes *irritability*. The infant's mood usually improves within a few weeks of starting treatment but may temporarily deteriorate when the drug is tapered off.

Benzodiazepines

Benzodiazepines (lorazepam, diazepam, and clonazepam) play an important role in the treatment of *status epilepticus* and are useful in the treatment of *febrile seizures*. However, a benzodiazepine prescribed as a maintenance AED often rapidly induces tolerance, and seizures typically recur within a few weeks to months. If the dose of the benzodiazepine is then increased, somnolence and even suppression of the patient's central respiratory drive may result; if the dose is then reduced, the seizures again become frequent. All of this will be avoided if a benzodiazepine is not prescribed to prevent epileptic seizures. Exceptions include children with a history of severe intractable epilepsy or an underlying degenerative disease for whom no other AED is effective.

Adverse effects of the newer AEDs

Gabapentin almost never causes serious adverse effects but often causes mild *neurocognitive impairment* (lightheadedness, fatigue, and difficulty concentrating). Starting gabapentin at a low dose is thus recommended. *Topiramate* also may cause cognitive slowing, and for this reason, "starting low and going slow" is also recommended. *Topiramate* and *zonisamide* may cause the patient to develop *kidney stones*. There have been a few case reports of *glaucoma* following the initiation of *topiramate* therapy. Glaucoma was reversible following discontinuation of the drug. *Topiramate* and *zonisamide* often cause *appetite suppression* and, rarely, *oligohidrosis* (decreased sweating) resulting in *heat intolerance*. For this reason, patients taking these drugs should be carefully monitored during warm weather, and these drugs should not be combined with carbonic-anhydrase inhibitors and anticholinergic drugs. *Levetiracetam*, a generally well-tolerated drug, occasionally causes a *change in mental status* (e.g., agitation, confusion). Overall, however, the newer AEDs are easier to manage and often better tolerated than phenytoin, phenobarbital, carbamazepine, or valproate.

General precautions for patients with epilepsy

Patients with epilepsy should not swim unless they have infrequent seizures, they wear a life vest, and an adult (who is a good swimmer) is present to watch them. Climbing to high places (e.g., rock climbing, ropes in gym) should be discouraged. A helmet should be worn when riding a bicycle. The adolescent and adult patient with epilepsy should not operate heavy machinery or work with high-voltage electrical equipment. Patients with very frequent or prolonged seizures may need stricter guidelines.

In most other ways, patients with a history of epilepsy should be encouraged to lead a normal life. There is no need for special modifications in school assuming that the patient does not have another disability (e.g., cerebral palsy that caused seizures). Team and individual sports are permitted.

Drugs that may lower the seizure threshold

Frequently prescribed medications that may cause a nonepileptic patient to have a seizure or provoke a seizure when taken by an epileptic patient include *antipsychotic drugs, tricyclic antidepressants, buproprion,* and *amphetamine-containing drugs* prescribed for ADHD. Methylphenidate has, at most, a weak epileptogenic effect.

Not all of these medications are contraindicated for patients with epilepsy. Tricyclic antidepressants and buproprion should be avoided, but patients with a history of epilepsy and ADHD often take an amphetamine-containing drug or methylphenidate, and patients with epilepsy and a psychiatric disorder are often prescribed an antipsychotic drug (in both cases, obviously, with an AED). In most cases, exacerbation of seizures does not result.

Polypharmacy

Treatment with a single AED prevents seizures in more than 70% of patients with epilepsy (12). The remaining 30% of patients have seizures that are more difficult to control. If a trial of three appropriate AEDs has not resulted in good control, a *second drug is usually added.* The AED that controlled the patient's seizures best and caused the fewest adverse effects generally is continued. Gabapentin or levetiracetam or, in many cases, topirimate or zonisamide can be safely added. Other AEDs may increase or decrease the plasma level of the original drug prescribed. In addition, certain AED combinations (e.g., valproate and phenobarbital) often result in toxicity and should be avoided. Patients who do not respond to a safe, well-established combination of two AEDs should be referred to a neurologist with specific expertise in the treatment of pediatric epilepsy.

The addition of a second drug results in good control for about 50% of patients whose seizures were not controlled by monotherapy. A third drug is less often helpful, and when three or more AEDs are taken, the danger of a drug interaction and toxicity is increased. When more than two drugs are required, the ketogenic diet or epilepsy surgery should be considered.

COMMON FORMS AND CAUSES OF PEDIATRIC EPILEPSY

The following section reviews common epilepsy syndromes occurring in infancy, childhood, and adolescence. Physicians should be aware that many other patients have cryptogenic seizures, for example, patients with unexplained complex partial seizures. Their seizures are diagnosed on the basis of the clinical presentation and the EEG and treated with an appropriate AED. The prognosis for these patients is less predictable than for many of the following disorders.

Common causes of partial seizures

Benign rolandic epilepsy

Benign rolandic epilepsy is the most common seizure disorder of childhood (13). The seizures usually start to occur during middle childhood, between 4 and 12 years of age. *Partial seizures during sleep,* causing awakening, inability to speak, and clonic movements of one arm or side of the face, are typically reported. The seizures also occur during the day in many cases. The nocturnal seizures often secondarily generalize; rarely this occurs during the day as well. Occasionally there is a *family history* of the same disorder, and asymptomatic relatives have characteristic EEG abnormalities.

Unilateral or bilateral *centrotemporal spikes* (see Fig. 6.3) are a classic and usually obvious feature of the EEG. If MRI reveals an abnormality that could explain the seizures, the seizures should be regarded as symptomatic, and the diagnosis of benign Rolandic epilepsy is effectively ruled out.

The seizures typically persist for several years and are *always outgrown* during late childhood or adolescence (13). The main issue concerns treatment. Since the seizures are eventually outgrown and status epilepticus rarely, if ever, occurs, some physicians do not initiate treatment with an AED (14). If the seizures are frequent or occur during the daytime, an AED is more often prescribed. The approach chosen depends on the frequency of the seizures and the attitude of the family. Any AED for partial seizures is likely to be effective.

A less common and probably related form of partial epilepsy causes visual symptoms, such as flashing lights or loss of vision; loss of consciousness; and sometimes tonic-clonic movements and is diagnosed on the basis of localized occipital lobe EEG discharges. This syndrome, which is often hereditary, is known as *benign occipital epilepsy*. Unlike benign Rolandic seizures, these seizures occasionally persist into adult life. The seizures can usually be controlled with an AED for partial seizures.

Symptomatic partial seizures

Brain tumors, arteriovenous malformations, areas of infarction, and many other structural abnormalities often cause *symptomatic partial seizures*. Most of these underlying conditions are described elsewhere in this book. Two conditions, neurocysticercosis and congenital cerebral malformation, are discussed here.

Neurocysticercosis

The cause of neurocysticercosis is the pork tapeworm, a parasitic nematode endemic to Central and South America. Neurocysticercosis should be considered whenever a patient who has lived in Central or South America presents with unexplained seizures.

Primary infection of the gastrointestinal tract by the parasite may be asymptomatic. Secondary seeding of the brain causes an intense inflammatory reaction, headaches, and seizures. During the acute phase of infection, contrast-enhanced MRI usually reveals one or more small cystic areas in the cerebral cortex and edema in a fairly large area of surrounding tissue. Seizures may also occur after the larvae have died months or years later, at which time calcified, nonedematous deposits are seen by CT or MRI. Treatment usually includes an antiparasitic drug, a corticosteroid, and an AED for partial seizures (15).

Congenital cerebral malformations

Many congenital cortical malformations, ranging from severe (for example, lissencephaly, characterized by an almost complete absence of cortical gyri and sulci) to subtle (focal areas of cortical dysplasia) occur. The etiology of these malformations is often genetic; the histological basis has become better defined (16,17).

Patients with a major congenital brain malformation are usually microcephalic and developmentally delayed. Some of these children have a dysmorphic appearance, which is most characteristic in cases of *holoprosencephaly* associated with midline facial defects. MRI will demonstrate the malformation. Genetic consultation is recommended. The usual outcome is characterized by mental retardation and spastic quadriplegia. Seizures commonly occur. An AED indicated for partial seizures is most likely to be effective, but the seizures are often frequent, and good control may be difficult to achieve.

In contrast, a localized area of cortical dysplasia (see Fig. 6.4) may first present with partial seizures. There may be no history of cognitive or motor delay. Patients whose seizures are not well controlled by AEDs may benefit from surgical resection of the dysplastic area of the cortex.

Common primary generalized epilepsy syndromes

Absence epilepsy

Childhood absence epilepsy is a common disorder. Absence seizures usually first present during middle childhood. These seizures often occur *many times a day*. The seizures take the form of *brief* (5 to 30 seconds) *staring spells*. Blinking, head nodding, and semi-purposeful hand movements (automatisms) may be noted during the seizures. In contrast to complex partial seizures, which are somewhat similar in appearance, a *postictal state is never described*; in other words, the child "snaps out of it" after each seizure. Children with absence seizures may also have occasional primary generalized tonic-clonic seizures or myoclonic seizures. In some cases, there is a family history of epilepsy.

The physical examination usually reveals no abnormalities. The child should be asked to *hyperventilate for 3 minutes*; this often *provokes an absence seizure* and essentially confirms the diagnosis. The EEG includes intermittent *generalized 3-Hz spike-wave* discharges (see Fig. 6.2). MRI is unnecessary if there is a positive response to hyperventilation or the EEG shows this pattern.

Childhood absence seizures usually stop occurring by the end of adolescence and often sooner. Absence seizures that last for a minute or longer and are associated with prominent automatisms (*atypical absence seizures*) and absence seizures that are first noted during adolescence (*juvenile absence seizures*) typically continue to occur throughout adult life.

Valproate, zonisamide, topirimate, or lamotrigine is prescribed to control the seizures. These drugs also control the myoclonic and generalized tonic-clonic seizures that may occur. Ethosuximide controls absence seizures but does not prevent other types of seizure.

Nonepileptic staring spells

Many children who do not have seizures "zone out" in the classroom. In many cases, these children are recognized to have a learning disability, are excessively shy or anxious, or are autistic. They may feel overwhelmed in a challenging or large-group setting and periodically retreat into a private world. These episodes of "zoning out" are usually less often noticed at home than at school, suggesting that they are not seizures. Nevertheless, it is often prudent to order an EEG.

Juvenile myoclonic epilepsy and other causes of myoclonus

Myoclonus is also discussed in Chapter 4. A myoclonic jerk is a lightning fast movement, usually of the upper extremities, that is usually a seizure if it occurs during wakefulness.

Juvenile myoclonic epilepsy (JME) usually presents during adolescence. Myoclonic jerks of the arms after awakening, sometimes mistaken for clumsiness, are often the first sign. Myoclonus also may involve the lower extremities, resulting in falls. Patients often have generalized tonic-clonic seizures as well as myoclonic seizures (see Case 6.1).

The physical examination typically reveals no abnormal findings. The EEG is characterized by *4- to 6-Hz generalized spike-wave or polyspike discharges.* MRI is not necessary given a typical history and EEG result.

The seizures are well controlled by valproate-based drugs. Topirimate, lamotrigine (18), and, in the authors' experience, zonisamide are also effective. The patient must be informed that this condition will require lifelong treatment with an AED.

Rarely, myoclonic seizures are a sign of a more serious neurological disorder. *Degenerative disorders* that can cause myoclonic seizures include Lafora body disease, Unverricht-Lundborg disease, ceroid lipofuscinosis, mitochondrial encephalopathy, and subacute sclerosing panencephalitis (a rare complication of measles infection). In such cases, the patient is said to have *progressive myoclonic epilepsy.* Any patient presenting with myoclonus and progressive ataxia, cognitive regression, or loss of vision should undergo a comprehensive evaluation for a neurodegenerative disorder (see Chapter 14).

Myoclonic jerks presenting together with chaotic eye movements (*opsoclonus*) suggest an occult *neuroblastoma.* This syndrome (*opsoclonus-myoclonus*) also can occur in the absence of an underlying cause. Urine catecholamines are elevated in cases of neuroblastoma. The idiopathic syndrome may be immune mediated and is responsive to corticosteroids.

Atonic seizures

Atonic seizures (drop attacks) are characterized by an *abrupt loss of both consciousness and muscle tone,* causing the patient to suddenly fall to the ground. Atonic seizures almost exclusively occur in the context of *Lennox-Gastaut syndrome.* Valproate and other drugs for primary generalized epilepsy are prescribed to these patients, but atonic seizures are often difficult to control. Patients often wear a *protective helmet* to prevent serious injury.

Infantile spasms

Infantile spasms present during the first 2 years of life and, usually, during the first year. The infant is noted to have *multiple episodes of repetitive head, trunk, or bilateral upper extremity flexion, or hyperextension.* A cluster of these seizures *on awakening* is often reported. A brief cry, staring or eye rolling, or a transient loss of consciousness often accompanies the abnormal movements. In other cases, the seizures are subtle and, in some cases, have been occurring for weeks or months before they are noticed and brought to medical attention.

The EEG is characterized by *hypsarrhythmia*: a disorganized background with continuous high-amplitude slow waves and multifocal spike activity (see Fig 6.7). Periods of generalized voltage suppression (*electrodecremental response*) occur during the seizures.

In more than one half of cases, patients with infantile spasms *have an identifiable underlying condition* affecting brain development (e.g., prenatal cerebral infarction, cerebral malformation, syndrome of congenital malformation, chromosomal anomaly, metabolic disorder), and these seizures are called *symptomatic* infantile spasms. If no underlying disorder is identified, the seizures are called *cryptogenic* infantile spasms. The prognosis tends to be better for patients with cryptogenic infantile spasms, but both types may lead to other forms of epilepsy and neurodevelopmental delays. *West syndrome* is defined by the triad of infantile spasms, developmental delay, and a hypsarrhythmic EEG.

MRI, karyotype, genetic testing suggested by the patient's physical examination, and metabolic studies (see Chapter 14) should be ordered unless there is an obvious cause for the seizures (for example, a history of a known genetic disorder or brain injury).

The standard treatment for infantile spasms remains a series of intramuscular injections of *adrenocorticotropic hormone*, or ACTH (Acthar Gel, Questcor). In addition to controlling the seizures, treatment with ACTH may improve the patient's developmental prognosis. Recent evidence (19) suggests that promptly treating cryptogenic infantile spasms with ACTH, as opposed to delaying treatment even by a few weeks, results in an improved prognosis.

ACTH injections are started while the patient is hospitalized. The initial dose has never been standardized; 20 to 80 IU daily is the usual range (20). Baram et al. (21) suggest that a dose of 150 IU/m^2 (body surface area) is most effective. If the seizures come under control within a few days of starting treatment, the same dose is maintained for 1 to 2 weeks. If treatment with ACTH has been successful in stopping the seizures, the patient is usually discharged from the hospital after about 1 week, and a slowly down-tapering (1 month) course of ACTH injections is continued at home under the supervision of a visiting nurse. If there is no improvement within a few days of starting the drug, the dose may be doubled if it was at the lower end of the therapeutic range initially. If there is still no improvement, the drug should be rapidly tapered off.

Adverse effects associated with long-term corticosteroid therapy (e.g., cushingoid features, hypertension, cardiomyopathy, gastric ulcers, diabetes mellitus, and infection) may occur during the course of treatment with ACTH. Blood pressure, plasma and urine glucose, electrolytes, stool occult blood must be carefully monitored, and infections should be treated aggressively.

In cases of infantile spasms caused by an underlying condition with an inherently poor prognosis, such as a severe brain injury or malformation (see Fig. 6.6), the long-term benefits of treatment with ACTH may not justify the risks. Other medications that may control the seizures include benzodiazepines, topirimate, valproate-based AEDs (although the risk of hepatotoxicity must be weighed), and zonisamide. These medications have not been shown to improve the long-term prognosis, although they have not been carefully studied in this respect. Vigabatrin is an AED prescribed in Canada and Europe that is often used to treat infantile spasms. Visual disturbances and cerebral white-matter changes were reported during clinical trials of vigabatrin in this country and precluded FDA approval.

Lennox-Gastaut syndrome

Lennox-Gastaut syndrome (LGS) is one of the most severe and refractory forms of childhood epilepsy. To meet criteria for LGS, a patient must have: (a) *seizures of multiple types* (including myoclonic, absence, tonic-clonic, and/or atonic seizures); (b) a history of *developmental delay* or *mental retardation*; and (c) an EEG showing a *generalized slow* (1.5 to 2 Hz) *spike-wave pattern*. In a substantial number of cases, the patient has a history of infantile spasms. Neurocutaneous disorders (especially tuberous sclerosis) and a wide range of other inherited and metabolic defects affecting neurological development are often diagnosed. The seizures tend to be difficult to control, and treatment with at least two AEDs is almost always required. Valproate is usually one of the AEDs prescribed. Felbamate is often especially effective and, therefore, is often prescribed despite the risks of aplastic anemia and hepatotoxicity.

Febrile seizures and illness-related seizures

Febrile seizures have been estimated to occur in 5% of children (1). The age of onset is usually between 1 and 3 years of age. The cause is still poorly understood. Genetic factors probably play a role (22). A febrile seizure is not more likely to occur with a high-grade fever compared with a low-grade fever.

Two to 10% of children with a history of febrile seizures will eventually have a *nonfebrile* seizure (23,24); this contrasts with the 1% lifetime risk of developing epilepsy for the general population. If the history reveals *family members with epilepsy, a "complex" feature* of the febrile seizure (e.g., duration >20 minutes, unilateral motor activity or lateral eye deviation during the seizure, or postictal Todd's paralysis), or *delayed development*, then the chance of a future nonfebrile seizure is further increased. A late age of onset (older than 3 years) of febrile seizures also may be associated with an increased chance that epilepsy will develop.

Diagnostic studies

The child with a history of a single, brief, otherwise uncomplicated febrile seizure does not require CT, MRI, or EEG. Recurrent or complex febrile seizures, a history of abnormal neurological development, and a family history of epilepsy are reasons to consider further testing, although a recent study (25) suggests that the yield of brain imaging is low even in cases of complex febrile seizures.

A seizure heralding the onset of meningitis is unusual. Nevertheless, when a child has had a first febrile seizure and is brought to the emergency room still febrile, the possibility of meningitis is often considered. A lumbar puncture (LP) is appropriate if the child does not recover quickly from the seizure or was noted to be unusually irritable or lethargic before the seizure. Some physicians recommend an LP for infants less than 1 year of age who have had a first febrile seizure. If an infant or child is seen in the emergency room for additional febrile seizures, an LP should be deferred unless there is a strong clinical suspicion of meningitis.

Management

A *diazepam rectal suppository* (Diastat, Valeant Pharmaceuticals), 2.5 to 10 mg, can be given to abort a febrile seizure. A prescription for this drug should be given to the family of the child with a history of febrile seizures because timely administration will often prevent the need for an emergency room visit (26), and the family usually finds it very reassuring to have a treatment available at home. Brief febrile seizures do not require administration of diazepam; a seizure lasting more than 5 minutes is usually treated.

Acetaminophen or ibuprofen is sometimes given preventively every 4 to 6 hours when a child with a history of febrile seizures develops a fever, although it is unclear how effective this is in preventing a febrile seizure.

Occasionally children who have had very frequent febrile seizures are prescribed phenobarbital or another AED to prevent future febrile seizures. The frequency and duration of the child's seizures, a family history of epilepsy, any abnormal test (MRI/EEG) results, the attitude of the parents, and the risk of adverse medication effects are factors to consider when deciding whether or not to initiate treatment. Preventive treatment for febrile seizures does not decrease the likelihood that a child will develop epilepsy.

Prognosis

Febrile seizures usually recur, and parents should be so informed. In the great majority of cases, the seizures stop occurring well before 6 years of age, and in most cases, before 3 years of age.

Nonfebrile, infection-associated seizures and vaccination

A seizure occasionally occurs during a nonfebrile infection such as viral gastroenteritis. According to a recent study (27), the chance of developing epilepsy following such a seizure is equivalent to the chance of developing epilepsy following a febrile seizure.

A vaccination may be followed by fever and, therefore, by a febrile seizure. However, a child's vaccination schedule should not be significantly modified because of a history of febrile seizures. In the case of a patient who has had many febrile seizures, vaccinations are sometimes given individually rather than in combination to reduce the chance that a fever will ensue.

Neonatal seizures

The brain of the neonate is largely unmyelinated, and therefore, some seizures in the newborn do not have a counterpart in children (28). *Multifocal clonic* seizures only occur in the neonate. *Focal clonic* seizures in the neonate are somewhat similar to partial motor seizures in older patients. *Subtle* seizures are roughly analogous to complex partial seizures. *Myoclonic seizures* take the same form regardless of age.

Several benign hereditary forms of epilepsy present during the first week of life (29). In most cases, the seizures are myoclonic and stop occurring within a few days to weeks. These syndromes are uncommon, and neonatal seizures should generally be assumed to have a serious cause. *Hypoglycemia*, which can cause permanent neurological damage, must be promptly treated. *Hypocalcemia, hypoxemic brain injury, intracranial bleeding, stroke* (see Case 10.1), *meningitis, and encephalitis* should be considered when a neonate has seizures. Less common causes include cerebral malformation, tumor, and metabolic disorders (see Chapter 14).

Hypoglycemia and hypocalcemia should be promptly corrected. If the seizures then stop occurring, no further testing may be necessary. Otherwise, LP, MRI or CT, and EEG should be ordered. In many cases, it is appropriate to order laboratory tests, such as urine organic acids and plasma and CSF lactic acid levels, to investigate the possibility that the neonate has a metabolic disease (see Chapter 14).

To control the seizures, *phenobarbital* is started with a loading dose of 20 mg/kg, followed by a maintenance regimen of 3 to 5 mg/kg/day. Up to two additional loading boluses of 10 mg/kg may be given if the seizures do not stop occurring. *Phenytoin* (15-mg/kg loading dose and 5-mg/kg/day maintenance dose) and/or a *benzodiazepine*, such as clonazepam or midazolam (30), are added if the seizures are not controlled by phenobarbital.

Patients with a history of neonatal seizures are typically discharged from the hospital while they are still taking phenobarbital or another AED. One or more follow-up EEG studies are usually ordered during the next 6 months. If the patient remains seizure free, the MRI did not reveal a structural abnormality, and the EEG does not show epileptiform activity, the AED is often successfully tapered off.

Status epilepticus

Status epilepticus means a seizure, or sequential seizures, *lasting longer than approximately one-half hour.* A *generalized tonic-clonic* seizure of this duration can be *fatal or cause permanent neurological injury* (31). *Absence status epilepticus* and *simple* and *complex partial status epilepticus* also occur but are less dangerous.

Generalized status epilepticus requires emergent intervention. The patient is brought to the emergency room or treated in the field by the emergency medical services. Airway support is provided, and cardiac monitoring is initiated. Serum glucose is measured by fingerstick; *hypoglycemia is promptly treated.* Other tests are temporarily deferred, as the focus is on stopping the seizure.

An *intravenously administered benzodiazepine*, either diazepam in 5-mg boluses or lorazepam in boluses of 0.1 mg/kg body weight, is promptly given. The patient is also given *an intravenous loading dose of phenytoin* (15 to 20 mg/kg) *or its isomer, fos-phenytoin* (Cerebyx, Eisai). Together with a benzodiazepine, this is usually sufficient to abort the seizure. A bolus of *phenobarbital* or *intravenous valproate* (Depakone, Abbott) is added if the seizure continues. Endotracheal intubation should be considered at this point if it has not been done yet.

In a large majority of cases, this regimen will prove effective. If the seizure persists, the patient is administered pentobarbital, midazolam, lidocaine, thiopental, or propofol (32). An anesthesiologist must monitor the patient. These drugs produce a comatose state and always stop a seizure. The patient is usually maintained on one of these drugs for at least a day and often longer in the intensive care unit. Mechanical ventilation must be continued.

Simple and complex partial status epilepticus are treated with intravenously administered phenytoin, valproate, phenobarbital, and/or a benzodiazepine. In cases of absence status epilepticus, either an intravenously administered benzodiazepine or valproate is effective.

In all cases of generalized status epilepticus, the *cause of the seizure* must be sought with appropriate laboratory studies (electrolytes, serum glucose, complete blood count, liver function tests, AED level, and toxicology screening). MRI and, usually, LP should be performed. The EEG is usually most informative if it is recorded a few days after the seizure.

NONPHARMACOLOGICAL TREATMENTS FOR EPILEPSY

Epilepsy surgery is considered in cases of intractable *partial* seizures. *Patients with idiopathic primary generalized epilepsy are never surgical candidates* because their seizures do not originate from a resectable part of the brain. The preoperative evaluation and surgery are performed at a center specializing in the neurosurgical treatment of epilepsy. The patient

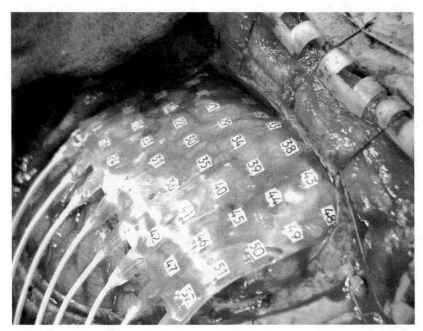

Figure 6.10 Subdural grid placement for seizure monitoring prior to surgery for partial epilepsy.
(Photograph Courtesy of Catherine A. Rubenacker, MD, Hackensack University Medical Center.)

usually undergoes EEG monitoring with intracranially placed electrodes (Fig. 6.10) to localize the origin of the seizures. *Functional imaging* studies (single-photon emission tomography) and *magnetoencephalography* may provide additional information useful in localizing the epileptogenic focus. The patient usually also undergoes preoperative *neuropsychological testing* during anesthesia of each cerebral hemisphere separately (*Wada test*) to evaluate the impact of the planned resection on speech, reasoning, and memory.

Surgical interventions vary from targeted subpial resections to removal of a large volume of cerebral cortex and underlying structures. The result is often a significant reduction in seizure frequency. Many patients are able to reduce their AED regimen, and complete cure results in a substantial number of cases. Mild, transient visual field defects are common following surgery on either temporal lobe. As long as preoperative neuropsychological testing has screened out patients judged as high risk, intelligence and cognitive performance are usually unaffected and may even be improved by surgery (33).

Commissurotomy, or dividing the corpus callosum, is often effective in reducing the severity of seizures in cases of refractory epilepsy. The procedure prevents the spread of epileptic discharges from one cerebral hemisphere to the opposite hemisphere. Commissurotomy often causes cognitive impairment and, therefore, is usually performed only when the patient has a prior history of significant mental retardation or other severe neurological impairments.

Vagus nerve stimulation is accomplished by means of a battery-powered stimulator implanted in the patient's neck. An electrical stimulus is delivered to the nerve at set intervals. Improved control of seizures may result.

Children with epilepsy are placed on a *ketogenic diet* if the response to multiple AEDs in combination has been unsatisfactory and epilepsy surgery is either not possible (as in cases of idiopathic primary generalized epilepsy) or has not resulted in better control. The ketogenic diet almost completely *eliminates carbohydrates from the diet and substitutes fats*. A nutritionist with appropriate training and experience must plan the diet. Some of the meals routinely recommended as part of the ketogenic diet may seem strange (e.g., four eggs, a stick of butter, and a glass of heavy cream for breakfast). The ketogenic diet requires getting used to and a high level of commitment on the part of the patient and family, but it can be beneficial (34). In many cases, one or more of the patient's AEDs can be tapered off, and, occasionally, the seizures stop occurring altogether. A preliminary study (35) suggests that a less drastic low-carbohydrate regimen (Atkins diet) may help control some patients' seizures.

QUESTIONS PARENTS OFTEN ASK ABOUT SEIZURES

Seizures are often terrifying to parents. Parents will have many questions to ask the doctor, usually including the following:

1. Can my child die from a seizure?

   The answer is that death from a seizure occurs extremely rarely, usually as the result of status epilepticus. There are also rare reports of patients with epilepsy who die mysteriously while asleep (36), perhaps as the result of a seizure that caused airway obstruction or triggered a fatal cardiac arrhythmia. The vast majority of seizures are not life threatening.

2. Does my child have epilepsy?

   Epilepsy is defined as a history of at least two seizures that were not provoked by a general medical cause (e.g., fever, hypoglycemia, side effect of a drug, etc.). If a person has an unprovoked seizure at 3 years of age and a second unprovoked seizure at 6 years of age, the child technically has epilepsy. However, this child's life is different from that of the patient who has a seizure every week. The point to make to parents is that epilepsy is a broad term that does not suggest the impact of the disorder on any given patient's life.

3. Are patients with epilepsy mentally retarded? Is my child going to become brain damaged if he has more seizures?

A significant brain injury often results in cognitive impairment and increases the chance of a future seizure. Thus many children with a history of a brain injury (patients with cerebral palsy) are mentally retarded or otherwise neurologically impaired and also have seizures, leading many people to associate mental retardation with epilepsy. However, most patients with epilepsy are of normal intelligence. Status epilepticus may cause permanent neurological damage; frequent complex partial seizures may be mildly deleterious to a patient's memory (7). Other seizures have not been shown to adversely affect intelligence or personality.

4. Will these seizures happen again, and if so, will my child grow out of them?

Seizures are more likely to recur in cases of abnormal neurological development and when the MRI or EEG is abnormal. In cases of an identifiable epilepsy syndrome, the recurrence risk is often well described. For example, childhood absence seizures are almost certain to recur, and Rolandic seizures also usually recur. A seizure caused by a medical disorder, such as hypoglycemia, is unlikely to recur if the medical condition that caused the seizure is appropriately managed.

Diagnosis of a specific disorder also may suggest the long-term prognosis. For example, benign Rolandic epilepsy is always eventually outgrown, whereas juvenile myoclonic epilepsy is a life-long condition. In cases of cryptogenic epilepsy, the risk of recurrence and the long-term prognosis are more difficult to predict.

5. What should I do if my child has another seizure?

A patient who is having a seizure should not be moved unless the patient is in a dangerous position, in which case he or she should be placed on the floor or on the ground on his or her back. **Nothing should be put into the patient's mouth. It is not possible for a patient to swallow his tongue during a seizure (or ever). A person who puts his or her finger into the mouth of a patient who is having a generalized tonic-clonic seizure risks losing his or her finger because, during the seizure, the patient's jaw clenches**.

The *time of onset* of the seizure should be noted, and the duration of the seizure should be timed on a watch. Although it will be difficult to be calm, the parent should try to carefully **observe the patient** during the seizure and remember as much as possible. Before the seizure started, was the patient ill or acting strangely? During the seizure, was one side of the body mostly involved (did one arm shake or stiffen more than the other arm)? Did the patient's eyes roll back or go to one side, or did the head turn to the right or left? Did the patient turn blue? Was the patient groggy or unarousable after the seizure ended? Did the patient bite his or her tongue or lose control of his or her urine or feces?

After the seizure ends, the patient may be rolled onto his side to prevent aspiration. If the patient is already seeing a doctor for seizures and has had appropriate diagnostic studies, it is not necessary to take the patient to the emergency room if the seizure lasted less than 5 minutes. The parents should call the physician who normally treats the patient. Longer seizures or recurrent seizures are reasons to call for an ambulance.

NONEPILEPTIC SEIZURE-LIKE PHENOMENA

Syncopal episodes and *breath-holding spells* (see Chapter 7) are often mistaken for epileptic seizures. The *lack of a postictal state* is the most reliable feature differentiating these phenomena from seizures. Tremor (see Chapter 4) is also sometimes mistaken for a seizure.

Tantrums and outbursts

Patients with a history of autism, ADHD, bipolar disorder, and other behavior disorders often are sent to the neurologist to make certain that their temper tantrums, outbursts, and episodes of agitation are not seizures.

Aggressive or agitated behavior may be noted during or after a complex partial seizure, but complex partial seizures are primarily characterized by *diminished responsiveness, automatisms, tonic eye deviation* or *unilateral clonic movements*, and a *postictal state*. In many cases of seizures presenting with behavioral manifestations, the patient's behaviors are usually stereotypic. If the patient has a history of behavioral outbursts and no other history suggestive of a complex partial seizure and the patient's behaviors are different during each episode, it is *unlikely that these episodes are seizures* (37). In questionable cases, EEG and MRI may be ordered to further investigate. However, the physician is reminded that the EEG in a fairly significant number of patients who do *not* have seizures is abnormal. A recent study (38) suggests that many physicians inappropriately order an EEG to evaluate phenomena that do not suggest a seizure.

Nonepileptic seizures

Nonepileptic seizures (NES) are seizure-like behaviors that do not correlate with epileptiform discharges. Also known as pseudoseizures, NES are *unconsciously motivated and result from psychological stress*. Patients with NES may have a history of depression or another psychiatric disorder. In some cases, physical or sexual abuse is reported. However, some of these patients also have a history of *epileptic* seizures. In the latter case, the NES may reflect the patient's dependency on a supportive medical system and a need for excessive attention. NES are diagnosed only after comprehensive diagnostic testing, including video/EEG monitoring. A formal psychiatric evaluation is necessary.

The following may be considered:

1. Repetitive tremulous or jerking movements of one arm or leg are *unlikely* to be seizures if they occur during a normal EEG recording.

2. A *generalized tonic-clonic seizure* always involves the entire cortex of both cerebral hemispheres and, therefore, *must entail complete loss of consciousness*. Thus, episodes of apparent tonic-clonic activity *on both sides of the body*, in a patient who is *awake*, are *unlikely* to be epileptic seizures.

3. *A lack of a postictal state following an apparent generalized tonic-clonic seizure* is highly suggestive of an NES.

4. A patient with a history of many apparent generalized tonic-clonic seizures who has *not bitten his or her tongue or become incontinent* during *any* of these events may be having NES.

5. NES often incorporate exaggerated behaviors such as *flailing, thrashing, and pelvic thrusting*. If a patient has a history of events of this kind and multiple EEG tracings are normal, the possibility of NES should be considered. However, *frontal and temporal lobe epileptic seizures can also cause bizarre movements*. Moreover, the EEG may be normal if the seizures originate from the orbitofrontal or mesiotemporal cortex. The diagnosis of NES versus one of these types of seizure is often very difficult to make; even experienced epileptologists have misdiagnosed these patients.

Provocation testing

A technique that is useful in making the diagnosis of NES is *provocation testing*. Provocation testing is controversial, and it is probably most ethical to obtain patient consent to receive medication, including placebos, a few days prior to testing. Well after consent is obtained, the patient is asked if they are willing to be given a drug that may elicit a seizure so that the seizure can be observed by a physician. They are also told that, if a seizure is provoked, they will receive an antidote to stop the seizure. If the patient agrees, the first "drug" (an injection of normal saline solution or an alcohol swab rubbed on the neck) is administered. The patient is then observed; if a "seizure" occurs, it is assumed to be nonepileptic. The "antidote" (also normal saline or an alcohol swab) is then given; an "aborted seizure" further supports the diagnosis of NES. Another technique to diagnose NES is to measure the plasma *prolactin level* immediately after a seizure (39). The prolactin level is often elevated after epileptic seizures but not after NES.

Related conditions

Malingering refers to a medical complaint or medical sign faked *for a specific purpose* (e.g., missing work, obtaining benefits or compensation, skipping a test in school). A faked seizure can be a form of malingering. Provocation testing is a useful tool in the evaluation of these patients.

A *conversion symptom* is a *physical symptom or sign produced unconsciously in direct response to a psychological stressor*. For example, a person might complain that he has suddenly become unable to move his arm a few days after losing his job. The neurological examination reveals findings (e.g., reflexes that are symmetrical) that are inconsistent with an organic cause, and the result of diagnostic testing, including MRI and EEG, is normal. The symptom often improves over time and with the aid of psychotherapy.

A *somatization disorder* (40) refers to a *lengthy history of multiple physical complaints* that, after careful investigation, are *not found to have a medical cause*. These patients usually have a long history of undiagnosed (but endlessly investigated) symptoms such as headache, back pain, and abdominal pain. Seizures are not a typical complaint.

Munchausen syndrome refers to the *conscious* production of *actual physical signs* (i.e., by the patient injuring or infecting himself) because the patient derives *enjoyment from the experience of receiving medical attention*. *Munchausen syndrome by proxy* is a notorious disorder of *parents* who *produce actual disease in their child* and then take the child to the medical community to investigate the cause. The parents presumably derive satisfaction from the experience of working with medical professionals to "diagnose" their child's medical problem. An appropriate legal authority must be contacted if Munchausen syndrome by proxy is suspected.

Seizures are frightening to parents and patients. A straightforward and empathic manner on the part of the physician, who should be knowledgeable about the seizure etiology, interpretation of test results, the likelihood of recurrence, the long-term prognosis, and treatment, is appreciated. A normal MRI study is reassuring to many people. Parents usually become less panicked after more than one or two seizures have occurred, and they realize that their child is not going to die or sustain permanent neurological damage as a result of the seizures. A good response to medication, even if there is an occasional breakthrough seizure, is also reassuring.

REFERENCES

1. Hauser WA. Epidemiology of epilepsy in children. In: Pellock JM, Dodson WE, and Bourgeouis BFD, eds. *Pediatric Epilepsy: Diagnosis and Therapy*. New York: Demos Medical Publishing; 2001:81–96.
2. Williamson PD, Spencer DD, Spencer SS, et al. Complex partial seizures of frontal lobe origin. *Ann Neurol.* 1985;18:497–504.
3. Quesney LF. Clinical and EEG features of complex partial seizures of temporal lobe origin. *Epilepsia.* 1986;27;(suppl 2):S27–S45.
4. Sveinbjornsdottir S, Duncan JS. Parietal and occipital lobe epilepsy: a review. *Epilepsia.* 1993;34:493–521.
5. Shinnar S, Berg AT, O'Dell C, et al. Predictors of multiple seizures in a cohort of children prospectively followed from the time of their first unprovoked seizure. *Ann Neurol.* 2000;48:140–147.
6. Berg AT, Shinnar S, Testa FM, et al. Status epilepticus after the initial diagnosis of epilepsy in children. *Neurology.* 2004;63:1027–1034.

7. Helmstaeder C, Kurthen M, Lux S, et al. Chronic epilepsy and cognition: a longitudinal study in temporal lobe epilepsy. *Ann Neurol.* 2003;54:425–432.
8. Gelisse P, Genton P, Kuate C, et al. Worsening of seizures by oxcarbazepine in juvenile idiopathic generalized epilepsies. *Epilepsia.* 2004;45:1282–1286.
9. Yerby MS. Teratogenicity of anticonvulsant medication. In: Pellock JM, Dodson WE, and Bourgeouis BFD, eds. *Pediatric Epilepsy: Diagnosis and Therapy.* New York: Demos Medical Publishing; 2001:357–372.
10. Browne TR, Holmes GL. *Handbook of Epilepsy.* Philadelphia: Lippincott; 2000:439.
11. Bryan A, Dreifuss FE. Valproic acid hepatic fatalities: III. U.S. experience since 1986. *Neurology.* 1996;46:465–469.
12. Browne TR, Holmes GL. *Handbook of Epilepsy.* Philadelphia: Lippincott; 2000:140.
13. Berkovic SF. Localization related epilepsies. In: Pellock JM, Dodson WE, and Bourgeouis BFD, eds. *Pediatric Epilepsy: Diagnosis and Therapy.* New York: Demos Medical Publishing; 2001:247–248.
14. Peters JM, Camfield CS, Camfield PR. Population study of benign Rolandic epilepsy: is treatment needed? *Neurology.* 2001;57:537–539.
15. Garcia HH, Pretell EJ, Gilman RH, et al. A trial of antiparasitic treatment to reduce the rate of seizures due to cerebral cysticercosis. *N Engl J Med.* 2004;350:249–258.
16. Mochida GH, Walsh CA. Genetic basis of malformations of the cerebral cortex. *Arch Neurol.* 2004;61:637–640.
17. Barkovich AJ, Kuzniecky RI, Jackson GD, et al. A developmental and genetic classification for malformations of cortical development. *Neurology.* 2005;65:1873–1887.
18. Prasad A, Kuzniecky RI, Knowlton RC, et al. Evolving antiepileptic drug treatment in juvenile myoclonic epilepsy. *Arch Neurol.* 2003;60:1100–1105.
19. Kivity S, Lerman P, Ariel R, et al. Long-term cognitive outcomes of a cohort of children with cryptogenic infantile spasms treated with high-dose adrenocorticotropic hormone. *Epilepsia.* 2004;45:255–262.
20. Haines ST, Casto DT. Treatment of infantile spasms. *Ann Pharmacother.* 1994;28:779–790.
21. Baram TZ, Mitchell WG, Tournay A, et al. High-dose corticotropin (ACTH) versus prednisone for infantile spasms: a prospective, randomized, blinded study. *Pediatrics.* 1996;97:375–379.
22. Nakayama J, Yamamoto N, Hamano K, et al. Linkage and association of febrile seizures to the IMPA2 gene on human chromosome 18. *Neurology.* 2004;63:1803–1807.
23. Berg AT, Shinnar S. Unprovoked seizures in children with febrile seizures: short-term outcome. *Neurology.* 1996;47:562–568.
24. Verity CM, Golding J. Risk of epilepsy after febrile convulsions: a national cohort study. *BMJ.* 1991;303:1373–1376.
25. Teng D, Dayan P, Tyler S, et al. Risk of intracranial pathological conditions requiring emergency intervention after a first complex febrile seizure episode among children. *Pediatrics.* 2006;117:304–307.
26. O'Dell C, Shinnar S, Ballaban-Gil KR, et al. Rectal diazepam gel in the home management of seizures in children. *Pediatr Neurol.* 2005;33:166–172.

27. Lee WL, Ong HT. Afebrile seizures associated with minor infections: comparison with febrile seizures and unprovoked seizures. *Pediatr Neurol.* 2004;31:157–164.

28. Volpe JJ. *Neurology of the Newborn.* Philadelphia: Saunders; 2001:185–206.

29. Pellock JM, Dodson WE, Bourgeouis BFD, eds. *Pediatric Epilepsy: Diagnosis and Therapy.* New York: Demos Medical Publishing; 2001.

30. Castro-Conde JR, Hernandez-Borges AA, Martinez ED, et al. Midazolam in neonatal seizures with no response to phenobarbital. *Neurology.* 2005;64:876–879.

31. Sahin M, Menache CC, Holmes GL, et al. Prolonged treatment for acute symptomatic refractory status epilepticus; outcome in children. *Neurology.* 2003;61: 398–401.

32. Van Gestel JPJ, Blusse van Oud-Albas HJ, Malingre M, et al. Propofol and thiopental for refractory status epilepticus in children. *Neurology.* 2005;65:591–592.

33. Krokman M, Granstrom ML, Kantola-Sorsa E, et al. Two-year follow-up of intelligence after pediatric epilepsy surgery. *Pediatr Neurol.* 2005;33:173–178.

34. Hemingway C, Freeman JM, Pillas DJ, et al. The ketogenic diet: a 3- to 6-year follow-up of 150 children enrolled prospectively. *Pediatrics.* 2001;108:898–905.

35. Kossoff EH, Kraus GL, McGrogan JR, et al. Efficacy of the Atkins diet as therapy for intractable epilepsy. *Neurology.* 2003;61:1789–1791.

36. Nouri S, Devinsky O, Balish M. Sudden unexpected death in epilepsy. http://www.emedicine.com/neuro/topic659.htm.

37. Delgado-Escueto AV, Mattson RH, King L, et al. The nature of aggression during epileptic seizures. *N Engl J Med.* 1981;305:711–717.

38. Matoth I, Taustein I, Kay BS, et al. Overuse of EEG in the evaluation of common neurological conditions. *Pediatr Neurol.* 2002;27:378–383.

39. Ahmad S, Beckett MW. Value of serum prolactin in the management of syncope. *Emerg Med J Online.* 2004;21:E3.

40. American Psychiatric Association. *Diagnostic and Statistical Manual of Mental Disorders, Text Revision.* 4th ed. Washington, DC: American Psychiatric Association; 2000:486.

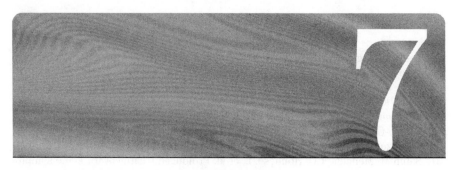

DIZZINESS, FAINTING, AND LOSS OF BALANCE

DIZZINESS

The first step in evaluating a complaint of dizziness (Table 7.1) is to determine what the patient means by "dizzy." The patient and parent should be asked:

1. Has the patient fainted or felt lightheaded?
2. Has the patient experienced a sensation of spinning, rocking, or movement ("Do you feel the room spinning?")
3. Has the patient's balance, gait, or coordination deteriorated?
4. Has the patient had episodes of feeling disoriented or removed from his or her surroundings?

FAINTING

Vasovagal episodes

Fainting spells (*vasovagal* or *neurocardiogenic syncopal episodes*) are common. Usually the patient, who is typically an older child or adolescent, briefly loses consciousness in a hot or crowded room (often in church) or when anxious or frightened (often during blood drawing). The patient is usually able to recall feeling lightheaded, falling, and waking up surrounded by concerned friends or family members. Prolonged postictal grogginess, such as is typical following many kinds of seizure, is *not* typical after a fainting spell. Tongue biting does not occur during a vasovagal spell, although urinary incontinence occasionally does. Observers frequently report *upward eye rolling and a few clonic jerks* during the period of unconsciousness. These observations are not, in and of themselves, suggestive of a seizure. However, if prolonged tonic-clonic activity was observed while the patient was unconscious or the patient was *groggy* for a prolonged

TABLE 7.1
Evaluation of dizziness: common causes

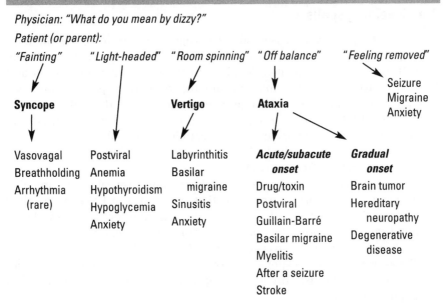

Physician: "What do you mean by dizzy?"
Patient (or parent):

"Fainting"	"Light-headed"	"Room spinning"	"Off balance"	"Feeling removed"
↓	↓	↓	↓	↘ Seizure
Syncope		**Vertigo**	**Ataxia**	Migraine
↓		↓		Anxiety
Vasovagal	Postviral	Labyrinthitis	*Acute/subacute*	*Gradual*
Breathholding	Anemia	Basilar	*onset*	*onset*
Arrhythmia	Hypothyroidism	migraine	Drug/toxin	Brain tumor
(rare)	Hypoglycemia	Sinusitis	Postviral	Hereditary
	Anxiety	Anxiety	Guillain-Barré	neuropathy
			Basilar migraine	Degenerative
			Myelitis	disease
			After a seizure	
			Stroke	

period after awakening, a seizure should be suspected, and magnetic resonance imaging (MRI) and electroencephalogram (EEG) should be ordered.

The pathophysiology of the spells is thought to involve autonomically mediated bradycardia. In many cases, there is a family history of individuals who faint.

Examination and testing

Vasovagal syncope is primarily a clinical diagnosis. The physical examination should include orthostatic blood pressure testing. The rest of the examination is typically normal. MRI and EEG are not necessary in typical cases, and blood tests such as a complete blood count rarely suggest a cause if the patient is asymptomatic between episodes. A cardiologist should evaluate the patient who has experienced many fainting spells to exclude arrhythmia or structural heart disease. A study (1) of adult patients admitted to a hospital for syncopal episodes demonstrates a significantly higher diagnostic yield from Holter monitoring and echocardiogram than from MRI and EEG.

There is no specific treatment. The patient's intake of fluids and sodium may be increased; this sometimes is helpful. Fainting spells usually become less frequent as the patient grows older but may continue to occur occasionally during adult life.

Breath holding spells

Breath holding spells are essentially vasovagal episodes in young children. The typical history is that of a toddler who becomes frightened or hurts himself, starts to cry, inhales deeply, and then loses consciousness and falls to the ground. The child may appear either cyanotic or pale (*cyanotic* vs. *pallid* syncope), and a few clonic jerks may occur while the child is unconscious. The child *awakens promptly* after a few seconds and usually cries. A postictal state does not occur after a breath-holding spell.

A history of relatives who had similar spells during childhood or who still have fainting spells is frequently elicited.

The physical examination of these children should reveal no abnormality. The spells do not require neurodiagnostic testing (MRI or EEG) unless they are prolonged, associated with focal neurological signs, or are followed by a definite seizure or a postictal state. A cardiologist is sometimes consulted, although an underlying cause is very rarely discovered.

Reassurance that the spells are not life threatening or dangerous is an important part of the visit. Breath-holding spells are usually outgrown by 3 to 4 years of age (2,3).

In rare instances, a patient has breath-holding spells that are followed by a generalized tonic-clonic seizure. EEG monitoring and MRI reveal no abnormality. Treatment with an antiepileptic drug is generally not effective for these patients, whose brains are thought to be exquisitely sensitive to hypoxemia. As in more typical cases of breath-holding spells, these spells eventually spontaneously stop occurring.

LIGHTHEADEDNESS

Mononucleosis, other viral infections and postviral syndromes, anemia, chronic anxiety, hypoglycemia, and hypothyroidism are common conditions that cause *lightheadedness*; laboratory tests for these disorders can be ordered. A cardiologist should be consulted if the problem persists. Lightheadedness is a common symptom of chronic fatigue syndrome (CFS), which is discussed in Chapter 2. A positive tilt table test helps to support the diagnosis of CFS (4,5).

VERTIGO

Vertigo is a subjective sensation of movement unrelated to the actual motion of the patient. The movement may be described as spinning, rocking, or unidirectional and may be experienced as movement of the patient or of the patient's surroundings.

Labyrinthitis

A *viral infection of the labyrinth* is assumed to be the cause of many cases of acute-onset vertigo in children and adolescents, although this etiology is generally not provable. Patients often also complain of *nausea, mild generalized headache, and fatigue.* Tinnitus is occasionally reported. Fever is not typical. The physical examination may reveal *nystagmus* (see Chapter 14) and, occasionally, mild *gait ataxia. Upper limb ataxia does not occur.* The nystagmus (see Chapter 14) associated with vertigo of vestibular origin is typically *rotary* (a subtle torsional movement of the globe) and *fatigable* (does not persist indefinitely).

Labyrinthitis is normally self-limited. Meclizine, 12.5 mg every 6 hours as needed, is prescribed for vertigo. A benzodiazepine may also be helpful. A short course of a corticosteroid (as for migraine; see Chapter 2) is prescribed in some refractory cases. An ear, nose, and throat (ENT) specialist should be consulted if the symptoms do not improve within 2 weeks.

Brainstem disease

If a patient is otherwise neurologically asymptomatic and the physical examination reveals no atypical findings, then the patient's vertigo is very unlikely to be caused by a lesion in the brainstem. MRI should be ordered, however, when the examination demonstrates limb ataxia, severe gait ataxia, mental status or cranial nerve abnormalities, or when the patient's symptoms do not begin to resolve within a week.

Benign paroxysmal vertigo

Toddlers and very young children may experience episodes of severe vertigo, loss of balance, and an inability to walk that last less than 5 minutes. Nystagmus may be noted during these episodes by the child's parents. Between episodes, the child is asymptomatic. This syndrome, known as *benign paroxysmal vertigo*, is thought to be a migraine variant, and a family history of migraine is often elicited. In stereotypic cases, MRI is unnecessary. The episodes become less frequent over time, but the patient may have migraine headaches when older (6).

Case 7.1

A 3-year-old girl, having gone to bed the previous night in good health, awakens and says she is now unable to stand. Her parents bring her to the office. No other symptoms are reported. She was ill with an upper respiratory infection a week prior to onset of her current symptoms. She is not taking any medications.

(continued)

The physical examination reveals no neck or back tenderness, adenopathy, fever, or rash.

The patient is alert but miserable. Examination of the cranial nerves reveals nystagmus. She wobbles from side to side when sitting up. When she reaches for objects with either hand, her arm movements are uncoordinated and an intention tremor is obvious. She can support her weight when standing, but her stance is wide-based. She sways and starts to fall when she tries to walk. Her deep tendon reflexes are obtainable. She cries when pin sensation is tested in her feet.

Her father goes home and reports that he has found no open medication containers. Urine toxicology is negative.

Diagnosis: *Acute postinfectious cerebellitis.*

Outcome: MRI of the brain was not ordered given a classic presentation of postinfectious cerebellitis. The child started to improve in 2 days and was back to normal in 2 weeks. She has had no recurrence of symptoms.

Other causes of vertigo

Basilar migraine is discussed in Chapter 2. *Sinusitis, otitis media, and structural disorders of the inner ear* can cause vertigo (7).

ATAXIA

Ataxia means *incoordination*. (*Apraxia*, by comparison, means difficulty *planning* or *conceptualizing* movements or speech.) Ataxia is usually caused by cerebellar disease (*cerebellar ataxia*). *Truncal* ataxia (unsteady gait, difficulty tandem walking) is differentiated from *limb* ataxia (incoordination of the extremities, abnormal heel-to-shin or finger-to-nose test). Midline cerebellar lesions cause truncal ataxia, whereas lateral cerebellar lesions cause limb ataxia.

Less frequently in pediatric patients, a disease process affecting the *peripheral nervous system or spinal cord* causes ataxia (*sensory ataxia*). The patient usually also complains of numbness and weakness in the legs or paresthesias. The neurological examination usually reveals lower extremity weakness, abnormal reflexes, and diminished pin and joint position sensation. The *Romberg test* (see Chapter 1) is often positive, but tests of cerebellar function do not yield abnormal findings.

Acute-onset cerebellar ataxia

Acute-onset cerebellar ataxia in a child, adolescent, or adult is often caused by *a medication, drug of abuse, or toxin. Barbiturates, benzodiazepines, antiepileptic drugs, antihistamines,* and *alcohol* are very likely to impair cerebellar function when taken in excessive quantity. *Toxicology screening* should be ordered. If there is uncertainty about the cause, the medicine cabinet and bottles of alcoholic beverages in the home should be checked.

Postinfectious cerebellar ataxia is common in young children. The syndrome classically follows chicken pox or varicella vaccination but may also occur after other viral infections. In many cases, there is no evidence of a preceding infection. The clinical presentation is often dramatic. Within minutes to hours, the child becomes very unsteady and often unable to walk. The examination reveals gait ataxia, *titubation* (wobbly side-to-side movements of the head and trunk), limb ataxia, or nystagmus. Ataxia is maximal at onset and gradually improves over several weeks. Eventual complete resolution after a few weeks is the usual outcome, although a mild degree of ataxia occasionally persists. MRI may be deferred as long as there is continuing improvement (8). Lumbar puncture is unnecessary in typical cases.

It may be challenging to distinguish childhood postviral cerebellar ataxia from conditions causing an acute change in gait (also see Chapter 13). *Guillain-Barré syndrome* (GBS) typically presents with rapidly progressive weakness, unsteadiness, and numbness or paresthesias in the legs or arms. *Absent* lower extremity deep tendon reflexes suggest GBS; reflexes may be diminished but should be obtainable in the child with postinfectious ataxia. *Transverse myelitis* often causes difficulty walking and unsteadiness. A sensory level, a Babinski sign, back pain, or a history of a disturbance of bowel or bladder function suggests transverse myelitis, whereas limb ataxia, nystagmus, and titubation suggest cerebellar disease.

Nonneurological conditions, such as *toxic synovitis* and *viral myositis*, should also be considered. *Pain, not weakness*; normal sensation, normal reflexes, and an absence of signs of cerebellar disease (limb ataxia or nystagmus) suggest a nonneurological cause.

Progressive cerebellar ataxia

A history of *progressive cerebellar ataxia* suggests a *posterior fossa brain tumor.* Other symptoms suggestive of a tumor include lethargy, vomiting, double vision, hemiparesis, or posterior headaches. *Contrast-enhanced MRI* should be ordered. *Cerebellar pilocytic astrocytoma* (see Fig. 2.3) is a common and usually curable cerebellar tumor; other lesions of the posterior fossa tend to be more difficult to treat.

Progressive cerebellar ataxia may also occur as the result of a *degenerative disease of the nervous system* (9), such as *Friedreich ataxia, ataxia-telangiectasia, leukodystrophies,* and one of the hereditary *familial cerebellar ataxias.* These conditions are discussed in Chapters 10 and 14.

Progressive sensory ataxia

Hereditary neuropathies, the most common of which is *Charcot-Marie-Tooth disease* (see Chapter 8), cause *progressive sensory ataxia*. Multiple sclerosis, spinal cord tumors, and Friedreich ataxia (which affects the spinal cord as well as the cerebellum) are other possible causes of progressive sensory ataxia in a child or adolescent.

Intermittent ataxia

Intermittent episodes of ataxia often are caused by *repeated episodes of drug or alcohol ingestion, basilar migraine,* or occur in the aftermath of *epileptic seizures.* Very rarely, recurrent episodes of ataxia result from a *metabolic disease,* classically the *intermittent form of maple syrup urine disease* and *Hartnup disease;* a quantitative plasma amino acid and urine amino acid profile, respectively, obtained while the patient is symptomatic, are ordered to diagnose these two conditions. *Familial periodic cerebellar ataxia* is a rare condition characterized by recurrent episodes of ataxia and a dramatic response to acetazolamide.

"DIZZINESS" AS SYMPTOM OF ANXIETY

Symptoms of lightheadedness, vertigo, and *a feeling of disorientation* are common complaints of patients with a history of *generalized anxiety.* These patients often *report feeling physically removed from their surroundings* and may say that, when they look at objects, the *objects appear further away than they really are (micropsia).* MRI and EEG should be ordered to investigate the possibility of a seizure originating from the temporal or frontal lobe. Micropsia is also sometimes a migraine aura. A psychogenic etiology is equally common, in our experience.

REFERENCES

1. Pies LA, Ganji JR, Jarandila R, et al. Diagnostic patterns and temporal tends in the evaluation of adult patients hospitalized with syncope. *Arch Intern Med.* 2001;161:1889–1895.
2. DiMario FJ. Prospective study of children with cyanotic and pallid breath-holding spells. *Pediatrics.* 2001;107:265–269.
3. Lombroso CT, Lerman P. Breathholding spells (cyanotic and pallid infantile syncope). *Pediatrics.* 1967;39:563–581.
4. Stewart J, Gewtiz MH, Weldon A, et al. Patterns of orthostatic intolerance: the orthostatic tachycardia syndrome and chronic fatigue. *J Pediatr.* 1999;135:218–225.
5. Stewart J, Gewtiz MH, Weldon A, et al. Orthostatic intolerance in adolescent chronic fatigue syndrome. *Pediatrics.* 1999;103:116.
6. Lindskog U, Odkvist L, Noaksson L, et al. Benign paroxysmal vertigo in childhood: a long-term follow-up. *Headache.* 1999;39:33–37.

7. Brower CM, Cotton RT. The spectrum of vertigo in children. *Arch Otolaryngol.* 1995;121:911–915.
8. Gieron Korthals MA, Westberry KR, Emmanuel PJ. Acute childhood ataxia: 10-year experience. *J Child Neurol.* 1994;9:381–384.
9. Subramony SH. Clinical aspects of hereditary ataxias. *J Child Neurol.* 1995;10:353–362.

8

DELAY OR REGRESSION OF MOTOR DEVELOPMENT ASSOCIATED WITH LOW MUSCLE TONE

Infants and children who are late to achieve motor milestones are often brought to the office or clinic by their parents for evaluation. In other cases, a history suggestive of developmental delay is obtained during a routine visit. Much more rarely, the physician is asked to evaluate a young patient with the more ominous history of a *loss* of previously acquired motor milestones. This chapter reviews causes of motor delay and regression that are associated with the finding of *low to normal muscle tone*. Congenital hypertonia, or increased muscle tone, is discussed in Chapter 10.

If a child is delayed in acquiring both *language and motor* milestones, the child is said to be *globally developmentally delayed*. A genetic or metabolic disorder is sometimes the cause. Delayed *language* acquisition is often an early sign of *autism* (see Chapter 9).

DELAYED MOTOR MILESTONES

The "normal age" at which infants and children are supposed to first roll over, sit up, or walk is an average. By definition, some individuals must fall within the right-hand tail of the bell curve reflecting the age, in the general population, at which infants and children achieve a given motor milestone. Most of these "delayed" patients do *not* have a serious neurological problem; they have simply learned to roll over, sit, stand, walk, or run at a later age than many of their peers. Other infants and young children are delayed in acquiring one or more of the many fine and gross motor milestones in the Denver II developmental inventory. Some of these children continue to be a little clumsy and have immature fine motor skills, causing difficulty using scissors, writing neatly with a pencil, or buttoning their clothes.

Mild gross and fine motor delays are very rarely the result of a serious underlying neurological disorder. Parents should not be needlessly panicked, and unnecessary tests should not be ordered on the basis of a history of borderline motor delay, failure to reach one or two milestones exactly on schedule, or mild gross and fine motor immaturity.

Hypotonia in the neonate, infant, and toddler

Table 8.1 is a list of the ages by which a patient should achieve the most important gross motor milestones. Infants and children who do not have head control by about 2 months, have not rolled over by 6 months, have not learned to sit without support by 10 months, or have not learned to walk by 16 months of age can be considered to be developmentally delayed. Once again, this does not necessarily mean that there is a serious cause for the child's delays; in most such cases, the child does not have a serious disorder.

The most common finding revealed by the physical examination of infants and young children with a history of delayed motor development is *hypotonia* ("low muscle tone"). Hypotonia is a nonspecific symptom that can, in theory, result from a disorder of the brain, spinal cord, peripheral nerves, or muscle. In the great majority of cases, hypotonia is a nonspecific sign of neurodevelopmental immaturity.

Signs of hypotonia in the young infant (also see Chapter 1 and Fig. 1.4) include *head lag* during the *pull-to-sit* maneuver, slippage through the examiner's hands on *vertical suspension*, and a tendency to "drape" when held in *horizontal suspension*. Hypotonic infants often lie on the examination table in the "frog-leg" position with hips and shoulders abducted. Decreased resistance to passive manipulation of the limbs is often noted, although some infants with truncal hypotonia have normal extremity tone.

Young *children* who have a history of delayed motor milestones also often have low muscle tone. These patients typically walk, run, hop, or skip

TABLE 8.1

Important gross motor milestones of infancy and childhood

Milestone	Age of acquisition
Head control	Before 2 months
Rolls over	Before 6 months
Sits without support	Before 10 months
"Cruises"	Before 1 year
First steps alone	Before 16 months
Walks well	Before 2 years
Runs	Before 3 years

clumsily, and "soft signs" (see Chapter 1) are noted during tests of fine motor function.

The first task is to make certain that there is not a serious condition causing the patient's hypotonia and delayed development. The physician should be especially concerned if (a) there is a history of developmental *regression or marked stagnation following normal development* as opposed to a mild delay; (b) there is a history of *severe developmental delay* (many months behind schedule in achieving multiple milestones); (c) there is a history of *seizures*; (d) the examination reveals *unobtainable deep tendon reflexes* or a *positive Gowers sign* (in children); or (e) the examination reveals *spinal or orthopedic abnormalities* or signs of a *syndrome of congenital malformation*.

Benign hypotonia with delayed motor milestones

Most patients who are late to acquire motor milestones have no serious underlying disorder and are eventually recognized to have *nonspecific developmental motor delay with hypotonia*. This common syndrome is also called *central hypotonia* or *benign congenital hypotonia*. The causes are poorly understood. The family history often reveals that a parent or sibling was late to walk or was clumsy as a child and thus suggests a genetic etiology. MRI and laboratory tests almost always yield unremarkable results and are unnecessary unless a specific disorder is suspected.

The prognosis is good. Motor milestones are eventually attained, and the child becomes able to walk, run, and generally function normally. If there is a long-term consequence, it is that the patient may remain a little clumsy and not become a star athlete ("picked last for softball"). Some of these children may also be delayed in developing fine motor abilities, but these skills too eventually improve in the great majority of cases (how many adults have poor fine motor abilities?).

Case 8.1

A 3-year-old girl is brought for evaluation because she was very late to learn to walk and still cannot run. Her parents state that she was floppy as a young infant and could barely hold her head up at 4 months of age. She had feeding problems in the nursery. Sitting up was attained at 15 months, and walking was attained at 2 and1/2 years. She has also been slow to acquire speech and is currently being evaluated for a special education class. Despite these handicaps, the child is gradually improving. She has not lost any motor or cognitive skills.

The physical examination reveals a thin little girl with an elongated face and a high-arched palate. There is no calf hypertrophy, and no orthopedic abnormalities are noted. Her speech reveals articulation problems. The cranial nerves are intact.

Resting extremity tone is low normal. She has generally decreased strength, graded at 4/5 in the proximal upper and lower extremities, but close to normal strength in the distal extremities and hands. Gowers sign is positive. Fine motor skills are age appropriate. Reflexes are normal. She is not ataxic.

Plasma CPK is within normal limits. A muscle biopsy specimen sent to a neuropathologist is reported to contain unusual rod-like structures in myocytes that are visible by electron microscope.

Diagnosis: *Congenital myopathy* (nemaline rod disease).

Outcome: The patient continued to make slow progress. She was placed in a special education class. Years later, at 20, she functions independently and attends a special education program at a local community college. She still reports weakness but no loss of motor abilities.

Physical therapy may be helpful, although it is probably not essential because virtually all of these children improve without treatment. Occupational therapy to improve pencil skills and a computer keyboard are often helpful for children with immature fine motor skills. Persistence of poor fine motor skills beyond about 7 years of age is unusual.

Sensory integration disorder

"Sensory integration disorder" is a diagnosis often made by occupational therapists to describe children who are clumsy, have immature fine motor skills and a history of behavioral problems, and are *excessively irritated by sensory stimuli*. Parents of these children often describe an aversion to loud noises, intolerance of clothing textures, and extreme dislike of particular foods and food textures.

Few pediatric neurologists believe that sensory integration disorder is a distinct entity. We note that many children diagnosed with attention-deficit hyperactivity disorder (ADHD), autism, or an anxiety disorder also have "sensory issues," or signs of *tactile hypersensitivity*. Therefore, we believe that "sensory symptoms" are nonspecific. In the authors' experience, many children said to have sensory integration disorder are anxious, and a family history of anxiety disorder is often elicited from the parents of these children.

Many therapies are suggested for and administered to these patients, including brushing the skin and other techniques claimed to desensitize the nervous system. These therapies typically involve many sessions, are often expensive, and imply to parents and children that there is a significant problem that requires treatment. Given the fact that few, if any, adult patients have sensory integration disorder, it seems reasonable to question whether these costly interventions for children are necessary.

OTHER CAUSES OF HYPOTONIA

Table 8.2 summarizes the clinical features of more serious disorders causing hypotonia.

TABLE 8.2

Specific conditions associated with hypotonia and motor delay/regression in infancy and childhood

Symptoms	Key signs	Condition; diagnostic tests (in italics)
Global developmental delay, history of abnormal facial appearance, limb or organ malformations	*Dysmorphic facial features*; microcephaly; eye, ear, limb, or organ anomalies	One of many **syndromes of congenital malformation**; *TORCH titers, karyotype; genetic consultation and testing*
Markedly delayed acquisition of early motor milestones, sometimes with regression; decreased movements; often a history of pneumonia	Severe hypotonia, *absent deep tendon reflexes*, tongue fasciculations, pectus excavatum	**Spinal muscular atrophy type I**; *specific genetic test; muscle biopsy (rarely needed)*
Hypotonia, lethargy, poor feeding in previously healthy infant	Depressed reflexes, poorly reactive pupils	**Infantile botulism**; *EMG; stool analysis for bacterium*
Marked developmental delay, hypotonia, history of seizures	Microcephaly (often), sometimes dysmorphic facial features	**Cerebral malformation**; *brain MRI*
Clumsiness, falling, loss of motor milestones in a previously normal 2- to 3-year-old boy	Obtainable deep tendon reflexes, calf hypertrophy, *positive Gowers sign*	**Duchenne muscular dystrophy**; *plasma CPK, genetic tests, muscle biopsy*
History of severe hypotonia at birth, developmental delay; often no regression; child attains milestones very late but often makes noticeable progress	Weakness, positive Gowers sign	**Congenital myopathy**; *muscle biopsy; CPK usually normal*
Slowly progressive weakness in older child or adolescent, usually in the legs; mild sensory loss	Pes cavus, absent reflexes; difficulty walking on toes/ heels; distal sensory loss	**Sensorimotor neuropathy** (usually Charcot-Marie-Tooth disease); *nerve conduction study, genetic testing*

Spinal muscular atrophy

When it *is impossible to elicit deep tendon reflexes* from a hypotonic infant who has not acquired motor milestones, the diagnosis of *spinal muscular atrophy* (SMA) should be considered.

The underlying process in SMA is the progressive degeneration of spinal motor neurons (anterior horn cells). Three forms of SMA are distinguished by the age of onset. Neonates and infants with *Werdnig-Hoffman disease* (SMA type I) are evaluated for diminished motor activity ("the baby isn't moving much") during the first few months of life. The mother may have reported decreased fetal movements during the pregnancy. These infants typically do not attain any motor milestones. They lie in the "frog leg" position and are found to be severely hypotonic ("dishrag floppy") when evaluated by pull-to-sit and vertical and horizontal suspension.

The *deep tendon reflexes should be unobtainable*. If reflexes can be elicited, the baby in all likelihood does not have SMA. *Tongue fasciculations*, reflecting denervation, are a classic finding but are not always noted. Since brain function is unaffected, infants with SMA are *alert and interactive*, which is often falsely reassuring to parents. There may be a *history of pneumonia* or *pectus excavatum* resulting from poor respiratory muscle function.

Other children with SMA have a history of normal early infantile (type II SMA) or childhood (type III SMA or *Kugelberg-Welander disease*) motor development that is eventually followed by stagnation and regression. Children with SMA type II typically become able to sit unsupported but never walk. Patients with SMA type III may become ambulatory, and regression sometimes does not commence until adolescence. Absence of deep tendon reflexes remains a key diagnostic finding, although hereditary diseases of the peripheral nerve (see following section, Hereditary Sensory-Motor Neuropathies) also can cause disappearance of reflexes and should be considered in cases presenting at a later age.

Genetic testing (1) has become the accepted method for diagnosing SMA. The commercially available genetic test for SMA is sensitive and specific and has made muscle biopsy, once required for diagnosis, unnecessary in almost all cases. The two genes causing the disease are on chromosome 5q. Inheritance is autosomal recessive. The genes are common and carried by one in 50 people. The existence of three forms of SMA is explained by variation in the production of a protein affecting the survival of motor neurons (2).

SMA type I is a devastating disease and a terrible diagnosis for parents to confront. Currently there is no specific treatment, but clinical trials of potentially useful medications are underway (2). Without intervention, SMA type I causes death from respiratory failure within 2 years and often sooner. Patients should be followed, when possible, at a center for childhood neuromuscular diseases. Tracheostomy is usually offered when respiratory function begins to decline. There are difficult associated ethical questions. Parents should be made aware of long-term outcome of the disease and the benefits of aggressive treatment so that the most informed decision can be made.

Survival for patients with types II and III SMA is much better than for patients with type I SMA, and patients with SMA type III may attain a normal life span.

Infantile botulism

Infantile botulism should be suspected when a *previously normal* infant becomes lethargic and hypotonic and has trouble feeding. *Hypotonia, depressed reflexes*, and *poorly reactive pupils* are important findings on examination. The etiology is an *anticholinergic toxin*, causing both neuromuscular and parasympathetic blockade, produced by the bacterium *Clostridium botulinum*. A history of honey ingestion, by which the bacterial spores can be introduced, is obtained in a small minority of cases. Usually the source of the infection is never discovered. The definitive diagnosis is made by *identification of Clostridium botulinum in the stool*. Electromyography (EMG; see Chapter 12) with *repetitive nerve stimulation* can provide supportive evidence but is technically difficult to perform.

Without intervention, death from respiratory failure often occurs, and mechanical ventilation is therefore usually necessary. Antibiotics are usually given but do not alter the prognosis, since the toxin persists at the synaptic junction for weeks. *Specific immune globulin* may be more effective. With appropriate care, full recovery often occurs, but the process can be very prolonged (3).

Muscular dystrophy

Duchenne muscular dystrophy (DMD) is an X-linked recessive degenerative neuromuscular disease primarily affecting boys. The causative gene may be partially expressed in the female heterozygote, resulting in less severe impairment (4). DMD results from the absence of a protein (*dystrophin*) in the cell membrane of skeletal myocytes. The absence of dystrophin causes myocyte instability, leading to the progressive deterioration and death of muscle cells. Fat and scar tissue replace muscle, sometimes causing enlargement or *pseudohypertrophy* (classically, of the gastrocnemius).

In typical cases of DMD, motor milestones are normally acquired during the first 2 or 3 years of life. At that point, *clumsiness, falling, difficulty climbing stairs, and poor exercise tolerance* start to become noticeable. By the time the child is brought to medical attention, the physical examination usually reveals difficulty running, a waddling gait, and a *positive Gowers sign* (see Chapter 1). Pseudohypertrophy may or may not be noted. Muscle tone is low to normal, and deep tendon reflexes should be obtainable.

The plasma *creatine phosphokinase* (CPK) level is *always* elevated, often above 3,000 mg/dL. The diagnosis of DMD is confirmed either by genetic testing, which is specific but does not detect some variants, or the finding of *absent dystrophin* by *muscle biopsy.*

The prognosis is one of gradual, relentless deterioration leading to loss of the ability to walk by 10 years of age and eventual wheelchair dependency. Many children develop lordosis or scoliosis. Most are mildly mentally retarded, since dystrophin is normally also expressed in neurons. Cardiac arrhythmia is a common complication that can be life threatening.

There is no specific treatment. Prednisone may confer a transient improvement in motor function (5). A recent study (6) suggests that creatine monohydrate is beneficial for some patients. Myoblast transplantation and gene therapy have not resulted in clinical improvement.

Referral to a center for childhood neuromuscular diseases is recommended so that supportive services can be coordinated. Cardiac function in particular must be closely followed. Physical therapy may improve quality of life, but life expectancy is often less than two decades even with the best care.

Becker muscular dystrophy is a similar X-linked recessive neuromuscular disorder that presents at about 10 years of age. The typical history is of arrest and slow regression of motor development. Clinical signs of myopathy (proximal weakness and Gowers sign) are noted. The plasma CPK level is elevated. Muscle biopsy, the most sensitive and specific test, reveals *chemically abnormal dystrophin*. A genetic test is available but, like the test for DMD, is not sensitive for all genetic variants. Longevity and quality of life are significantly better than for patients with DMD.

Several rare forms of muscular dystrophy are transmitted by *autosomal recessive* inheritance and, therefore, affect girls and boys in equal numbers (7). The clinical presentation may resemble either DMD or Becker muscular dystrophy. A *muscle biopsy specimen* is required for diagnosis and should be examined by a neuropathologist familiar with these disorders.

Congenital myopathies

The *congenital myopathies* are a heterogeneous group of disorders presenting with *severe hypotonia at birth* and subsequently *delayed motor development*, but their course is characterized by less striking regression, no regression, or, in some cases, gradual improvement. The cause is always an inherited defect in myocyte structure. Several distinct forms, *each distinguished by a unique ultrastructural appearance of myocytes* that is visible by electron microscopy, have been identified (8,9). The genetic inheritance pattern is complex and varies even for each form of congenital myopathy.

Affected neonates are often severely hypotonic at birth and may die without respiratory support. Poor survival is more characteristic of some forms of congenital myopathy (e.g., *myotubular myopathy*) than other forms. If they survive the neonatal period, patients with a congenital myopathy often slowly improve but attain motor milestones very late. As children, they have trouble running, jumping, and climbing. The physical examination usually reveals proximal weakness, a waddling gait, and a positive Gowers sign. Pseudohypertrophy is not noted. Some syndromes, such as *nemaline rod disease*, are associated with a dysmorphic facial appearance.

The plasma CPK level and EMG are typically normal. The diagnosis of a congenital myopathy can only be made by examination of a *muscle biopsy* specimen by a neuropathologist.

Some degree of weakness persists throughout life, but regression does not always occur. Some types of congenital myopathy are associated with low intelligence. Patients with *central core disease* are susceptible to *malignant hyperthermia*, and therefore, anesthetics cannot be administered to these patients without special precautions.

Hereditary sensory-motor neuropathies

Hereditary sensory-motor neuropathies is a group of hereditary disorders of the *peripheral nerve axon or myelin sheath* that are characterized clinically by *slowly progressive weakness of the legs* and, to a lesser degree, weakness in the upper extremities. Patients also often report mild to moderate distal sensory loss. Most patients with *Charcot-Marie-Tooth disease* (CMT), the most common disease of this group, do not experience symptoms until the second decade or later. Rarer forms of hereditary sensory-motor neuropathy may present during middle or even early childhood (10). Symptoms are very *gradual in onset* (over the course of many months to years). The physical examination usually reveals *pes cavus* resulting from atrophy of the plantar muscles, distal extremity weakness, difficulty walking on the toes and heels and hopping on one foot, trace to absent deep tendon reflexes, and diminished pin sensation. There may be mild gait ataxia due to loss of proprioception (sensory ataxia). A *positive Romberg sign* (see Chapter 1) is often noted.

Confirmation of the diagnosis of a specific disease entity within this group usually entails genetic testing, which is specific but currently not sensitive for all variants. *Sural nerve biopsy* is performed if genetic testing is inconclusive. Physical therapy and orthotics may be helpful. Some patients eventually become wheelchair dependent.

Syndrome of hypotonia and severe developmental delay

A small percentage of infants with a history of hypotonia and delayed motor development do not make any substantial progress. Most of these patients are also delayed in achieving cognitive milestones. Some have seizures. However, developmental regression does not occur. Magnetic resonance imaging (MRI) and laboratory tests for a genetic, metabolic, or degenerative disorders yield no abnormal findings. In the past, these children were said to have "hypotonic cerebral palsy." The pathogenesis of this syndrome, for which there are surely multiple causes, is not understood. Treatment is supportive (Table 8.3).

Table 8.3

Hypotonia in the neonate: common causes

Cause	Diagnostic test
Common:	
Benign congenital ("central") hypotonia	None; all tests normal.
Hypoxic-ischemic encephalopathy	Evidence of muscle, heart, or other organ injury (elevated CPK or LFTs liver function test); low umbilical cord blood pH; sometimes abnormal CT (edema) or EEG.
Hypotonia associated with congenital anomalies ("syndromic" appearance); typical examples include Down and Prader-Willi syndromes	Karyotype; specific genetic testing based on clinical presentation; genetic consultation.
Uncommon to rare:	
Cervical spinal cord injury	Cervical spine MRI.
Neuromuscular diseases	Specific tests for spinal muscular atrophy, congenital myopathy, myotonic dystrophy, glycogen storage disease, myasthenia gravis on basis of clinical presentation (see text). Muscle biopsy often necessary.
Metabolic and degenerative disorders; peroxisomal disorders.	See Chapter 14 and text; many diagnosed by neonatal screening.
Hypothyroidism	Usually diagnosed by neonatal screening; thyroid function tests.

HYPOTONIC NEONATE

There is considerable overlap between disorders causing neonatal and infantile hypotonia. Although other causes of neonatal hypotonia must be carefully excluded, in many cases, the eventual diagnosis made is that of benign or "central" hypotonia.

Hypoxic-ischemic encephalopathy

Neonatal *hypoxic-ischemic encephalopathy* (HIE) occurs as the result of perinatal cardiorespiratory insufficiency. There is usually a history of low Apgar scores. Most neonates with HIE are poorly responsive, exhibit decreased movements, and are hypotonic. A smaller number of patients are "hyperalert" and jittery. Focal abnormalities such as asymmetrical movements are a worrisome sign suggesting infarction.

Either *low umbilical cord blood pH* or an *elevation of hepatic enzymes or* CPK suggesting hypoxemic damage to muscle, heart, or liver is required for the diagnosis of HIE. If there is no evidence of acidosis or of damage to other organs, another cause should be sought for the neonate's neurological condition. In more severe cases of HIE, computed tomography (CT) demonstrates generalized cerebral edema or focal areas of infarction. The electroencephalogram (EEG) may be abnormally slow or contain epileptiform activity or, in the worst cases, is a burst-suppression tracing.

Neonates with HIE who become more alert within the first few days of life have the best prognosis. Prolonged unresponsiveness, seizures, and focal neurological deficits are poor prognostic signs (11).

Hypotonia associated with congenital anomalies

Many hypotonic neonates are diagnosed with a specific *syndrome of congenital malformation*. Characteristic signs of *Down syndrome* include upslanting palpebral fissures, a low nasal bridge, low-set ears, wide-spaced nipples, and simian creases. Hypotonia in these patients may be mild or severe. The diagnosis is confirmed by routine karyotype. Atlantoaxial instability occurs in cases of Down syndrome and, in rare cases, has resulted in a cervical spinal cord injury. During childhood, a cervical spine x-ray should be reviewed for signs of instability if a patient with Down syndrome wishes to participate in sports. Almond-shaped eyes, a small down-curved mouth, small hands and feet, and small genitalia suggest *Prader-Willi syndrome*. A fluorescent in situ hybridization (FISH) probe can confirm the presence of the gene on chromosome 15 causing this disorder.

Many other syndromes of congenital malformation are associated with generalized hypotonia. TORCH (toxoplasma, rubella, cytomegalovirus, herpies, syphilis) infection is a possibility. A large number of other patients have a dysmorphic appearance or are found to have malformed internal organs but, despite extensive evaluations, are not diagnosed with a specific syndrome. In most such cases, *hypotonia should be considered to be a nonspecific feature of the underlying disorder*. Tests for a neurological or degenerative etiology should not be ordered unless there are aspects of the history or examination (for example, seizures, a midline facial defect, or an abnormal state of arousal) specifically suggesting involvement of the nervous system. Some neuromuscular diseases, such as congenital myopathies (discussed earlier), are associated with dysmorphic features. However, muscle biopsy is not appropriate for the great majority of "syndromic" infants. A geneticist should be consulted if the diagnosis remains uncertain.

Cervical spinal cord injury

A neonate presenting with *flaccid quadriplegia* may have a *cervical spinal cord injury*. In many cases, there is a history of a *difficult delivery* (vaginal or cesarean) resulting in *excessive traction on the neonate's neck*. An infant with an acute cervical spinal cord injury *does not move and is profoundly hypotonic*. Deep tendon reflexes are often not obtainable in the arms and may be either normal or absent in the lower extremities. A swollen bladder is often palpated. If the spinal cord is damaged at an upper cervical level (C5 or above), the result is often *respiratory failure*, since the phrenic nerve originates from C3-5.

Mechanical ventilation is required in cases of respiratory failure. MRI is ordered to assess the cervical spine. If a cervical spinal cord injury is demonstrated, a corticosteroid should be started. A neurosurgical consultation should be requested.

The prognosis correlates with the extent of injury. In cases of transection, the patient may remain permanently quadriplegic and require a tracheotomy.

Neuromuscular diseases in the neonate

A number of hereditary neuromuscular diseases may present in the neonatal period. Neonates with SMA type I (discussed earlier) are immobile and profoundly hypotonic. Deep tendon reflexes are unobtainable, and tongue fasciculations may be noted. The mother may have noticed decreased fetal movements during the third trimester. There may be associated *arthrogryposis* (contractures of the hands or feet); however, arthrogryposis can be caused by other neuromuscular disorders. The DNA test for SMA should be ordered. Treatment is supportive.

The cause of *transitory neonatal myasthenia* is *the antiacetylcholine receptor antibody* carried by the baby's mother and passed to the fetus (12). The diagnosis relies on a *history of myasthenia gravis in the mother*. Affected infants often require mechanical ventilation during the first several weeks of life but recover if supportive care is maintained. The prognosis is good, since symptoms do not recur. Medication for myasthenia gravis is not necessary.

Neonates with congenital myotonic dystrophy (CMD) are hypotonic and may have difficulty breathing and feeding. A "fish-mouth" appearance (caused by facial muscle weakness) is common. CMD is an autosomal dominant disorder usually inherited through the mother (for reasons too complex to detail here, paternal inheritance causes less severe manifestations) (13). If a hypotonic neonate's mother has been diagnosed with myotonic dystrophy, the neonate probably has CMD. CMD may also be suspected if the family history suggests adult-onset myotonic dystrophy: cataracts, diabetes, frontal balding, cardiac conduction defects, or mental retardation in maternal relatives.

The diagnosis of CMD is confirmed by *genetic testing*. The prognosis tends to be poor, with significant mortality resulting from respiratory insufficiency during infancy and a high incidence of mental retardation among patients who survive the neonatal period (14).

Congenital myopathies are discussed earlier. Some forms are fatal in the neonatal period or infancy. However, patients with several forms will survive if supportive care is maintained and make steady developmental progress during childhood.

Pompe disease, a *glycogen storage disease*, should be suspected if a hypotonic neonate is found to have *cardiomegaly*. *Muscle biopsy* is necessary for diagnosis. There is no treatment, and infants with this disease usually die during the first year of life as the result of heart failure.

Other causes of hypotonia in the neonate

Hypothermia, lethargy, hoarse cry, hypotonia, and an open posterior fontanelle are signs of *neonatal hypothyroidism*. In many other cases, the neonate appears normal and hypothyroidism is diagnosed by a neonatal screening test. Ongoing treatment with thyroid hormone is essential to prevent mental retardation (cretinism).

Peroxisomal disorders are a group of rare conditions presenting with seizures, cerebral malformations, a characteristic craniofacial appearance, and malformations of the liver and kidneys as well as global hypotonia (15). The archetypal disorders are *Zellweger syndrome* and *neonatal adrenoleukodystrophy* (not related to childhood-onset adrenoleukodystrophy, discussed in Chapter 10). Peroxisomal disorders are associated with an *elevation of the plasma very long–chain fatty acid level*, which is a good initial screening test. Assays of erythrocyte membrane components, bile acid pathway products, and fibroblast plasmalogen levels sent to a specialized laboratory are required to confirm the diagnosis. The prognosis is generally poor, and treatment is primarily supportive. Seizures are controlled with an antiepileptic drug.

REFERENCES

1. Stewart H, Wallace A, McGaughran J, et al. Molecular diagnosis of spinal muscular atrophy. *Arch Dis Child.* 1998;78:531–535.
2. Hirtz D, Iannaccone S, Heemskerk J, et al. Challenges and opportunities in clinical trials for spinal muscular atrophy. *Neurology.* 2005;65:1352–1357.
3. Cherringon M. Clinical spectrum of botulism. *Muscle Nerve.* 1998;51:1427–1432.
4. Norman A, Harper P. A survey of manifesting carriers of Duchenne and Becker muscular dystrophy in Wales. *Clin Genet.* 1989;36:31–37.
5. DeSilva S, Drachman DB, Mellits D, et al. Prednisone treatment in Duchenne muscular dystrophy. *Arch Neurol.* 1987;44:818–822.
6. Tarnopolsky MAA, Mahoney DJ, Vajsar J, et al. Creatine monohydrate enhances strength and body composition in Duchenne muscular dystrophy. *Neurology.* 2004;62:1771–1777.
7. Brown RH. Dystrophin-associated proteins and the muscular dystrophies: a glossary. *Ann Rev Med.* 1997;48:457–466.
8. Cwik VA, Brooke MH. Disorders of muscle: dystrophies and myopathies. In: Berg BO, ed. *Principles of Child Neurology.* New York: McGraw Hill; 1996:1677–1679.
9. Volpe JJ. *Neurology of the Newborn.* Philadelphia: Saunders; 2001:686–689.

10. Lyon G, Adams RD, Kolodny EH. *Neurology of Hereditary Metabolic Diseases of Children*. New York: McGraw Hill; 1996:219–233.
11. Dixon G, Badawi N, Kurinczuk JJ, et al. Early developmental outcomes after newborn encephalopathy. *Pediatrics*. 2002;109:26–33.
12. Gardnerova M, Eynard B, Morel E, et al. The fetal/adult acetylcholine receptor antibody ratio in mothers with myasthenia gravis as a marker for transfer of the disease to the newborn. *Neurology*. 1997;48:50–54.
13. Gharehbaghi-Schnell EB, Finsterer J, Korschineck I, et al. Genotype-phenotype correlation in myotonic dystrophy. *Clin Genet*. 1998;53:20–26.
14. Ashizawa T. Myotonic dystrophy as a brain disorder. *Arch Neurol*. 1998;55:291–293.
15. Lyon G, Adams RD, Kolodny EH. *Neurology of Hereditary Metabolic Diseases of Children*. New York: McGraw Hill; 1996:30–39.

AUTISM AND LANGUAGE DISORDERS

A toddler who does not follow verbal directions by 18 months, or who is not using words to communicate by 2 years of age should be evaluated by his doctor. Every pediatric intern is taught, appropriately, to order a *hearing test* in this situation. In practice, a disorder of peripheral hearing is rarely revealed. Once the child's hearing has been established to be normal, the next question raised often concerns the possibility that the child may have an *autistic spectrum disorder* (ASD). We are not aware of any studies reporting the prevalence of autism among language-delayed children. In a typical pediatric neurology practice, autism is often diagnosed in these cases; in the authors' experience, about 50% of language-delayed children fall in the autistic spectrum. However, this high number probably reflects selection bias (with more mildly affected children not being referred to the neurologist).

Nonautistic children who are late to acquire language have a better prognosis, although delayed language acquisition often precedes a speech disorder and puts the child at risk for a language-based learning disability.

NOMENCLATURE OF AUTISM

The terms *autistic spectrum disorder* (ASD) and *pervasive developmental disorder* (PDD) mean the same thing. PDD is the basis for the *Diagnostic and Statistical Manual of Mental Disorders, 4th Edition* (DSM-IV) classification, which is important since the diagnosis of *autistic disorder*, the prototypical condition, relies on DSM-IV criteria (1). *Asperger syndrome* is also a DSM-IV diagnosis.

ASD is a better term to use in discussions with family members. Parents often become overly focused on which of the five types of PDD their child has, which matters less than the child's behavior and development. Moreover, one form of PDD described in the DSM is a condition that has nothing to do with autism. Rett syndrome (see Chapter 11) is a fatal degenerative disorder that often initially causes delayed language acquisition and may transiently resemble an ASD. Children with Rett syndrome rapidly deteriorate neurologically, develop seizures, and become mentally retarded, spastic, and ataxic. Life span is about 20 years. Rett syndrome does not, in the authors' opinion, belong in the DSM-IV. The remaining two disorders, Heller's syndrome and PDD–not otherwise specified, are best thought of as belonging to a general spectrum of autistic conditions.

DIAGNOSIS OF AUTISM

Autism is generally characterized by *impaired language skills*, *poor social relatedness*, and a pattern of behavior that is *excessively rigid and inflexible*.

LANGUAGE

Most children with an ASD *have a poorly developed capacity for language.* In severe cases, the autistic child never learns to speak at all or masters only a few words or phrases. More typically, a toddler learns a few words by about 15 months of age and then stops talking (*autistic regression*). Speech may re-emerge months or years later, but the child's use of language rarely reaches age-appropriate norms. Typical features of these children's speech are a limited ability to engage in conversations, echoing or parroting responses (*Examiner*: "What color is your train?"; *Child*: "Your train"), articulation problems, and abnormal *prosody* (flat, nasal, or singsong voice quality).

Children with an ASD often speak in excessively concrete phrases devoid of descriptive, personal, or emotional content. They are often unable to talk about the "big picture." They may describe their favorite television show, movie, story, or activity in a way that fails to communicate the plot or the overall purpose. Instead the autistic child fixates on specifics, such as the color of a book character's clothing, the events in a single scene, or a cursory description of what a character does ("Harry Potter has a wand"). When asked to elaborate, the child will repeat the descriptions. A *limited capacity for imaginative play* (with toys or play acting) also strongly suggests the diagnosis of autism.

Asperger syndrome

Patients with *Asperger syndrome* do not have a history of delayed language milestones. These children speak much more fluently than most other autistic individuals, although their speech is often subtly abnormal in terms of prosody, and their use of language in social situations may be stilted or odd. In addition to acquiring language milestones on schedule, many children with Asperger syndrome are exceptionally good readers (are *hyperlexic*) at an early age. During the last few years, Asperger syndrome has become an "in-vogue" diagnosis inaccurately applied to *any* child with a mild autistic syndrome. According to DSM-IV criteria, if a child has a history of delayed language milestones or significant language impairment, then the child does *not* have Asperger syndrome (1).

SOCIALIZATION

All autistic patients are socially disabled. Young autistic children often play alone or do not progress beyond parallel play. *Poor eye contact* is a classic sign of autism suggesting a limited capacity for social relatedness. Many older autistic children never desire friendships or have "friendships" that are parallel play based. People with an ASD often *are not demonstrative*; in other words, they do not share their interests or enthusiasm with other people. Autistic individuals may *lack a capacity for empathy*, for example, for an individual who is injured or upset. However, the stereotype of the autistic child who has no affection for his parents or others is false. Many of these children are very attached to their parents and siblings (sometimes excessively so) or may be indiscriminately affectionate (for instance, hugging a doctor or nurse whom they have never previously met).

Some autistic people eventually show some interest in making more age-appropriate friendships, but their poor social skills and failure to pick up on interpersonal cues prevent them from interacting easily. Socialization is also often impaired by impulsive, aggressive, or idiosyncratic behaviors and by excessive anxiety, especially in novel situations and large groups.

ADAPTABILITY AND STEREOTYPED BEHAVIORS

Autistic children *do not adapt well to changes in their routine*. The autistic child may become disoriented and upset if the morning drive to his school does not follow an identical same route every day; if he has a new teacher; if his clothing is not always of a particular color or type; if a specific food is not served in a specific way every night; or if the toys or furniture in his room are rearranged. When the child's routine or a familiar daily setting is changed, his behavior may worsen for weeks.

A parent or teacher often reports that the child often makes odd, repetitive, *stereotypic movements* such as flapping the hands, wiggling fingers, and walking on tiptoes. The autistic child's *interests* also tend to be stereotyped. The child may watch the same videotape over and over every day, never losing interest. The child may be obsessed with a particular type of toy (e.g., toy trains) to the exclusion of all other toys, may have an unusual hobby or interest (e.g., reading maps for hours), or may be entranced by a class of ordinary object (e.g., doorknobs, faucets, blinds). *Spinning objects*, such as wheels and tops, fascinate many autistic children. Parents of autistic children refer to these obsessional and repetitive behaviors as "*stimming*" (for self-stimulating). In the case of patients with Asperger syndrome, stereotypic behaviors are often more sophisticated and may take the form of an eccentric or exaggerated interest (reading only books about insects or playing a particular video game to the exclusion of all other interests).

Autism versus obsessive-compulsive disorder

The autistic child's stereotypic, repetitive behaviors resemble the habits of patients with obsessive-compulsive disorder (OCD; see Chapter 5), and therefore, many parents refer to their autistic child's behaviors as "OCD behaviors." In fact, these behaviors differ from those associated with OCD in an important way. The thoughts and behaviors of the patient with OCD are *ego-dystonic*, sources of *discomfort* that drive the patient to seek medical help. In contrast, many autistic children appear to derive *comfort* from their habits (which are thus said to be *ego-syntonic*). This difference may partially explain why the stereotypic behaviors of autistic patients often do not respond to serotonin-selective reuptake inhibitors, which are drugs that are effective for OCD.

Case 9.1

A 12-year-old boy, who was diagnosed with ADHD at age 6, is referred for consultation regarding his medication. He often appears distracted in the classroom. He has been taking methylphenidate since age 8. The medication has never been very effective, although he takes a high dose. A trial of an amphetamine-based drug was also not successful, and the drug was discontinued because of side effects.

Prenatal and perinatal history is unremarkable. Gross motor milestones were normally acquired. Language skills were attained by 2 years of age. The boy read well at age 4 and continues to enjoy reading, although his teacher feels that his reading comprehension is weak. Despite his apparent distractibility, his grades are good. He has always been well behaved in the classroom.

When younger, the child did not enjoy imaginative play but did act out scenes from television shows verbatim. He has never had many friends but is unconcerned about his lack of a social life. He gets very upset if his routine is disrupted, for example, if he does not leave for school by 7:15 every morning. He has long been fascinated by the study of ancient history and possesses a large number of books on the subject.

The physical examination reveals immature fine motor skills and clumsiness while hopping on either foot but no focal neurological deficits. Eye contact is not sustained, and his speech is flat and nasal. The patient makes odd finger movements from time to time.

(continued)

A learning evaluation demonstrates excellent comprehension of a paragraph that is read to him, yet below-average reading comprehension. He has trouble understanding metaphors. When he is asked to explain what "the grass is always greener on the other side" and other common sayings mean, he consistently replies "I can't give you the dictionary definition."

Diagnosis: *Asperger syndrome.*

Outcome: The patient was prescribed atomoxetine, which helped him stay more focused in school. A trial of fluoxetine was later prescribed to address his obsessional behaviors, but it only made him irritable and aggressive; the drug was discontinued. He attends a social skills class but makes no friends. At 20, he still resides with his parents.

Autistic savants

In rare cases, autistic children are extraordinarily gifted. Such children may play a musical instrument at a virtuoso level with little training or perform impossibly complicated mathematical calculations without paper and pencil. These patients are called *autistic savants*. Depictions of these patients in the media aside, they are not typical. Much more commonly in cases of autism, cognitive testing reveals *unusual, incongruous deficits or learning disabilities*. A given cognitive skill may be well developed, yet a related aptitude is poorly developed.

The spectrum of autism

Autism is a *spectrum* of disorders. Many children do not exhibit the full range of features. The diagnosis of an ASD in milder cases usually is made at a later age. This is especially true for autistic children with a well-developed capacity for language (Asperger syndrome). Observation during a series of office visits may be necessary to diagnose a subtle ASD as opposed a behavioral disorder. Referral to a child psychologist may be helpful if the diagnosis remains uncertain. In some cases, the child is ultimately simply said to have an "autistic flavor." Some of these children are diagnosed with a *nonverbal learning disability* (see Chapter 3). The relationship of autism to syndromes currently classified as "psychiatric," such as schizoid personality disorder, is interesting and not well-researched.

ETIOLOGY

Autism can result from a variety of neurodevelopmental defects. Patients with many disorders characterized by abnormal brain development, including Down syndrome, fragile X syndrome, and neurofibromatosis type I are often autistic, suggesting that autism is a developmental/behavioral outcome and not a single disorder.

Although the cause of idiopathic autism (i.e., autism that is not caused by a recognized underlying disorder) is not determined in a large majority of cases, autopsy studies of these patients have reported abnormal development of the cerebellum, amygdala, hippocampus, and cerebral cortex (2–5). Other studies suggest atypical chemical and metabolic activity in the brain (6,7). Functional imaging studies suggest that autistic children use different parts of the brain to perform cognitive tasks than nonautistic children use (8–10).

Autism is more common in boys than in girls. There is a history of an *autistic sibling* in about 5% of cases. Other family members may have a history of *delayed language acquisition*. In the authors' and several colleagues' experience, there is often a history of one or more individuals in the child's family diagnosed with an anxiety or mood disorder (especially *bipolar disorder*) or schizophrenia. It has even been theorized that autism, in some cases, results from a mood disorder that, due to early age of onset, adversely affects brain development (11,12).

Similar conditions

Children with a history of *delayed language acquisition* may be socially withdrawn and make poor eye contact. Many of these children are capable of fantasy play and do not exhibit stereotypic tendencies. The most appropriate diagnosis for these patients is language delay causing social shyness. *Children raised in a setting of social deprivation, such as an orphanage,* may appear autistic. *Depression* in young children can mimic autism (see Chapter 5). Young children with *attention-deficit hyperactivity disorder* (ADHD) may have poor social skills and behave inappropriately and sometimes make poor eye contact as a result of being distracted easily. However, they typically enjoy social interaction and do not have a history of stereotypic or idiosyncratic behaviors. Many autistic children are exceedingly anxious; however, a history of excessive anxiety but of normal language acquisition and a normal interest in making friends is not suggestive of autism but, instead, is suggestive of an *anxiety disorder*. The resemblance of *OCD* to autism is discussed earlier. A history of normal early cognitive development distinguishes psychiatric disorders such as schizophrenia from autism.

Diagnostic testing

Autism is a clinical diagnosis that cannot be confirmed or excluded by any laboratory test. Testing is only for the purpose of finding an underlying cause and reveals a cause infrequently. A *DNA test for fragile X syndrome* is ordered if the autistic patient is a boy. If the examiner suspects Down syndrome, neurofibromatosis type I, or another congenital disorder predisposing to autistic behaviors, a confirmatory genetic test can be ordered.

A *karyotype with high-resolution band analysis* (to detect small deletions) is also often ordered. The value of other tests is debatable. Magnetic resonance imaging (MRI) of the brain may reveal subtle anatomical abnormalities such as slightly enlarged cerebral ventricles or an underdeveloped cerebellum. These findings do suggest that there is abnormal development of the brain but are nonspecific and do not reveal the cause. The yield of tests for metabolic diseases (e.g., organic acids, amino acids, etc.; see Chapter 14) is low, and these tests should not be ordered unless the physician strongly suspects a metabolic condition on other grounds. Electroencephalogram (EEG) is ordered if there is a history of seizures, which have been found to occur in up to 40% of cases of autism (13).

Landau-Kleffner syndrome (LKS) (14) is a rare childhood disorder characterized by *regression of receptive language ability* (auditory verbal agnosia) and *epileptiform discharges*, sometimes occurring with clinical seizures, *during sleep*. Stereotypic behavior, poor eye contact, and poor social relatedness are *not* typical in cases of LKS. In LKS, an EEG recorded during sleep reveals epileptiform discharges. The striking loss of receptive language ability in cases of LKS occurs later in life and should not be confused with the mild early-childhood language regression reported in typical cases of idiopathic autism. LKS often responds to treatment with a corticosteroid (15).

INTERVENTIONS

Behavioral modification

Autistic children should be formally evaluated by the state Early Intervention program or their school district's Child Study Team. *Applied behavior analysis* (ABA) *with discrete trials*, an intensive behavioral modification method that encourages the child to socially interact and use language, is currently the preferred behavioral/educational therapy for autistic children. *ABA is the only therapy for autism that has been shown to be beneficial in controlled studies* (16,17), and although it does not appear to help all patients, ABA should be routinely recommended. Unfortunately, an ABA program is prohibitively expensive for many families, and many states do not yet provide or cover the cost of ABA.

Speech therapy is almost always a part of the treatment plan for an autistic child. Many autistic children receive physical and occupational therapy; given a choice, these services are less important than speech therapy and ABA. A *special classroom or school* is generally recommended. Higher functioning children often can be partially or even completely mainstreamed. Psychotherapy or social skills classes may be beneficial for higher functioning autistic patients, especially patients with Asperger syndrome. Autistic children may respond to behavior modification techniques, taught by a trained child psychologist to the parents, to address specific problems (e.g., unwillingness to toilet train).

Medication

Medication is often prescribed to reduce the intensity of behaviors associated with autism (18). Autistic patients often become agitated or may act impulsively and endanger themselves or others. An antipsychotic drug, such as risperidone, quetiapine, haloperidol, thioridazine, or aripiprazole, is often prescribed to these patients. Other patients respond to a mood-stabilizing drug such as valproate, carbamazepine, oxcarbazepine, or lamotrigine. Alpha-2 agonists (guanfacine and clonidine) also are useful. These drugs are discussed in Chapters 3, 5, and 6. Physicians should be aware that *children with an ASD tend to react unpredictably to psychiatric drugs.* In some cases, these drugs are strikingly effective and well tolerated, and in other cases, the same medications are ineffective or cause undesirable changes in behavior.

Some children with an ASD are *distractible*, and their ability to focus may be improved by a stimulant medication for ADHD (methylphenidate or an amphetamine-based drug). Atomoxetine is often effective if a stimulant medication is not. In other cases, these drugs make patients irritable or aggressive. Some autistic patients who are *withdrawn or anxious* respond well to a tricyclic antidepressant or a serotonin-selective reuptake inhibitor (SSRI). In most cases, treatment with an SSRI does not reduce the frequency or intensity of an autistic child's stereotypic behaviors.

Epidemiology, popular theories about autism, and nontraditional treatments

The incidence of autism may be increasing. This possibility was dramatically suggested by reports from the California Department of Developmental Disabilities documenting a large increase in the number of reported cases of ASD during the 1990s and until 2002 (although a slight decrease was subsequently reported). It is still not clear whether the reported increase reflected better diagnosis and enhanced awareness of the disorder (19) compared with in the past. Some autistic patients might previously have been diagnosed as mentally retarded, psychiatrically disturbed, or simply labeled eccentric. Epidemiological research is conducted by the Centers for Disease Control Autism and Developmental Disabilities Monitoring (ADDM) Network, and the Centers of Excellence for Autism and Developmental Disabilities Research and Epidemiology (CADDRE), which maintain surveillance in 18 states using consistent criteria. Their findings may help determine whether or not autism is truly increasing in frequency.

Reports of an increase in the number of cases of autism as well as the understandable desperation of parents have led to the emergence of a number of popular theories about the cause of autism and an interest in unconventional treatments.

Many parents of autistic children believe that their child's disorder was caused by a routine immunization. The measles, mumps, and rubella (MMR) vaccination is usually blamed. Many parents note, correctly, that autistic tendencies often become evident at about the same age that the MMR is first administered (about 1 year of age). However, epidemiological studies conducted in several countries (20–23) do not support a link between the MMR vaccination and autism. These studies do not demonstrate an increased incidence of autism following MMR vaccination compared with the incidence in nonvaccinated children of the same age or an increase in the incidence of autism during the years immediately following the introduction of the MMR vaccine in the United States in 1971.

Although these studies do not implicate the MMR vaccine, an immunological process could still be the cause of some cases of autism. Exposure to a common virus carrying a new mutation might trigger an antibody response that could damage developing brain neurons during early childhood. Serious immune-mediated neurological complications do occur, albeit rarely, following an immunization or a viral infection, as in cases of acute demyelinating encephalomyelitis (ADEM; see Chapter 13). However, ADEM is a dramatic disease often presenting with fever, seizures, and coma and often causes focal neurological deficits that may become permanent. No such signs and symptoms precede typical cases of autism, and therefore, an immune-mediated process causing this disorder would have to be much subtler.

Many parents believe that thimerosal, a mercury-containing preservative used in vaccines, causes autism. Some parents have even gone so far as to administer a course of a chelating medication to their autistic child in order to remove mercury that they believe is damaging their child's brain. A large Danish study, showing only a continuing increase in the incidence of autism following the removal of thimerosal from vaccines, argues against a relationship between thimerosal and autism (24). More recent studies from the United Kingdom (25,26) also show no relationship. The use of chelating medications should be strongly discouraged given the serious adverse effects that may be caused by these drugs.

Some parents report that their autistic child has chronic diarrhea. A "leaky gut" (in some cases blamed on the MMR vaccination) is theorized to cause the diarrhea and is said to worsen or cause autism by allowing neurotoxic chemicals into the bloodstream. A gluten-free diet is sometimes suggested for these children to improve behavior and enhance neurological development. There are, at this point, no convincing data supporting or refuting the efficacy of a gluten-free diet, which is usually difficult for practical reasons to maintain.

Another popular theory suggests that colonization of the intestine with the fungal organism *Candida* leads to the formation of abnormal organic acids that damage the brain and thereby cause autism. As a result, some autistic children have been prescribed a long course of an antifungal drug. *Candida* is a routinely cultured intestinal organism; why colonization should produce a devastating neurological syndrome in some children and not in other children has not been convincingly explained.

Injections of secretin, a neurotransmitter, have been used to treat autistic children based on anecdotal reports of clinical improvement. Several controlled studies (27; for results of Food and Drug Administration phase III clinical trial, see the *New York Times*, January 6, 2004) have failed to show any benefit from this therapy. Hyman and Levy (28) review many other unconventional therapies.

Autism is a devastating disorder. Physicians should be sympathetic to parents' need to explore exotic theories and treatments. Additionally, we need to expect that many parents will report that these treatments are "working," since children with autism often make progress during the normal course of their development. We should offer the best possible scientific information to families and discourage dangerous treatments, but we should refrain from being high-handedly dismissive of odd-sounding theories and therapies. After all, we do not know what causes most cases of autism, and we have no cure to offer patients and families.

Prognosis

Autism is a life-long disorder. Although speech often improves during childhood, most patients never are able to have normal friendships and remain rigid and unable to adapt to change. Medication to treat symptoms of anxiety or distractibility or to control aggressive outbursts often continues to be necessary. Some autistic adults are employable. Most must live in a supervised setting or with their parents.

PRIMARY DISORDERS OF LANGUAGE

Language disorders of childhood include speech apraxia (poor articulation), stuttering, word-finding difficulty, poorly developed social use of language (semantic pragmatic deficit), and auditory comprehension disorder. The latter syndrome is discussed in Chapter 3 because these children are often diagnosed as a result of a school-related problem.

Webster and Shevell (29) review the neurobiology of these disorders. A history of delayed language milestones is common. Some of these children also have a history of delayed motor development. The physical examination may reveal "soft signs."

Language disorders are usually formally characterized and treated by a speech pathologist or speech therapist. MRI, EEG, and other medical tests are generally of little value.

Selective mutism is defined as a *total lack of speech in specific situations* (e.g., in school or with strangers) (30). Many children diagnosed with selective mutism are anxious or shy. A history of delayed language milestones or a speech disorder is also common. Selective mutism can be confused with an autistic spectrum disorder. Treatment consists of psychotherapy, speech therapy, or a medication to alleviate anxiety such as an SSRI.

MENTAL RETARDATION

Mental retardation (MR) is usually diagnosed during childhood following a history of markedly delayed cognitive development. The diagnosis of MR requires a full-scale IQ below 70. Patients display poor adaptive as well as intellectual skills. *Mild, moderate, severe, and profound* MR are respectively identified by an IQ of 50 to 70, 35 to 50, 20 to 35, and below 20. Patients with an IQ of 70 to 80 fall in the borderline range.

Examination and diagnostic testing

The patient's skin should be examined for signs of a neurocutaneous disorder. Dysmorphic features suggest a syndrome of congenital malformation. A geneticist is often consulted.

The diagnosis of MR relies *on psychological testing* demonstrating an IQ below 70. A *fragile X DNA test* should be ordered if the patient is male. The plasma lead level should be checked. *Karyotype with high-resolution band analysis* to look for microdeletions is often ordered. MRI usually does not contribute to the diagnosis in cases of mild or moderate MR, but in cases of severe and profound MR, MRI may show evidence of a hypoxemic brain injury, focal infarction, or a congenital brain malformation. A degenerative or metabolic disorder is rarely the cause of mental retardation, but the state neonatal screening panel should be checked to make certain that slowly progressive diseases, such as phenylketonuria, have been ruled out.

Patients with mild MR are capable of about a sixth grade level of education and can be employed in a supervised setting. As adults, they often live with their parents or in a group home. Patients with moderate MR acquire communication and self-care skills and can be trained to perform simple, repetitive tasks. They must reside in a highly supervised environment. Patients with severe MR may learn some adaptive and self-help behaviors and can be taught to speak a few words. Patients with profound MR cannot speak or care for themselves, are capable of few useful behaviors, and require constant supervision. Most are nonambulatory, and spastic quadriparesis is common. Many are blind or visually impaired. Life expectancy is typically under 20 years.

Many patients with MR have autistic tendencies. Other behavioral problems associated with MR include outbursts, mood swings, excessive anxiety, hyperactivity, and psychosis. Behavioral modification or treatment with a neuroleptic, stimulant, antidepressant, or mood-stabilizing medication may be helpful.

REFERENCES

1. American Psychiatric Association. *Diagnostic and Statistical Manual of Mental Disorders, Text Revision.* 4th ed. Washington, DC: American Psychiatric Association; 2000;69–84.
2. Bauman M, Kemper T. Histoanatomical observations of the brain in early infantile autism. *Neurology.* 1985;35:866–974.

3. Casanova MF, Buxhoeveden DP, Switala AE, et al. Minicolumnar pathology in autism. *Neurology*. 2002;58:428–432.
4. Haas RH, Townsend J, Courchesne E, et al. Neurological abnormalities in infantile autism. *J Child Neurol*. 1996;11:84–92.
5. Aylward EH, Minshew NJ, Goldstein G, et al. MRI volumes of amygdala and hippocampus in non-mentally retarded autistic adolescents and adults. *Neurology*. 1999;53:2145–2150.
6. Friedman SD, Shaw DW, Artru AA, et al. Regional brain chemical alterations in young children with autism spectrum disorder. *Neurology*. 2003;60:100–107.
7. Purcell AE, Jeon OH, Zimmerman AW, et al. Postmortem brain abnormalities of the glutamate neurotransmitter system in autism. *Neurology*. 2001;57:1618–1628.
8. Luna B, Minshew NJ, Garver KE, et al. Neocortical system abnormalities in autism. *Neurology*. 2002;59:834–840.
9. Huhl D, Bolte S, Feineis-Matthews S, et al. Functional imbalance of visual pathways indicates alternative face processing strategies in autism. *Neurology*. 2003;61:1232–1237.
10. Herbert MR, Harris GJ, Kristen KT, et al. Abnormal asymmetry in language association cortex in autism. *Ann Neurol*. 2002;52:588–596.
11. DeLong CR. Autism: new data suggest a new hypothesis. *Neurology*. 1999;52:911–916.
12. Chugani DC, Muzik O, Behen M, et al. Developmental changes in brain serotonin synthesis capacity in autistic and nonautistic children. *Ann Neurol*. 1999;54:287–295.
13. Danielsson S, Gillberg IC, Billstedt E, et al. Epilepsy in young adults with autism: a prospective population-based follow-up study of 120 individuals. *Epilepsia*. 2005;46:918–923.
14. Landau WM, Kleffner FR. Syndrome of acquired aphasia with convulsive disorder in children. *Neurology*. 1957;7:523–530.
15. Sinclair DB, Snyder TJ. Corticosteroids for the treatment of Landau-Kleffner syndrome and continuous spike-wave discharge during sleep. *Pediatr Neurol*. 2005;32:300–306.
16. Maurice C, ed. *Behavioral Intervention in Young Children with Autism*. Austin, TX: Pro-Ed; 1996.
17. Lovaas OI. Behavioral treatment and normal educational and intellectual functioning in young autistic children. *J Consult Clin Psychol*. 1987;55:3–9.
18. Kwok WM. Psychopharmacology in autism spectrum disorders. *Curr Opin Psychiatry*. 2003;16:529–534.
19. Coury DL, Nash PL. Epidemiology and etiology of autistic spectrum disorders difficult to determine. *Pediatr Ann*. 2003;32:696–700.
20. Taylor B, Miller E, Farrington CP, et al. Autism and measles, mumps, and rubella vaccine: no epidemiological evidence for a causal connection. *Lancet*. 1999;353:2026–2029.
21. Makela, A, Nuorti JP, Heikki, P. Neurologic disorders after measles-mumps-rubella vaccination. *Pediatrics*. 2002;110:957–963.
22. Kaye JA, del Mar Melero-Montes M, Jick H. Mumps, measles, and rubella vaccine and the incidence of autism recorded by general practitioners: a time trend analysis. *BMJ*. 2001;322:460–463.
23. Gillberg C, Steffenberg S, Schaumann H. Is autism more common now than ten years ago? *Br J Psychiatry*. 1991;158:403–409.

24. Madsen KM, Lauritsen MB, Pedersen CB, et al. Thimerosal and the occurrence of autism: negative ecological evidence from Danish population-based data. *Pediatrics.* 2003;112:604–606.
25. Heron J, Golding J, the ALSPAC Study Team. Thimerosal exposure in infants and developmental disorders: a prospective cohort study in the United Kingdom does not support a causal association. *Pediatrics.* 2004;114:577–583.
26. Andrews N, Miller E, Grant A, et al. Thimerosal exposure in infants and developmental disorders: a retrospective study in the United Kingdom does not support a causal association. *Pediatrics.* 2004;114:584–591.
27. Dunn-Geier J, Ho HH, Auersperg E, et al. Effect of secretin on children with autism: a randomized controlled trial. *Dev Med Child Neurol.* 2000;42:796–802.
28. Hyman SL, Levy SE. Autistic spectrum disorders: when nontraditional medicine is not enough. *Contemp Pediatr.* 2000;17:101–116.
29. Webster RI, Shevell, MI. Neurobiology of specific language impairment. *J Child Neurol.* 2004;19:471–481.
30. Krysanski VL. A brief review of selective mutism literature. *J Psychol.* 2003; 137:29–40.

10

CEREBRAL PALSY (STATIC ENCEPHALOPATHY) AND RELATED PROBLEMS

CEREBRAL PALSY

Cerebral palsy (CP) is a general term for a *nonprogressive motor impairment* accompanied, usually, by *spasticity*. CP always results from a prenatal, perinatal, or neonatal brain injury, although in many cases, the timing of the injury cannot be determined. In some cases, MRI cannot detect the injury to the brain.

CP is also a term loosely, and questionably, used to characterize a range of nonprogressive upper motor neuron syndromes of infancy and childhood. For example, a spastic 6-year-old boy in a wheelchair may be said (by his parents or even physician) to have "CP resulting from bacterial meningitis at age 2," "CP caused by untreated hydrocephalus," or even "CP after removal of a brain tumor." *Static encephalopathy* is a more accurate term for these nonprogressive syndromes that often clinically resemble typical cases of congenital CP.

Etiology

The cause of CP in a patient who was born at term after a normal pregnancy is often never discovered. A history of a difficult delivery or perinatal cardiorespiratory distress is *not* commonly reported. As every pediatric resident quickly learns during his or her first rotation in the delivery room, the "umbilical cord wrapped around the neck," notorious in the popular imagination, is a routine occurrence and only exceptionally results in a hypoxemic injury to the brain. A low ($\leq$3) Apgar score at 1, 5, and even 10 minutes generally does not predict the development of CP (1). A viral infection during pregnancy might disrupt fetal brain development but almost never can be proven to be the cause of CP in a particular patient.

In some cases, however, there is a history of toxemia, tobacco or cocaine use, or another potential cause of placental insufficiency, and in other cases, a specific disorder known to affect brain development can be identified. Some TORCH (toxoplasma, syphilis, rubella, cytomegalovirus, or herpes) infections cause a CP-like syndrome. In most such cases, the patient exhibits characteristic facial dysmorphisms, ophthalmological or otological problems, microcephaly, or cerebral calcifications visible by computed tomography (CT). Uncommon brain malformations identified by magnetic resonance imaging (MRI), such as lissencephaly and holoprosencephaly, often cause motor delays and spasticity. These patients often are microcephalic, are dysmorphic in appearance, and have seizures.

The etiology of CP in children who were born prematurely or who required mechanical ventilation in the neonatal intensive care unit is better understood. A characteristic radiological finding, *periventricular leukomalacia* (PVL), resulting from an injury to cerebral white matter lying adjacent to the lateral cerebral ventricles, is well described. The periventricular area consists of axons of cortical upper motor neurons that project to the lumbar spinal cord, where they synapse on spinal motor neurons that supply the lower extremities. *Spastic weakness of the legs* (a classic upper motor neuron finding; see Chapter 1) thus typically results from PVL.

Physiological factors contributing to the development of PVL include fragile periventricular blood vessels, a poorly developed capacity for cerebrovascular autoregulation, an inadequate reaction to injury by immature astrocytes, and a high brain water content in the brain of the neonate (2,3). Maternal infection resulting in cytokine-mediated neurological injury in the fetus has also been suggested to be the cause of some cases of PVL (4).

Clinical manifestations

The classic clinical syndrome caused by PVL is *spastic diplegia*. In the mildest cases, the toddler or child may be unaffected other than having *tight heel cords*. Tight heel cords restrict the child's ability to dorsiflex the foot and cause tripping and falling. Children with tight heel cords often *walk on their tiptoes* and are unable to walk on their heels. Some of these children were late to learn to walk. On examination, the foot cannot be dorsiflexed beyond 90 degrees. Percussion of the Achilles tendon while the foot is held in dorsiflexion may elicit clonus.

Toe walking is also a common stereotypic behavior of *autistic children* and can also be a *habit of a normal child* that has no neurological significance. Tightness of the heel cords is not noted in typical cases of autism or habitual toe walking.

Tightness of the thigh adductors is another common manifestation of spastic diplegia. An early sign, during infancy, may be a "catch" when the thigh is passively abducted. The examiner may, in these cases, obtain a *crossed adductor reflex* (adduction of both thighs when the medial surface of one thigh is struck with the reflex hammer). *Spread of reflexes* may also be noted, so that when one deep tendon reflex is obtained, the entire limb will briskly respond. When tight heel cords accompany adductor tightness, the patient's gait is usually compromised. These patients may walk with a *circumducting gait*. Other patients develop more extensive spasticity affecting multiple muscle groups in the lower extremities, further impairing ambulation or preventing ambulation altogether. Disabling *joint contractures* develop in many cases.

Other presentations of CP

In some cases of CP, a parent initially brings their baby for evaluation because the infant has been *delayed in acquiring the early motor milestones* of head control, rolling over, or sitting up. During the first few months of life, the physical examination of these patients usually reveals *hypotonia* that can be demonstrated by the pull-to-sit test or vertical and horizontal suspension (see Fig. 1.4). These patients may be indistinguishable from infants with benign or central hypotonia (see Chapter 8). However, the clinical presentation begins to differ at between 3 and 6 months of age, when spasticity in the extremities and sometimes the trunk is first noted. The delayed appearance of spasticity can be explained by the normal delay in the myelination of the brain and spinal cord during infancy. When spasticity has developed, passive flexion of a limb often elicits excessive resistance followed by a give-way or *clasp-knife* response. Tight heel cords or adductor tightness may also be noted. Arching of the back (*opisthotonic posturing*), a tendency to hold the hands in a "fisted" position, stiffness or "scissoring" of the legs, and mild to coarse tremors of the extremities (*tonic spasms*) are other common manifestations of spasticity.

Infants with CP who were born at term typically develop spasticity of all limbs (quadriparesis). MRI may reveal generalized attenuation of the cerebral white matter, cortical atrophy, or, in the most severe cases, multifocal infarcts. Many of these patients never become ambulatory, and spasticity in the upper extremities makes it difficult for them to use their hands. Joint contractures are often a significant problem for these patients.

As children with CP grow older, *truncal hypotonia* often persists, even though the extremities become progressively spastic. It is not unusual to see a child or adolescent with immobile, spastic extremities and joint contractures, yet whose truncal hypotonia precludes an upright posture in the wheelchair. Limb muscles and axial muscles are supplied by different brainstem and spinal pathways, resulting in this mixed picture.

Choreoathetoid CP was once common in children who had had *kernicterus* as infants and is still occasionally seen. Patients present with athetoid (writhing) or dystonic movements primarily of the upper extremities. MRI may reveal the injury to the basal ganglia. Antipsychotic medications (see Chapter 4) are used to treat the movement disorder. Choreoathetoid CP has become rare as a result of the aggressive treatment of neonatal hyperbilirubinemia.

Diagnostic studies

Practice-parameter guidelines for children with CP have recently been published (5), and suggestions for diagnostic studies are included. PVL can be detected in the neonate by *cranial ultrasound*. Most lesions associated with CP, including PVL, multifocal infarction, and white matter attenuation, can be demonstrated by CT (Fig. 10.1). MRI is better for identifying abnormalities in the cerebral gray matter such as congenital malformations. If the imaging study reveals a congenital malformation or calcification or if the patient has a dysmorphic appearance, then karyotype, TORCH titers, and appropriate genetic studies should be ordered. EEG should be ordered if the patient is suspected of having seizures.

Management

Patients diagnosed with CP should be followed at a center for children with neurological disabilities so that appropriate services can be coordinated. Physical therapy, speech therapy, occupational therapy, and social work

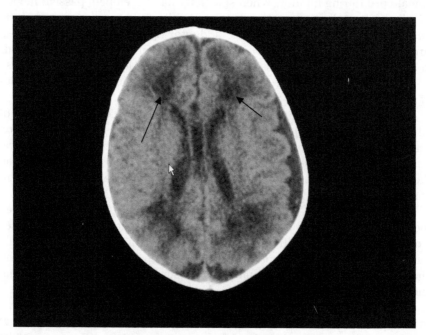

Figure 10.1 CT showing **periventricular leukomalacia** in a female neonate. Arrows show areas of infarction. (Courtesy of Howard Seigerman, MD, and Eliot Lerner, MD, The Valley Hospital.)

services, as well the services of an orthopedic surgeon, general surgeon, neurologist, urologist, and gastroenterologist, should be available.

A daily regimen of range-of-motion exercises and a fitted *ankle-foot orthosis* (AFO) to maintain the foot in a position of dorsiflexion are often prescribed to address heel cord tightness. Orthotic appliances to minimize thigh adduction and to prevent joint contractures at the knees, wrists, and elbows are worn by more severely disabled patients.

Lioresal, dantrolene, or clonazepam is sometimes prescribed to diminish spasticity, but the usefulness of these drugs is limited by a high incidence of sedation. A surgically implanted intrathecal lioresal (Baclofen) pump allows for lioresal to be administered in lower doses, significantly reducing somnolence (6).

Intramuscular injections of botulinum toxin (Botox, Allergen), a neuro-muscular junction (anticholinergic) agent, are given to treat spasticity. Injections are usually given every 3 months. The site of the injections must be carefully selected to provide comfort and increased range of motion but not impair useful motor function. Botulinum toxin also cannot be used in too many muscle groups because of the danger of causing systemic toxicity. Immunity to the toxin eventually develops, and switching to a different serotype may become necessary.

Some patients benefit from tendon-lengthening surgery and other proce-dures to improve range of motion at the ankle, knee, wrist, or elbow prevent or delay the development of joint contractures. Selective rhizotomy (dorsal nerve root section) is sometimes performed to decrease spasticity in one or more limbs.

Associated problems

Many general medical problems are associated with CP. The tonic muscle activity associated with spasticity requires a high metabolic rate that often leads to *cachexia. Neuroendocrine dysfunction* may result in *growth retar-dation* and *precocious puberty. Hip displacement* is a common complication of adductor spasticity. *Pressure sores and skin infections* often result from immobility and long hours spent in a wheelchair. *Kyphosis* and *scoliosis* (causing restricted lung capacity), diminished intercostal and accessory respiratory muscle strength, and poor ability to regulate secretions predis-pose the patient to episodes of *pneumonia.* In many cases of CP, the *ability to swallow is impaired,* and a gastrostomy tube for feeding must be placed to prevent aspiration. *Gastroesophageal reflux* is also common. *Urinary tract infections* result from frequent bladder catheterization. Largely as a result of these complications, life expectancy is only about 20 years for patients with severe CP.

Many patients with CP have *seizures* that should be differentiated from nonepileptic *tonic spasms* (resulting from spasticity). A history of tonic-clonic movements, a change in the patient's level of consciousness, tonic eye deviation, nystagmus, or cyanosis suggests an epileptic seizure. An electroencephalogram (EEG) may help to differentiate seizures from tonic spasms. In most cases of CP, seizures are partial and can be controlled with an appropriate antiepileptic drug (AED).

UNCOMMON CAUSES OF CHILDHOOD STIFFNESS

Hypocalcemia and *hypomagnesemia* can cause increased muscle tone (*tetany*). *Neuromyotonia, Schwartz-Jampel syndrome, startle disease*, and *stiff-person syndrome* are rare neuromuscular conditions causing muscle stiffness (7–9).

NEONATAL STIFFNESS AND JITTERINESS

Hypertonicity and tremulousness during the *neonatal* period usually do not result from spasticity. An abnormally low plasma glucose, calcium, phosphorus, or magnesium level and drug withdrawal (from chronic prenatal opiate exposure) should be excluded by appropriate laboratory tests. Many jittery neonates simply have an immature nervous system, and their tremors improve during the first few weeks of life. In rare cases, a serious neurological disorder, such as a leukodystrophy, is found to be the cause, but in these cases, abnormal findings other than hypertonicity can usually be elicited.

PRENATAL AND PERINATAL STROKE

Not all risk factors for prenatal and perinatal stroke (focal infarction) have been identified, but a large number of predisposing conditions are recognized. Intrauterine growth retardation and preeclampsia increase the risk of prenatal and neonatal stroke according to one study (10). Prothrombotic tendencies are discovered in a substantial number of cases (11). Agenesis of a cerebral artery is sometimes determined to be the cause.

The initial manifestation of a *peri*natal stroke is often *seizure activity* during the first few days of life. An imaging study is ordered and reveals an abnormal-appearing area in the cerebral hemisphere contralateral to the seizure, consistent with infarction. In contrast, neonates with a history of a focal cerebral infarction that occurred weeks or months *before delivery* often exhibit no symptoms at birth and present with *hemiparesis during infancy*. A parent at some point usually notices that the infant does not use one upper extremity as much as the other. One arm is clearly favored when reaching and holding, and the other arm is held at the side. In some cases, there is also involvement of the lower extremity. Spasticity sometimes develops. The deep tendon reflexes are usually brisk on the affected side, and a Babinski sign may be noted.

Diagnostic testing

Depending on the age of the infarction, MRI may reveal an area of ischemia, atrophy, or a cystic cavity (*porencephalic cyst*) in the cerebral hemisphere contralateral to the motor deficit (Fig. 10.2). Magnetic resonance angiography (MRA) is recommended to visualize possible anomalies of the cerebral vessels predisposing to infarction. Laboratory tests should include complete blood count, lactic acid (elevated in mitochondrial disorders), sickle-cell preparation, and plasma homocysteine level (which, when elevated, predisposes to thrombosis). A hematologist will generally order *tests to exclude prothrombotic risk factors* (Factor V Leiden mutation, Protein C and S deficiency, antithrombin III deficiency, and other disorders). A cardiologist is often consulted, and electrocardiogram (EKG), echocardiogram, and possibly Holter monitoring are ordered. In many cases, however, no cause for the stroke is discovered (12).

Prognosis

A prenatal or perinatal stroke often does not lead to hemiparesis, aphasia, or a disabling cognitive impairment in childhood. Presumably, the prognosis following an early cerebral infarction is favorable because of the plasticity of the developing brain. In many cases, the unaffected hemisphere assumes many

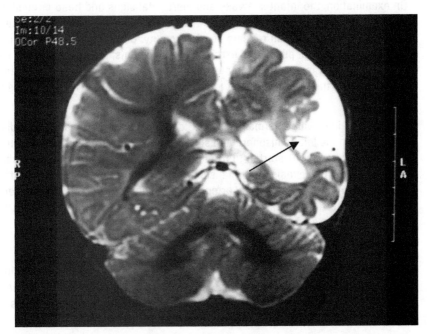

Figure 10.2 MRI showing a **chronic left hemispheric infarct** in a 6-month-old infant. (Courtesy of Howard Seigerman, MD, and Eliot Lerner, MD, The Valley Hospital.)

functions originally assigned to the hemisphere in which the stroke occurred. If the stroke involved the left hemisphere, the patient often becomes left handed. In most cases, language abilities used for everyday communication are unimpaired. However, more subtle cognitive deficits can often be demonstrated by neuropsychological testing (13,14). During the first several years of life, these children usually receive physical, occupational, and speech therapy. Some patients require an orthotic device, botulinum toxin injections, or surgery to treat spasticity. However, most patients are ambulatory. Patients whose stroke involved the cerebral cortex are at risk for focal seizures, which can be controlled with an AED.

Case 10.1

A hospital nurse notes that the right arm of a 2-day-old female neonate is spasmodically jerking. The baby appears alert, and no other abnormal behaviors or signs are noted. The baby is transferred to the neonatal intensive care unit for evaluation of suspected seizures. Phenobarbital is started.

The patient had been born by cesarean section following an uncomplicated 35-week twin pregnancy. She weighed 5 lbs at birth, and her Apgar scores were normal. She has been feeding well and has had no other medical problems.

On examination, the infant is awake and alert. Vital signs and head circumference are normal. The anterior fontanelle is flat. Examination of the skin, facies, heart, lung, and abdomen reveals no abnormality. Cranial nerve examination demonstrates normal pupils and extraocular movements; facial movements are symmetric; suck is strong. Motor examination reveals decreased tone and movements of the right upper and lower extremity. The Moro reflex is absent on the right.

CT of the brain is within normal limits. EEG demonstrates abnormally sharp discharges from the left hemisphere and slowing of the background rhythm on the same side. Acyclovir is started to treat possible herpes encephalitis. MRI performed 1 day later reveals abnormal signal in the left frontoparietal area in the distribution of the middle cerebral artery. Lumbar puncture does not reveal pleocytosis or other abnormalities. Polymerase chain reaction (PCR) and viral culture for herpes are negative. Acyclovir is discontinued.

Diagnosis: *Acute temporal lobe infarct (ischemic stroke).*

Outcome: All laboratory studies, including those ordered by the consulting hematologist to evaluate prothrombotic risk factors, yield no abnormal findings. Echocardiogram and EKG are normal. MRA of the cerebral blood vessels is normal.

The baby is discharged from the hospital at 3 weeks of age and is still taking phenobarbital. She is followed closely and receives early intervention services.

At 3 months of age, she still does not move the right arm as much as the left. However, she achieves head control, rolls over, and sits up on schedule. She remains seizure free. An EEG is repeated at 6 months and demonstrates slowing over the right temporal lobe but no epileptiform discharges. Phenobarbital is discontinued.

By 15 months, the patient has learned to walk, but her gait appears asymmetric. Her right heel cord is tight, and the deep tendon reflexes are brisk on the right. An ankle-foot orthosis is prescribed by her orthopedist. She continues to be followed in clinic, and by 3 years of age, her gait is virtually normal. At this point, she is starting to scribble on paper using her left hand. At 5 years, her speech is normal to most observers, although she seems to have some trouble following multistep directions. She does well in school until first grade, when reading skills are slow to develop.

LEUKODYSTROPHIES

The leukodystrophies comprise a group of uncommon to rare hereditary diseases that result in loss of motor function and, in most cases, hypertonicity. Unlike CP, the leukodystrophies are *degenerative diseases*. Leukodystrophies may also present with or lead to the development of ataxia, cognitive deterioration, seizures, and many other neurological problems. The underlying process in all of the leukodystrophies is the *progressive destruction of myelin*. The biochemical cause and the clinical presentation differentiate these disorders.

Although a leukodystrophy may first present during infancy, childhood, adolescence, or even adult life, some presentations are most typical. *Krabbe disease* classically presents during the neonatal or early infantile period (15). Patients are *irritable, hypertonic*, often *blind*, make no developmental progress, and fail to thrive. Progression to a vegetative state or death is rapid. The most common presentation of *metachromatic leukodystrophy* (MLD) is of arrest of motor and cognitive development during late infancy or early childhood, followed by gradual regression. In cases of middle childhood–onset *adrenoleukodystrophy* (ALD), striking behavioral symptoms, such as hyperactivity or psychosis, may precede other signs of neurological deterioration, and these children may initially be thought to have attention-deficit hyperactivity disorder (ADHD) or a psychiatric disorder. Dysarthria, ataxia, spasticity, loss of ambulation, blindness, and dementia eventually follow. *Adrenal insufficiency* is caused by ALD and may precede or follow the neurological manifestations. *Pelizaeus-Merzbacher disease* is a rare X-linked leukodystrophy that may present during infancy or childhood, often with abnormal eye movements as the first sign, followed by a degenerative course. *Canavan disease* and *Alexander disease* are diseases of the cerebral white matter that usually present during infancy. These infants are often *macrocephalic*.

Diagnostic tests

In cases of leukodystrophy, *MRI* reveals *abnormal-appearing cerebral white matter* (Fig. 10.3). Specific clinical findings and tests may be diagnostically helpful. As a result of involvement of the *peripheral as well as central nervous system*, patients with MLD, ALD, and sometimes Krabbe disease (but not the other leukodystrophies) are found to have *diminished deep tendon reflexes despite generalized hypertonicity*, and *prolonged nerve conduction velocities* (see Chapter 12). The plasma *very long–chain fatty acid* level is elevated in ALD. ALD may cause adrenal failure, and plasma electrolytes and the cortisol level should be closely followed. An elevated *urine sulfatide* level is suggestive of MLD, although is nonspecific and also occurs in cases of mucopolysaccharidosis (see Chapter 14). Genetic testing is available for ALD and MLD. The diagnosis of Krabbe disease can be definitively

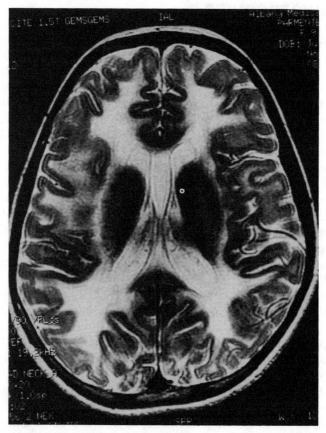

Figure 10.3 MRI of **metachromatic leukodystrophy** in a 9-year-old girl, showing diffuse white matter changes.

made by *enzyme assay of cultured fibroblasts from a skin biopsy*, demonstrating a deficiency of the enzyme *galactocerebroside beta galactosidase*. A genetic test is also available. An elevated *urine N-acetylaspartic acid* level is diagnostic of Canavan disease. Pelizaeus-Merzbacher disease can be diagnosed by a genetic test. Brain biopsy is currently necessary to diagnose Alexander disease, but genetic testing may soon be available.

Treatment

All of the leukodystrophies cause global neurological deterioration leading to a vegetative state or death, although the rate of deterioration varies (younger patients, as a rule, have the worst prognosis). *Genetic counseling is essential.* ALD and Pelizaeus-Merzbacher disease are X-linked recessive disorders, and the other leukodystrophies are autosomal recessive disorders. Prenatal testing for many of these conditions is available.

Orally administered medium-chain fatty acids (Lorenzo's oil) may benefit patients with ALD (16,17), especially if started early in the course of the disease. Patients with MLD and ALD have benefited significantly from bone marrow transplantation (18,19). Bone marrow transplantation also may slow the course of Krabbe disease. Gene therapy is being attempted for Canavan disease.

ERB PALSY
Clinical presentation

An otherwise healthy neonate with an immobile, floppy arm usually has *Erb palsy*. Erb palsy results from an *injury to the upper brachial plexus*, resulting in flaccid weakness of muscles supplied by the fifth and sixth cervical nerve roots. The classic history is that of a large-for-gestational age baby, often the infant of a diabetic mother, who was born following a prolonged vaginal delivery, sometimes complicated by shoulder dystocia. *The affected extremity is usually immobile, flaccid, adducted, and internally rotated.* The *Moro response is asymmetric.* The biceps reflex is absent (although it is difficult to obtain even in a normal neonate), but the brachioradialis reflex is intact.

If the *lower part of the brachial plexus* (C7-T1) is also involved, *complete paralysis* of the extremity with abolition of all deep tendon reflexes and ipsilateral *Horner syndrome* results. Horner syndrome is defined by the triad of ptosis (drooping of the eyelid), meiosis (absent pupillary dilatation), and anhidrosis (diminished facial sweating) and is caused by an interruption of the cervical sympathetic pathway. Horner syndrome may be partial (i.e., ptosis only) or complete.

In a small number of cases of neonatal brachial plexus injury, involvement of higher cervical (C3-4) efferents causes *unilateral paralysis of the diaphragm* presenting with *asymmetrical respirations.*

Diagnostic studies

Erb palsy is a clinical diagnosis. Sometimes a shoulder x-ray shows an *ipsilateral clavicular fracture.* In the relatively rare case of Erb palsy that does not resolve after 2 to 3 months, electromyography and MRI of the brachial plexus are ordered. In cases of partial diaphragmatic paralysis, *fluoroscopy* is used to observe the movements of the diaphragm.

Prognosis and treatment

In most cases of Erb palsy, upper extremity function improves to normal or near normal (20). *Physical therapy* is provided during the period of recovery to prevent the development of joint contractures. A good outcome is generally to be expected. In a small percentage of cases there is no improvement or very limited recovery of function. These patients may be candidates for surgery, which entails removal of scar tissue at the injury site and reanastomosis of damaged nerves with a sural nerve graft. Both the timing and efficacy are controversial (21,22).

Diaphragmatic paralysis may or may not spontaneously improve. Surgical plication of the diaphragm or a diaphragmatic pacemaker is considered in refractory cases.

TORTICOLLIS IN INFANCY

Torticollis, or head tilt, may be fixed or intermittent. Many cases of *fixed* torticollis in the neonatal period are the result of intrauterine positioning. The infant's head is tilted to one side and cannot be easily moved to the midline. There are no other complaints or abnormal neurological findings. Head position usually normalizes over the course of several months. Physical therapy may help. In some cases, torticollis is caused by a fibrous contracture of the sternocleidomastoid muscle (23) and is treated surgically.

When torticollis is associated with one or more *focal neurological abnormalities, hypotonia, or spasticity,* or if there is a history of *developmental delay,* a serious cause needs to be excluded. A *tumor in the brainstem or cervical spine* may be the cause, and therefore, MRI should be ordered. A malformation of the cranial base or of a cervical vertebra, which is often better seen by CT, can also cause torticollis.

Intermittent torticollis in the infant is sometimes associated with a family history of *migraine.* Episodes of torticollis may last several days and are separated by periods during which no torticollis is noted. The episodes eventually stop occurring. The patient may be at increased risk for developing migraine headaches when older.

Sandifer syndrome refers to repeated episodes of abnormal head or neck positioning caused by *gastroesophageal reflux disease* (see Chapter 4). The episodes will stop occurring if the underlying cause is effectively treated.

REFERENCES

1. Freeman JM, Nelson KB. Intrapartum asphyxia and cerebral palsy. *Pediatrics.* 1988;82:240–249.
2. Volpe JJ. *Neurology of the Newborn.* Saunders: Philadelphia; 1995:291–299.
3. Volpe JJ. Cerebral white matter injury of the premature infant: more common than you think. *Pediatrics.* 2003;112:176–180.
4. Graham EM, Holcroft CJ, Rai KK, et al. Neonatal cerebral white matter injury in preterm infants is associated with culture positive infections and only rarely with metabolic acidosis. *Am J Obstet Gynecol.* 2004;191:1305–1310
5. Ashwal S, Russman BS, Blasco PA, et al. Practice parameter: diagnostic assessment of the child with cerebral palsy. Report of the Quality Standards Subcommittee of the American Academy of Neurology and the Practice Committee of the Child Neurology Society. *Neurology.* 2004;62:851–863.
6. Buonaguro V, Scelsa B, Curci D, et al. Epilepsy and intrathecal baclofen therapy in children with cerebral palsy. *Pediatr Neurol.* 2005;33:110–113.
7. Shillito P, Molenar PC, Vincent A, et al. Acquired neuromyotonia: evidence for autoantibodies directed against K+ channels of peripheral nerves. *Ann Neurol.* 1995;38:713–722.
8. Giedion A, Boltshauser E, Briner J, et al. Heterogeneity in Schwartz-Jampel chondrodystrophic myotonia. *Eur J Pediatr.* 1997;156:214–223.
9. Kissel AJ, Ebel RJ. Stiff-person syndrome: stiff opposition to a simple explanation. *Neurology.* 1998;51:11–14.
10. Wu Y, March WM, Croen LA, et al. Perinatal stroke in children with motor impairment: a population-based study. *Pediatrics.* 2004;114:612–619.
11. Lynch JK, Han CJ, Nee LE, et al. Prothrombotic risk factors in children with stroke or porencephaly. *Pediatrics.* 2005;116:447–453.
12. Volpe JJ. *Neurology of the Newborn.* Philadelphia: Saunders; 2001:315–323.
13. Nass R, DeCoudres Peterson H, Koch D. Differential effects of congenital left and right brain injury on intelligence. *Brain Cogn.* 1989;9:258–266.
14. Janowsky JS, Nass R. Early language development in infants with cortical and subcortical brain injury. *J Dev Behav Pediatr.* 1987;8:3–7.
15. Lyon G, Adams RD, Kolodny EH. *Neurology of Hereditary Metabolic Diseases of Children.* New York: McGraw Hill; 1996:66–76; 344–345.
16. Moser HW. Lorenzo's oil. *Lancet.* 1993;341:544.
17. Moser HW, Raymond GV, Lu SE, et al. Follow-up of 89 asymptomatic patients with adrenoleukodystrophy treated with Lorenzo's oil. *Arch Neurol.* 2005;62:1073–1080.
18. Lyon G, Adams RD, Kolodny EH. *Neurology of Hereditary Metabolic Diseases of Children.* New York: McGraw Hill; 1996:66–76; 359–360.
19. Bayever E, Ladisch M, Philippart M, et al. Bone marrow transplantation for metachromatic leukodystrophy. *Lancet.* 1985;1:471–473.

20. Hoeksma AF, ter Steeg AM, Nelissen RG, et al. Neurological recovery in obstetric brachial plexus injuries: an historical cohort study. *Dev Med Child Neurol.* 2004;46: 76–83.
21. Al-Qattan MM. The outcome of Erb's palsy when the decision to operate is made at 4 months of age. *Plast Reconstr Surg.* 2000;106:1461–1465.
22. Terzis JK, Papaconstantinou KC. Management of obstetric brachial plexus palsy. *Hand Clin.* 1999;15:717–736.
23. Tatli B, Aydini N, Caliskan M, et al. Congenital muscular torticollis: evaluation and classification. *Pediatr Neurol.* 2006;34:41–44.

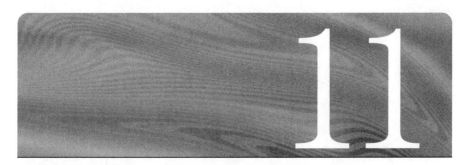

ABNORMALITIES OF CRANIAL SIZE AND SHAPE, HYDROCEPHALUS, AND SPINAL DYSRAPHISM

HEAD CIRCUMFERENCE

The head circumference (HC) (Fig. 11.1) should **always** be measured between the points *glabella* (junction of the frontal and nasal bones, between the eyebrows) and *inion* (external occipital protuberance). **Incorrect or inconsistent technique is a common cause of "abnormal" HC and "change" in the rate of head growth**. When a patient is said to have a large or small head, the physician should first *remeasure and plot the HC with all previous measurements on a standard curve*. In cases of premature birth, the age of a patient should be adjusted downward by the number of weeks the patient was born prior to term. When the patient's HC measures unusually large or small, the maternal and paternal HC should also be measured, since head size is often a familial trait (Table 11.1).

NONPROGRESSIVE MICROCEPHALY

Microcephaly is defined as an HC *more than two standard deviations below the mean* for the patient's age and gender. In cases of *nonprogressive* microcephaly, the HC remains at approximately the same percentile as the patient grows older. Causes include *familial trait, prenatal or perinatal cerebral ischemia, TORCH* (toxoplasma, rubella, cytomegalovirus, and herpes) *infection, cerebral malformation, chromosomal anomalies*, and a large number of *syndromes of congenital malformation*.

Laboratory studies to evaluate nonprogressive microcephaly often include TORCH titers, karyotype, and tests for congenital disorders that are suggested by the patient's physical examination (i.e., on the basis of dysmorphisms or organ anomalies). When the cause is a major cerebral malformation or global cerebral ischemia, motor development is delayed, and generalized

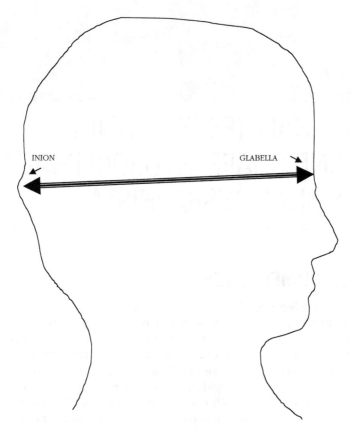

INION

GLABELLA

Figure 11.1 Tape placement for measurement of head circumference.

spasticity usually develops. Magnetic resonance imaging (MRI) should be ordered in such cases.

Head growth reflects brain growth. Although patients with familial microcephaly are often of normal intelligence, a large percentage of other microcephalic children are cognitively impaired or mentally retarded.

PROGRESSIVE MICROCEPHALY

Arrest or slowing of brain growth causing *progressive microcephaly* may occur after cardiac arrest or near drowning, may be a sign of a degenerative neurological disease, or may be the result of a serious medical condition (e.g., AIDS, congenital cyanotic heart disease, cancer). In all of these cases, the HC is noted to fall into progressively lower percentiles as the child grows older.

TABLE 11.1

Common causes of microcephaly and macrocephaly

Finding	Causes
Nonprogressive microcephaly	Familial trait
	Chromosomal anomaly, genetic disorder, or other syndrome of congenital malformation
	Global cerebral atrophy caused by prenatal or perinatal ischemia
	TORCH infection
	Cerebral malformation
Progressive microcephaly	Rett syndrome, other degenerative diseases
	Severe medical illness (cancer, cyanotic heart disease, etc.)
	Aftermath of prolonged cardiorespiratory arrest in infancy
Nonprogressive macrocephaly	Mismeasurement
	Familial trait
	Benign enlargement of subarachnoid space ("external hydrocephalus")
	Neurocutaneous syndrome (neurofibromatosis type I, tuberous sclerosis)
	Sotos syndrome
	Megalencephaly
	Many other genetic disorders
Progressive macrocephaly	Mismeasurement
	Hydrocephalus
	Degenerative diseases

TORCH, toxoplasma, rubella, cytomegalovirus, and herpes infection.

A gene located on the X chromosome that is lethal in the homozygous state (1) causes *Rett syndrome,* which is one of the most common neurodegenerative diseases. The disease is lethal in utero to the male, and therefore classic Rett syndrome *affects only girls.* Recent evidence, however, suggests that a variant gene might be linked to other developmental and behavioral disorders presenting in males and females (2).

Girls with Rett syndrome usually develop normally during the first year of life. During the *second year,* developmental milestones are delayed, especially language skills, which either are never acquired or are acquired and then lost. The child becomes progressively withdrawn and may transiently appear autistic (see Chapter 9). Purposeful movements of the hands are lost

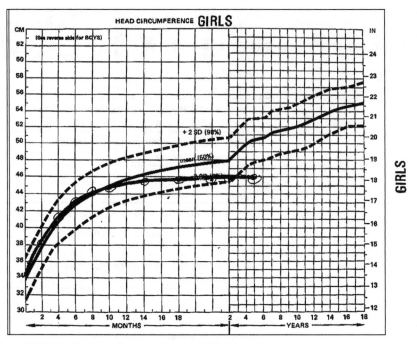

Figure 11.2 Head circumference in case of **Rett syndrome.**

next, and a characteristic *"hand-wringing"* habit often develops. During the next few years, the child becomes ataxic and begins to have epileptic seizures. An irregular breathing pattern is often noted. The eventual outcome is characterized by severe mental retardation and spastic quadriparesis.

Progressive microcephaly revealed by the HC curve is a classic early finding in cases of Rett syndrome (Fig. 11.2). A decline in HC should always bring to mind the possibility of this disorder in the case of a female toddler with a history of developmental stagnation or regression commencing in the second year. The diagnosis of Rett syndrome, which until 10 years ago was based entirely on the clinical presentation, can be confirmed by commercially available *genetic testing*. Life expectancy is about 20 years. There is no specific treatment. Seizure control is usually possible with an antiepileptic drug (AED) for primary generalized seizures (see Chapter 6).

NONPROGRESSIVE MACROCEPHALY

Macrocephaly is defined as an HC *more than two standard deviations above the mean for the patient's age and gender.*

Many infants and young children who have a large head simply have a large head. This is often a *familial trait*, and in such cases, at least one parent's HC is at or above the 90th percentile.

MRI or computed tomography (CT) is often ordered to evaluate children with a large head, although is not necessary if the patient's development has been normal, macrocephaly has not been progressive, and the neurological examination yields no abnormal findings. The imaging study often reveals a widened space between the frontal lobes and the calvarium and sometimes a mild degree of ventricular enlargement. This appearance is often unfortunately referred to in the accompanying report as "external hydrocephalus," which is a phrase that tends to terrify parents. *Benign enlargement of the subarachnoid space* is a much less intimidating and more accurate term for this normal variant, which has no adverse neurological or developmental implications. A follow-up imaging study is unnecessary.

Patients with neurofibromatosis type I, tuberous sclerosis, and many other hereditary and congenital disorders are often macrocephalic. Children who are macrocephalic, have a large body habitus, have a history of developmental delay, and exhibit other features of gigantism (e.g., coarse facial features, large hands and feet) are said to have *Sotos syndrome*. This is a syndrome of diverse etiology (3). Growth hormone levels are not elevated in these patients.

The rare cerebral malformation known as *hemimegalencephaly* is associated with nonprogressive macrocephaly, seizures, and focal neurological deficits. Asymmetrical development of the extremities may be noted. MRI shows asymmetrical development of the cerebral hemispheres and an abnormal appearance of the cortical sulci in the affected hemisphere.

Case 11.1

A 7-month-old healthy male infant has a large-appearing head. At birth, his HC was at the 50th percentile. At 2 months, the HC was at the 75th percentile. At 4 months, the HC was at the 90th percentile, and at 6 months, it was at the 95th percentile. The baby has attained all of his motor and cognitive milestones on schedule. There is no history of lethargy, vomiting, or "sunsetting" of the eyes.

Another physician has ordered an MRI scan that the parents bring with them. They are frightened because the radiologist's report mentions hydrocephalus.

The baby is alert and inquisitive, smiles at the examiner, and babbles. The head circumference is measured from glabella to inion and is at the 90th percentile for age and sex. The father's head circumference is also measured and is at the 95th percentile.

The head is normal in shape. The baby's anterior fontanelle is flat and closing. The examination of the cranial nerves, truncal and extremity muscle tone, movements, and reflexes is entirely normal for age. The baby sits up well, reaches, and transfers objects from one hand to another.

(continued)

The MRI images were reviewed with the family. They demonstrate enlargement of the subarachnoid space and mild symmetrical ventricular dilatation. The official report mentions external hydrocephalus.

Diagnosis: *Borderline macrocephaly, probably familial; benign enlargement of the subarachnoid space; previous mismeasurement of the infant's head circumference.*

Outcome: In retrospect, the baby's mother recalls that a different nurse measured the baby's head circumference at each visit to the doctor. The diagnosis was discussed with the family, who was told that the MRI shows a normal and benign variant and not a form of true hydrocephalus and that there is no cause for concern. Subsequently, the patient has had a normal course of development.

PROGRESSIVE MACROCEPHALY

Hydrocephalus: clinical presentation

Cerebrospinal fluid (CSF) (Fig. 11.3) is produced by the *choroid plexus* in the lateral ventricles. The CSF flows through the foramen of Monroe into the third ventricle and via the Sylvian aqueduct into the forth ventricle, which lies in the brainstem. CSF exits the fourth ventricle through the foramen of Luschka and Magendie into the subarachnoid space. From this point, most of the CSF is propelled rostrally by venous pulsations to the cerebral convexities, and thereby passes through the arachnoid granulations and is absorbed into the venous blood within the superior sagittal sinus. CSF also is propelled caudally and thereby surrounds the spinal cord and cauda equina.

All forms of *obstructive hydrocephalus* are caused by a *blockage of the normal flow of CSF*. If the site of obstruction is within one of the *ventricles, a foramen, or the Sylvian aqueduct*, the patient is said to have *noncommunicating hydrocephalus*. If the cause of the obstruction is impaired absorption of CSF by the *arachnoid granulations*, the patient is said to have *communicating hydrocephalus*.

The head circumference enlarges dramatically in cases of hydrocephalus in a neonate or infant because the cranial sutures are patent. A neonate born with hydrocephalus is usually found to have a *grossly enlarged cranium*. In some cases, the condition was diagnosed by prenatal ultrasound. On examination, open cranial sutures, bulging anterior fontanelle, and prominent cerebral veins are often obvious.

Hydrocephalus presenting during infancy causes a *rapid increase in the HC* which, when plotted on the standard HC curve, forms a line that crosses multiple percentiles. The infant may be lethargic or irritable. *Downward deviation of the eyes*, caused by pressure on the midbrain nucleus of cranial nerve III, is often noted. The infant may be hypertonic, especially in the legs, and the deep tendon reflexes are often brisk.

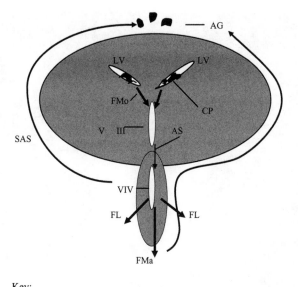

Key:

AG	Arachnoid granulations
AS	Aqueduct of Sylvius
CP	Choroidplexus
FL	Foramen of Luschka
FMa	Foramen of Magendie
FMo	Foramen of Monroe
LV	Lateral ventricle
SAS	Subarachnoid space
V III	Third ventricle
V IV	Fourth ventricle

Figure 11.3 Normal flow of cerebrospinal fluid (CSF).

In the *child and adolescent,* obstructive hydrocephalus *does not lead to enlargement of the HC* since the cranial sutures are fused. These patients usually present with symptoms and signs of *elevated intracranial pressure,* such as lethargy, vomiting, papilledema, brisk deep tendon reflexes, or abducens nerve palsy.

Imaging studies

A clinical presentation of this kind requires *urgent evaluation with CT or MRI,* preferably with *contrast enhancement,* to detect a tumor or vascular malformation potentially causing the blockage to CSF flow. If the patient is an infant with a patent anterior fontanelle, cranial ultrasound is sometimes an adequate preliminary study.

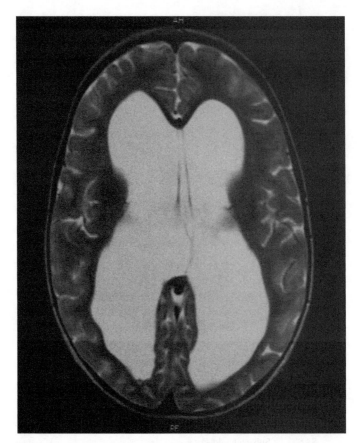

Figure 11.4 MRI showing **communicating hydrocephalus** in a 1-year-old boy. (Courtesy of Ajax George, MD, New York University School of Medicine.)

When viewing the imaging study, the physician must note the pattern of ventricular dilatation. *Communicating* hydrocephalus (Fig. 11.4) causes dilatation of all four ventricles, whereas *noncommunicating* hydrocephalus results in dilatation *only of the ventricle(s) rostral to the obstruction.* For example, dilatation of the lateral and third ventricles with a small or normal sized forth ventricle indicates an obstruction of the Sylvian aqueduct (Fig. 11.5). Especially in cases of noncommunicating hydrocephalus, the imaging study must be carefully examined for evidence of a tumor or vascular malformation that may be causing the obstruction.

Causes of hydrocephalus

The most common cause of noncommunicating hydrocephalus in the neonate and young infant is *aqueductal stenosis*, a blockage of the Sylvian aqueduct that obstructs CSF flow between the third and fourth ventricle. This condition

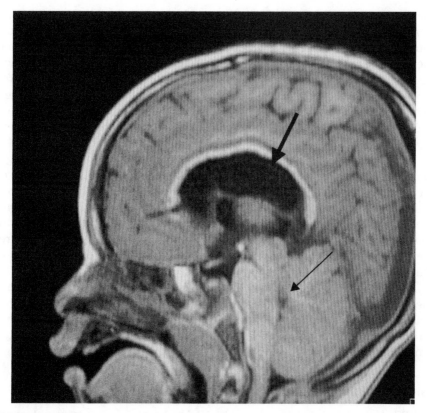

Figure 11.5 MRI showing **aqueductal stenosis** in a 3-year-old boy with noncommunicating hydrocephalus.
Note Small Fourth Ventricle (*small arrow*) and Enlarged Third Ventricle (*large arrow*).
(Courtesy of Ajax George, MD, New York University School of Medicine.)

is often an inherited X-linked recessive trait (4). Other important causes of noncommunicating hydrocephalus during infancy are midline, intraventricular, or posterior fossa *brain tumors* and *vein of Galen malformations*, the latter typically presenting with the syndrome of *high-output cardiac failure*.

The most common cause of communicating hydrocephalus in the neonate is *intraventricular hemorrhage* (5). Other potential causes of communicating hydrocephalus (at all ages) are *subarachnoid hemorrhage* and *bacterial meningitis*.

Treatments and complications

Infants with untreated hydrocephalus may become permanently neurologically disabled (mentally retarded and quadriplegic) or develop epilepsy (6). If tonsillar herniation results, the patient may die. Therefore, *surgery* is performed in cases of rapidly progressive hydrocephalus. A *ventriculoperi-toneal shunt* (VPS) is placed to divert CSF from a point rostral to the obstruction to the peritoneal cavity. An *external reservoir* for CSF is often inserted beneath the patient's scalp, allowing for future assessments of shunt function and easy access to CSF. In other cases, a *third ventriculostomy* allows for CSF flow from the third ventricle directly into the subarachnoid space underlying the midbrain without the need for a VPS. The result of surgery is typically a decrease in ventricular size during the next few months, improvement in the infant's clinical status, and gradual normalization of the HC.

Posthemorrhagic hydrocephalus in the neonate may occur following a germinal matrix hemorrhage. The treatment chosen depends on the rate of ventricular enlargement. If ventricular expansion appears to plateau, close follow-up with *daily HC measurements and a weekly cranial ultrasound study* may be sufficient. In cases of slowly progressive ventricular expansion, *serial lumbar punctures or ventricular taps* are sometimes effective in preventing further progression. *Surgery* is performed in cases of rapid ventricular enlargement or a poor response to other treatments (5).

In some cases, ventricular enlargement in a child does not progress beyond a point (*arrested hydrocephalus*). These patients are closely followed with serial imaging studies. If no clinical signs of raised intracranial pressure are noted on examination and ventricular size remains stable, surgery is often not necessary.

Shunt obstruction and infection

A VPS can become obstructed or colonized by bacteria years or even decades after it was inserted. The most common symptoms of shunt malfunction are nonspecific and include headache, vomiting, malaise, and low-grade fever. Nevertheless, a reliable rule of thumb is that *if a child with a VPS presents with unexplained constitutional symptoms, shunt malfunction is likely.* The location of the obstruction or infection may be at the rostral opening of the shunt within the ventricular system, along the shunt pathway, or at the caudal end of the shunt in the peritoneal cavity.

A neurosurgeon should be consulted. CT or MRI is ordered, and the result is compared to previous films to determine whether or not the ventricles have enlarged in size. A series of plain x-rays ("shunt series") is ordered to examine the course of the VPS from the neck to the peritoneal cavity to see if any components have become disconnected. A nuclear medicine study ("shunt-o-gram"), in which a radioisotope is injected into the shunt reservoir, is sometimes ordered to assess the adequacy of CSF flow from the shunt to the peritoneum. The neurosurgeon will usually obtain a sample of CSF from the reservoir for culture. The most frequently cultured organism is *Staphylococcus epidermidis*. In cases of infection or obstruction, the shunt is usually replaced after the patient has received a course of an appropriate antibiotic.

Related disorders

A *Dandy-Walker malformation* is characterized by *enlargement of the lateral ventricles, agenesis of the cerebellar vermis, and a posterior fossa CSF cyst* that communicates with the fourth ventricle (Fig. 11.6). The head is often elongated (dolichocephalic). Patients with a Dandy-Walker malformation are often mentally retarded. Cranial nerve palsies, ataxia, and spasticity are common. Treatment includes a VPS and a second, connecting shunt that drains the posterior fossa cyst.

Joubert syndrome refers to a group of disorders that share a midbrain-hindbrain malformation, in most cases including a *hypoplastic cerebellum*. Most patients are profoundly disabled. Patients with Joubert syndrome often exhibit an *irregular respiratory pattern*. They require constant care and rarely survive longer than a few years.

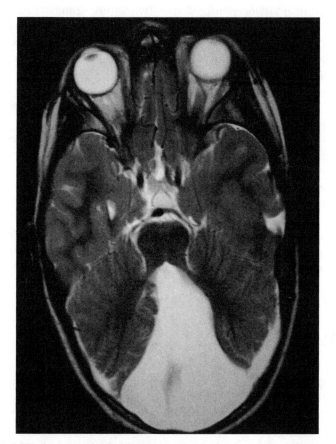

Figure 11.6 MRI showing **Dandy-Walker malformation** in a 7-year-old boy.
Note Large Posterior Fossa Cyst and Elongated (Dolichocephalic) Head. (Courtesy of Ajax George, MD, New York University School of Medicine.)

Degenerative disorders

Degenerative diseases may cause progressively macrocephaly as a result of abnormal intraneuronal storage. In most cases, the diagnosis of a degenerative disease is suspected on the basis of developmental arrest or regression, well before the child becomes macrocephalic. Tay-Sachs disease, mucopolysaccharidoses, and Alexander and Canavan diseases are among the diagnostic possibilities (see Chapters 10 and 14).

CRANIOSYNOSTOSIS

Craniosynostosis results from the premature closure of one or more of the cranial sutures. Abnormal enlargement of the cranium is perpendicular to the orientation of the closed suture. *Sagittal* stenosis causes the head to appear *brachycephalic* (wide and foreshortened), whereas *coronal* stenosis causes an elongated or *dolichocephalic* shape. Two-suture craniosynostosis is also fairly common (7). *Flattening of the occiput* or *plagiocephaly* is usually the result of an infant regularly *sleeping in a supine position* to help prevent sudden infant death syndrome (8) and rarely results from premature closure of the *lambdoid* suture.

The physical examination may reveal a *bony ridge along the closed suture*(s). The head is misshapen (as above). Signs of raised intracranial pressure and focal neurological findings are unusual.

Craniosynostosis is usually a sporadic condition, although familial cases are reported (9). Rarely, a thyroid defect or disorder of calcium or phosphorus metabolism causes craniosynostosis; usually there are other signs of a metabolic disturbance in these cases. Craniosynostosis is sometimes associated with syndromes of congenital facial dysmorphism and digital malformation, as in cases of *Apert* and *Carpenter syndromes*.

Craniosynostosis can usually be diagnosed by a series of *plain skull films*. *CT of the head with three-dimensional reconstruction* is often ordered but may require conscious sedation and entails more radiation exposure. Many neurosurgeons find plain films adequate. Surgery is performed to prevent elevated intracranial pressure and improve cosmetic appearance.

SPINAL DYSRAPHISM

Failure of the posterior neuropore to close during the first month of fetal life leads to a group of developmental abnormalities collectively known as *spinal dysraphism*. In cases of *spina bifida occulta*, the posterior arch of one or more lumbar vertebrae does not close, but the spinal cord and nerve roots remain in place. External stigmata may include a lumbosacral tuft of hair, lipoma, or dimple. A *meningocele* occurs when *meningeal tissue, but not spinal cord or nerve root tissue*, is extruded through the defect. In cases of *myelomeningocele* (MMC), the *spinal cord and nerve roots* are also extruded.

The extent of neurological disability correlates with the degree of involvement of neural structures and tissue. Patients with spina bifida occulta and many patients with meningocele are, therefore, neurologically asymptomatic, although a tethered spinal cord is a potential complication during childhood (see Chapter 14). MMC virtually always is associated with a significant neurological disability. Although the survival rate and prognosis for infants with a lumbar MMC has improved as a result of improvements in surgical management (10,11), many of these patients never become able to walk and do not achieve bowel or bladder control. In cases of lumbar MMC, the upper extremities function normally. Cervical MMC, on the other hand, usually results in quadriplegia. MMC is generally associated with hydrocephalus and upward protrusion of the cerebellum, a complex known as a *Chiari II malformation* (Fig. 11.7). This condition requires a VPS, and therefore, CT or MRI of the *brain* is ordered in all new cases of MMC.

When dermatological stigmata of spina bifida occulta are noted in an infant during the first 6 months of life, *ultrasonography of the lumbar area* is usually ordered. In rare cases, a sinus tract extends from a sacral dimple to

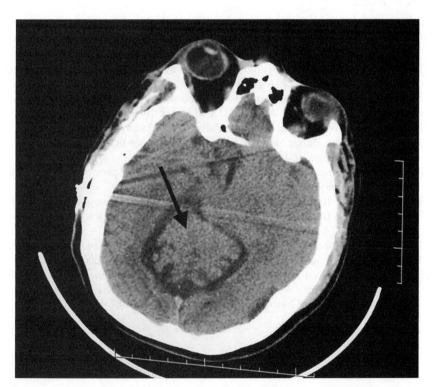

Figure 11.7 CT showing upward protrusion of cerebellum (*arrow*) in case of **Chiari II malformation.**

(Courtesy of Howard Seigerman, MD, and Eliot Lerner, MD, The Valley Hospital.)

the meninges and predisposes the patient to meningitis. Ultrasonography is also ordered to make certain that the infant will not have a tethered spinal cord in the future. After 6 months of age, the posterior vertebral elements are ossified and may be visualized by a *routine radiographic study* of the lumbar spine. Spinal MRI is the definitive study but is unlikely to reveal an abnormality if either of the previously mentioned studies is normal.

The primary care provider usually sees children with a history of MMC months to years after the spinal defect was repaired. Most patients are nonambulatory. The physician should make certain that the child has appropriate orthotics and a wheelchair that "fits" (i.e., that does not cause pressure sores). *Urinary tract infections* resulting from self-catheterization are a persistent problem. Many patients require antibiotic prophylaxis and a procholinergic medication to improve bladder function. The diagnosis of bladder dysfunction caused by spinal cord disease is discussed in Chapter 14. Most patients with MMC also have a VPS and must be monitored for signs of shunt malfunction.

REFERENCES

1. Gura T. Gene defect linked to Rett syndrome. *Science.* 1999;286:27.
2. Robinson R. Rett syndrome: a new range of phenotypes described in a Wartenberg lecture. *Neurology Today.* 2004;July:39–42.
3. Opitz JM, Weaver DW, Reynolds JF Jr. The syndromes of Sotos and Weaver: reports and review. *Am J Med Genet.* 1998;79:294–304.
4. Halliday, H, Chow CW, Wallace D, et al. X-linked hydrocephalus: a survey of a 20 year period in Victoria, Australia. *J Med Genet.* 1986;23:23–31.
5. Volpe JJ. *Neurology of the Newborn.* Philadelphia: Saunders; 1995:431–463.
6. McCullough DC, Balzer-Martin LA. Current prognosis in overt neonatal hydrocephalus. *J Neurosurg.* 1982;57:378–383.
7. Chumas PD, Cinalli G, Arnaud E, et al. Classification of previously unclassified cases of craniosynostosis. *J Neurosurg.* 1997;86:177–181.
8. Hutchison BL, Hutchison LA, Thompson JM, et al. Plagiocephaly and brachycephaly in the first two years of life: a prospective cohort study. *Pediatrics.* 2004;114:970–980.
9. Jacobsen RI. Abnormalities of the skull in children. *Neurol Clin.* 1985;3:117–145.
10. Volpe JJ. *Neurology of the Newborn.* Philadelphia: Saunders; 2001:9–15.
11. Marlin A. The initial treatment of the child with myelomeningocele: a practice survey of the American Society for Pediatric Neurosurgery (ASPN). In: Marlin A, ed. *Concepts in Pediatric Neurosurgery.* Basel: Karger; 1990;7–14.

COMMON NEUROLOGICAL COMPLICATIONS OF TRAUMA

BUMPS TO THE HEAD

Sooner or later, every toddler bumps his head. These minor accidents rarely result in a serious injury but are often frightening to the family. Many years later, parents bringing their child for evaluation of a neurological, behavioral, developmental, or school problem may recall the bump on the head and wonder whether it caused the current problem.

The meninges and cerebrospinal fluid prevent injury to the brain in the great majority of cases of minor head trauma. Parents may be reassured that, if the child did not experience a loss of consciousness or exhibit signs of neurological or developmental deterioration following the accident, the possibility that the accident caused the current problem is remote.

CEREBRAL CONCUSSION

A *cerebral concussion* refers to a *transient disturbance of neurological function caused by a blow to the head* in the *absence of an intracranial abnormality demonstrable by a brain imaging study.* Falls and bicycle accidents are common causes of concussion in children. Sports-related injuries often result in a concussion in adolescents.

The most common symptoms of a brain concussion are headache, vomiting, disorientation, impairment of short-term memory, and drowsiness. Concussion is graded on a scale of I to III (Table 12.1) (1). In most cases, observable changes in mental status do not persist for more than a few minutes or hours and rarely persist for more than 24 hours. Headaches, lightheadedness, concentration problems, and malaise tend to be more persistent; this complex is called *post-concussive syndrome.* In young children, multiple episodes of vomiting after a concussion may occur, and in some cases, the child needs to be hospitalized for intravenous fluids in order to prevent dehydration.

TABLE 12.1

Grading of concussion and recommendations for return to athletic activities

Grade I concussion	Grade II concussion	Grade III concussion
1) Transient confusion 2) No loss of consciousness 3) Symptoms resolve in less than 15 minutes	1) Transient confusion 2) No loss of consciousness 3) Symptoms last more than 15 minutes	1) Any loss of consciousness a) Brief (seconds) b) Prolonged (minutes or longer)
Recommendation:	**Recommendation:**	**Recommendation:**
Remove from contest; examine at 5-minute intervals for return of mental status abnormalities at rest and with exertion; may return to play in 15 minutes if remains asymptomatic	Remove from contest for day; examine repeatedly on-site; re-examination next day by a trained person; return to sports after 1 week if asymptomatic at rest and with exertion	Transport to emergency room; cervical spine immobilization if suspected neck injury; neurological examination with appropriate imaging study; admit to hospital for abnormal imaging results or persistently abnormal examination; allow a minimum of 2 weeks before return to sports, depending on neurological exam and symptoms at rest and with exertion

Adapted from Quality Standards Subcommittee of the American Academy of Neurology, 1997 (1).

Examination and diagnostic testing

The physical examination should follow the guidelines for patients with headaches and head injuries (see Chapters 1 and 2) and should include a *mental status assessment* (see next section). The physician should always look for signs of a *basilar skull fracture* in patients who have had a head injury. Focal neurological findings, if noted, suggest a cerebral contusion, intracranial hematoma, or spinal injury.

Mental status assessment

The *assessment of mental status* is an important part of the examination of the patient who has had a head injury. The following evaluation is derived from the standard adult mental status examination and is applicable primarily to adolescents, who are the patients most often seen for concussion; the examination may be modified for younger patients. The patient's *general level of alertness and behavior* is noted first. *Orientation* to *name*, *place* (for young patients, "the doctor's office"; for older patients, the name of the city or town), and *date* (day of the week and month, or the season for younger children) is assessed. The patient may be *asked about his or her activities during the current day or previous night, such as what he or she ate for breakfast and dinner, what program he or she watched on television,* or *recent news or sports events.* The older patient is *asked to spell the word "world" forward and backward and to count backward from 100 by sevens* to test his concentration ability. The patient's ability to *repeat a phrase* (for older children and adolescents, "no ifs, ands, or buts"), to *name common objects* (watch, collar, and glasses), and to *follow multistep directions* is tested to evaluate the integrity of language functions (see Chapter 3). The older patient is asked to *recall three dissimilar words* (e.g., "green, feather, honesty") *immediately after presentation and after 5 minutes* to assess short-term memory.

Many patients who have had a concussion are evaluated in the emergency room, where a noncontrast *computed tomography (CT) scan of the head* is often ordered. In cases of concussion, the result, by definition, is within normal limits. The patient is normally discharged if he or she is alert, has a normal mental status examination, and exhibits no focal deficits. If the patient was never seen in the emergency room and is seen during the next few days in the office because he is still experiencing symptoms, the patient is also often sent for a CT scan, which, in the great majority of cases, does not reveal any intracranial abnormality.

The physician is often asked when the patient can return to playing sports. Table 12.1 summarizes the recommendations of the American Academy of Neurology.

Case 12.1

A 16-year-old adolescent male, after consuming 12 cans of beer at a party, loses his balance while walking along the top of a high retaining wall and falls 15 feet, face first, onto concrete. He is brought unconscious to the emergency room by the emergency medical services.

On examination, his vital signs are normal. Ecchymoses around the orbits and generalized facial edema are obvious. Battle sign is absent. No fluid leak from the nose or ears is noted, and the patient's nasal mucous does not test positive for glucose when tested with a urine dipstick. The patient is unresponsive when his name is called and when his shoulder is shaken, but he moans in response to sternal rubbing. His pupils are briskly reactive. The doll's eyes maneuver yields normal responses. Gag is normal. He withdraws each extremity in response to nailbed pressure. Reflexes are symmetrical. Toes are downgoing. No abnormal posturing is noted.

(continued)

Cervical x-rays and CT of the neck are normal. Head CT does not demonstrate intracranial bleeding or a skull fracture but does show nasal and orbital fractures. Rib and clavicular fractures are demonstrated by other radiological studies. Serial hematocrit readings are normal and consistent. Urinalysis does not reveal blood.

He is admitted to the intensive care unit (ICU). The following day, he is responsive to voice and briefly opens his eyes. A repeat CT scan of the head is ordered and shows patchy areas of bleeding in the right frontoparietal region and both occipital lobes.

Diagnosis: *Cerebral contusion.*

Outcome: The patient stayed in the ICU for 2 weeks and made a gradual recovery. He was maintained on phenytoin for 2 weeks for seizure prophylaxis. He was sent to a rehabilitation hospital for a month where he continued to improve. At discharge, he was alert, and the neurological examination revealed no focal deficits. However, during the next 6 months, he was seen several times in the office because of headaches, memory complaints, difficulty concentrating, and behavioral outbursts. He was eventually prescribed a mood-stabilizing drug (oxcarbazepine) and nortriptyline for headache prophylaxis. He was not able to attend school for the remainder of the year because of these symptoms.

Postconcussive syndrome

Patients who complain of waxing and waning headaches, nausea, lightheadedness, photophobia, malaise, and difficulty concentrating, which persists for days to weeks after a concussion, are said to have *postconcussive syndrome.* No abnormal physical findings are noted. There is no specific treatment, but the condition is self-limited, and patients may be reassured than they will feel better within a few weeks if not sooner. Patients should not exercise until they are asymptomatic at rest. Quickly resuming strenuous activity often results in a worsening of symptoms. In some cases, the physician will order or repeat a brain imaging study, which is almost always normal. Daily use of analgesics (e.g., ibuprofen) for more than 10 days after a concussion should be *discouraged to prevent the occurrence of medication-overuse headaches.* Nortriptyline or gabapentin (see Chapter 2) may be prescribed if the patient has persistent headaches.

Skull fracture

A linear, nondisplaced *skull fracture* is a fairly common consequence of a head injury in an infant or young child. In many cases, the patient has fallen off of a bed onto the hard floor. Swelling is noted over the fracture, usually in the parietal region. The patient may be irritable but is alert, and no neurological deficits are typically noted on examination. A plain skull radiograph will reveal the fracture. CT of the head is appropriate in cases of a displaced or large skull fracture or if the neurological examination is not normal.

If the bone adjacent to the fracture is not displaced, no intervention is necessary since the fracture will spontaneously heal. The child may wear a protective helmet for a few weeks. Depressed skull fractures require neuro-surgical consultation, although if the dura mater is intact, surgery is generally not performed. The possibility that the child has been abused should be considered, especially if the circumstances of the accident are unclear or other signs of trauma are present.

An ophthalmologist or ear, nose, and throat specialist should evaluate orbital fractures.

Trochlear nerve palsy

The trochlear nerve traverses a long course within the cranium, making it vulnerable to trauma. Trochlear nerve palsy can be a delayed complication of head injury. Symptoms and signs may not be noted until several days after the accident and include *double vision* and *head tilting* when the patient looks downward and inward, such as while he or she reads. A careful examination of the patient's extraocular movements is necessary to demonstrate the palsy. The condition is self-limited in most cases.

MORE SERIOUS NEUROLOGICAL CONSEQUENCES OF HEAD INJURY

Falls from a great height, a blow to the head from a blunt object, and high-velocity automobile or pedestrian-struck accidents are the most common causes of serious traumatic brain injury.

Cerebral contusion

A *cerebral contusion* is an area of *localized capillary bleeding* (a "bruise") on the surface of or within the brain. The contusion is usually either directly beneath the area of impact (*coup*) or on the opposite side of the brain (*contracoup*). A cerebral contusion usually causes a *marked and persistent change in the patient's mental status and, often, one or more focal neurological deficits* or *seizures*.

A CT scan (Fig. 12.1) showing localized bleeding in the cerebral cortex or white matter confirms the diagnosis of a cerebral contusion. CT may not be abnormal until *2 to 3 days following the injury*, and therefore, *repeat studies* are *often necessary* in the case of a patient with a persistently abnormal mental status or focal neurological findings following a head injury.

H   C

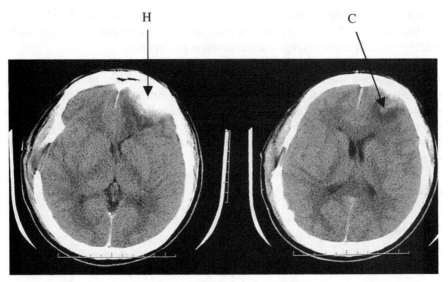

Figure 12.1 CT of a **subdural hematoma** (*H*) and a **cerebral contusion** (*C*) in a 20-year-old male.

(Courtesy of Howard Seigerman, MD, and Eliot Lerner, MD, The Valley Hospital.)

The patient with a cerebral contusion is prescribed phenytoin for 2 weeks to prevent seizures. The value of longer term antiepileptic therapy has not been established. A corticosteroid, usually dexamethasone, is often started to reduce cerebral edema, although it may not be that effective and is not uniformly recommended. Standard measures for elevated intracranial pressure (ICP) are suggested (see Chapter 2).

The prognosis relates to the size and location of the injury. Seizures, focal neurological deficits, amnesia, and psychiatric problems (organic brain syndrome) may follow large cerebral contusions. If the frontal lobes were involved, the injury may cause disinhibited behavior or a flattened affect. Temporal lobe injuries are associated with seizure, memory impairment, and exaggerated emotional responses (Kluver-Bucy syndrome).

Epidural and subdural hematoma

An *epidural hematoma* is a result of bleeding from the middle meningeal artery following a fracture of the temporal bone. The textbook presentation encompasses three phases: 1) loss of consciousness immediately following a blow to the temporal area; 2) temporary recovery of consciousness ("lucid interval"); and 3) deterioration to coma and death. In fact, *only the third phase consistently occurs. Any patient with a history of a significant blow to the temporal area should be sent for a CT scan. A lens-shaped collection of blood* underlying the temporal bone (Fig. 12.2) confirms the diagnosis of an

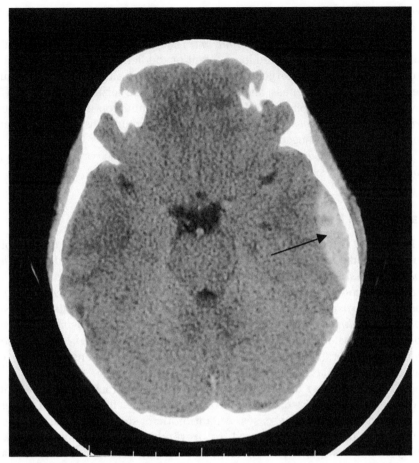

Figure 12.2 CT of an **epidural hematoma** in an 8-year-old boy.
(Courtesy of Howard Seigerman, MD, and Eliot Lerner, MD, The Valley Hospital.)

epidural hematoma. *Immediate surgical evacuation of the hematoma is necessary in order to prevent herniation and death.* Many patients who have had prompt surgery fully recover.

A *subdural hematoma* caused by bleeding from a cerebral or bridging vein may occasionally develop following an accidental head injury in a child or adolescent. Signs and symptoms include the relatively gradual onset of drowsiness and headache, hemiparesis, and focal seizures. CT reveals a crescent-shaped hyperdense mass, usually overlying the frontoparietal convexity. Surgical drainage is required to evacuate moderate-sized and large hematomas, but small collections of blood may gradually be resorbed, and these patients can sometimes avoid surgery. They are followed with serial imaging studies. A corticosteroid is sometimes started but has not been proven to be beneficial. Patients are prescribed phenytoin for seizure prophylaxis.

Child abuse (*shaken baby syndrome*) should be suspected when a subdural hematoma is discovered in an infant or toddler. These patients usually are brought to the emergency room because of altered mental status (lethargy, unresponsiveness, and poor feeding). Focal seizures may occur. CT reveals a subdural hematoma. Funduscopic examination may demonstrate *preretinal hemorrhages*, and a series of skeletal radiographs may show fractures varying in age, suggesting abuse.

A *disorder of coagulation* should be excluded if abuse or a head injury is not the cause of a subdural hematoma.

Basilar skull fracture

A fracture of the occipital bone, petrous bone, sphenoid bone, or ethmoid bone is called a *basilar skull fracture*. Characteristic signs include *bruising over the mastoid process* (Battle sign), purple *discoloration around the orbits* ("raccoon eyes"), and *blood behind a tympanic membrane*. In some cases a *cerebrospinal fluid (CSF) leak* from the nose or ear results. *CSF tests positive for glucose* when tested with a urine dipstick, whereas *nasal mucus does not*. Occasionally, *extraocular palsy or pupillary dysfunction* (caused by an injury to cranial nerves III–IV), *anosmia* (loss of the sense of smell), or carotid sinus fistula follows a basilar skull fracture.

CT usually either demonstrates the fracture or intracranial air. Patients are generally hospitalized, and a neurosurgeon is consulted, although surgery is not performed in many cases. An antibiotic is sometimes started when a CSF leak has been discovered, to prevent meningitis. However, since many CSF leaks spontaneously stop, some physicians recommend that an antibiotic not be started so that bacterial resistance does not develop.

Axonal shearing injury

An *axonal shearing injury* usually results from a violent torsional movement of the brain. The most common causes are high-velocity automobile accidents and accidents in which a pedestrian or bicyclist is struck by an automobile. Because of their different density, the cerebral gray and white matter accelerates at different rates and *axons may be broken off at the gray matter/white matter junction during the violent movement*. Consciousness is immediately lost, and the patient is transported to the hospital in a coma. The initial brain imaging study is either unrevealing or shows small hemorrhages at the gray matter/white matter junction. Weeks to months later, magnetic resonance imaging (MRI) reveals areas of local or widespread cortical atrophy as a result of retrograde neuronal degeneration. Patients with large axonal shearing injuries are usually permanently neurologically disabled. Focal deficits, seizures, and organic brain syndrome may result. In the worst cases, the outcome is death or survival in a persistent vegetative state.

Malignant cerebral edema

Malignant cerebral edema is a rare but serious syndrome that may follow head trauma. A patient may have had an apparently minor head injury and presents with signs of a concussion. For unclear reasons, severe cerebral edema rapidly develops, leading to coma and, in some cases, even death. These patients require aggressive measures for elevated ICP. A neurosurgeon should be consulted.

COMA

Coma is a state of *unresponsiveness to sensory stimuli*. A coma can result from nontraumatic causes (e.g., severe metabolic or endocrine disturbance, infection, medication, stroke, or tumor) and from major head trauma. Bedside tests to assess the comatose patient are listed in Table 12.2. The comatose patient is stimulated by *voice* (calling the patient's name loudly), *tactile stimulation* (shaking the patient's shoulder), and, if necessary, *pain* (pressure on the nailbed with the barrel of a pen or briskly rubbing the sternum with the knuckles). The examiner should note whether the patient *withdraws the extremity* in response to a *painful stimulus to the nailbed*. If the patient fails to withdraw one extremity or two extremities on the same side in response to painful stimulation, a contralateral brain injury should be suspected. The examination of the comatose patient should also include an evaluation of *pupillary responses to light*, the *doll's eyes* response, the *corneal reflex*, the *gag response*, and, in some cases, *caloric testing* and *apnea testing* (see Table 12.2). The *deep tendon and plantar reflexes* should be checked for symmetry. *Decorticate* and *decerebrate* posturing should be recognized. Decorticate posturing, resulting from a lesion at the level of the midbrain, is characterized by flexion of the arms at the elbows and extension of the lower extremities. Decerebrate posturing caused by a lesion in the pons is characterized by reflexive extension of arms and legs. The reader is referred to Plum and Posner's classic monograph (2) for a comprehensive discussion of the evaluation of coma.

The *Glasgow Coma Scale* (GCS) (Table 12.3), is often administered as an initial assessment to comatose patients and other patients who have had a head injury. The GCS has prognostic value; patients with a GCS score of 11 or greater were found, in a large study, to have an 82% chance of making a good recovery, whereas patients with an initial score of 4 or less had an 87% chance of dying or surviving in a persistent vegetative state (3). The scale is modified for infants. The GCS is not used to reassess the patient at any point after the initial evaluation.

TABLE 12.2

Bedside tests for comatose patients

Test and technique	Purpose
Response to voice and tactile stimulation: call patient's name loudly; shake patient's shoulder	Assess responsiveness
Response to pain: test response to nailbed pressure in each extremity; brisk sternal rub with knuckles	Assess responsiveness; elicit signs of a focal deficit (e.g., if no withdrawal of one extremity or both extremities on one side)
Pupillary reaction to light	Assess papillary size, response, symmetry; evaluate midbrain integrity
Doll's eyes maneuver: head is turned from one side to the other, eyes should go opposite way	Assess brainstem integrity; the pons coordinates lateral eye movements
Corneal reflex: lightly rub cornea with a gauze pad; eyelid should close	Assess trigeminal nerve, facial nerve, and brainstem (pons and midbrain)
Gag response: stimulate pharynx with a cotton swab; patient should respond	Assess brainstem integrity (caudal medulla)
Caloric testing: 60 cc of cold water injected into external auditory canals, check for extraocular movements (*nystagmus*)	Nystagmus should result; assess brainstem integrity (rostral medulla)
Apnea testing: patient's ventilator is disconnected for up to 20 minutes (generally only for brain death exam) to check for respiratory effort; the patient is given 100% oxygen by cannula while ventilator is disconnected	Apnea should stimulate respiratory response. Assess brainstem integrity (pons and medulla)
Deep tendon reflexes; check for Babinski sign	Assess for symmetry; asymmetry suggests a focal deficit
Posturing: sternal rub may elicit decorticate or decerebrate posturing (see text)	Decorticate posturing indicates a lesion at or above the midbrain; decerebrate posturing indicates a pontine lesion

Patients in a coma caused by a serious head injury are initially treated as cases of increased ICP (see Chapter 2). In some cases, a surgeon places an *ICP monitor* to provide information useful in regulating the ventilator and dosing medication (e.g., corticosteroids, mannitol). Patients are also sometimes placed in a *barbiturate-induced coma* to decrease cerebral metabolism, cerebral perfusion pressure, and cerebral edema.

TABLE 12.3
Glasgow coma scale

Adults (often also used for children)			Infants		
Eye opening	Spontaneous	4	**Eye opening**	Spontaneous	4
	To speech	3		To speech	3
	To pain	2		To pain	2
	None	1		None	1
Verbal	Oriented	5	**Verbal**	Coos, babbles	5
	Confused	4		Irritable	4
	Inappropriate words	3		Cries to pain	3
	Nonspecific sounds	2		Moans to pain	2
	None	1		None	1
Motor	Follows commands	6	**Motor**	Normal spontaneous movements	6
	Localizes pain	5		Withdraws to touch	5
	Withdraws to pain	4		Withdraws to pain	4
	Abnormal flexion	3		Abnormal flexion	3
	Abnormal extension	2		Abnormal extension	2
	None	1		None	1

From Jennet B, Teasdale G. Aspects of coma after severe head injury. *Lancet.* 1977;1:878–881, and James HE: Neurologic evaluation and support in the child with an acute brain insult. *Pediatr Ann.* 1986;15:16–22.

Persistent vegetative state

A *persistent vegetative state* refers to an absence of environmental awareness or self-awareness, with intact brainstem functions and sleep-wake cycles, lasting for more than 1 month. Emotional responses (e.g., crying or laughing) may be noted but do not result from any external stimulus. The prognosis is generally poor, although occasionally a patient may awaken after a lengthy vegetative state.

Brain death

Brain death is defined as a *complete and permanent cessation of brain function. Any* sign of brain activity, including *even slight responsiveness to pain, any cranial nerve activity* (e.g., complete or partial pupillary response, doll's eye response, gag response, nystagmus in response to caloric testing, decerebrate or decorticate posturing, or respiratory effort), or even *a seizure* **excludes the diagnosis of brain death**. In most cases, *apnea testing* is an important part of the brain death examination. *If the patient is* *able to breathe without the aid of a mechanical ventilator*, the patient is by definition *not brain dead*. Criteria for brain death tend to be strictest for younger patients, with multiple examinations over a period of up to 48 hours required for infants (4).

Drugs and toxins that suppress pupillary responses and the central respiratory drive can cause a temporary state resembling brain death. *Therefore, it is essential to allow any substance that might affect brain activity (especially barbiturates and benzodiazepines) to clear from the patient's system prior to making a diagnosis of brain death.* This may, in some cases, delay the diagnosis of brain death for several days.

The diagnosis of brain death generally requires confirmatory testing. The *EEG* should show *no* sign of cerebral activity (*flat* EEG tracing). A nuclear medicine scan measuring *regional cerebral blood flow* is also sometimes ordered and, in cases of brain death, should demonstrate no radioactive tracer uptake by the brain, in other words, no brain metabolism.

NECK INJURY

Neck injuries often occur during a contact sport or as a result of an automobile accident. The patient is usually immobilized on a backboard in a neck brace by the emergency medical services and transported to the emergency room. A complete series of cervical radiographs is taken. If a fracture or dislocation is revealed, a neurosurgeon or orthopedic surgeon should be consulted for recommendations. Neck immobilization (cervical collar) or surgery may be appropriate. The choice of treatment primarily depends on the stability of the fracture and the danger of spinal cord involvement. MRI is ordered in many cases.

MRI of the cervical spine must be ordered whenever *weakness, sensory loss, or sphincter dysfunction* follows a neck injury. Important MRI findings include disc herniation or displacement of a vertebral body *causing spinal cord compression or transection, spinal cord contusion,* and *bleeding within the cord parenchyma* (hematomyelia). In these cases, neurosurgical or orthopedic consultation should be requested. The patient is admitted to the intensive care unit. A Foley catheter is placed, and the patient's heart rate and blood pressure are continually monitored. Spinal injuries can damage autonomic pathways, resulting in urinary retention or arrhythmia. A high-dose corticosteroid protocol (methylprednisone, 30 mg/kg body weight loading dose, followed by 4 mg/kg/hr for 23 hours) has traditionally been prescribed in cases of spinal cord injury. Based on recent studies, this protocol is no longer recommended in cases of nonpenetrating spinal cord injury (5,6). Many patients with a nonpenetrating cord injury ultimately make a good recovery. Spinal cord transection is a devastating condition often resulting in paraparesis, paraplegia, quadriplegia, and/or permanent loss of bowel or bladder control.

Spinal cord concussion

If MRI reveals no abnormality in the spinal canal, neurological symptoms following an injury to the neck are probably the result of a *spinal cord concussion*. As in cases of a cerebral concussion, the symptoms of a spinal cord concussion (e.g., numbness, tingling, weakness, or gait or sphincter dysfunction) are *transient*. Many patients are nevertheless hospitalized overnight. Some physicians have administered a corticosteroid as a precaution; based on the studies cited earlier (5,6), this is no longer recommended. A full recovery within 24 hours is to be expected. Persistent deficits are a reason to order a second MRI and to consider a brain imaging study as well.

Neck sprain, whiplash injury, and stingers

Patients with a history of a neck injury and normal radiological studies who experience neck *pain* but report *no neurological symptoms* are said to have "neck sprain," which is a nonspecific term for a mild musculoskeletal injury. If the accident was associated with transient hyperextension of the neck, it is often called a "whiplash injury." Treatment is supportive and consists of rest, anti-inflammatory medication, or a cervical collar. Physical therapy and sometimes nortriptyline or gabapentin may be helpful for the patient with persistent neck pain. Recent studies (7–9) indicate that the average duration of whiplash symptoms is much greater in some countries than in other countries, suggesting the importance of cultural expectations and psychological factors in the recovery process.

Athletes call posttraumatic, burning (neuropathic) pain that travels down the arm a "*stinger.*" The symptoms are usually of fairly short duration. If a patient has a history of multiple episodes, MRI and/or CT of the cervical spine or brachial plexus may be ordered to look for a bone deformity compressing a nerve root.

BACK INJURY

Back pain after a fall, weight lifting, or heavy physical labor is often the result of a mild musculoskeletal injury and is called "back strain." Back strain is the likely diagnosis if the patient with posttraumatic back pain reports no neurological symptoms (e.g., weakness or paresthesias) and the pain does not radiate to a lower extremity. Rest and ibuprofen or naproxen is usually sufficient treatment. If the pain is severe or persistent or if the patient has fallen onto his or her back, a series of plain radiographs of the lumbar spine should be ordered to look for a vertebral fracture. In cases of vertebral fracture, *percussion of the spine* often demonstrates tenderness. In other cases, the x-ray film will show *spondylolisthesis*, or dislocation of a lumbar vertebral body.

If posttraumatic back pain *radiates to the thigh or leg* or if the patient reports symptoms of weakness, sensory loss, or paresthesias in a lower extremity, *compression of a nerve root* by a herniated nucleus pulposus ("herniated disc") is likely to be the cause. In many such cases of *radiculopathy* (nerve root compression), the *straight leg-raising test* (see Chapter 1) exacerbates the pain. Other signs suggestive of lumbar radiculopathy include asymmetry of the patellar or Achilles tendon reflex, weakness in one lower extremity, inability to walk on the toe or heel on the affected side, and unilaterally decreased sensation to pinprick. MRI of the lumbosacral spine (Fig. 12.3) will usually demonstrate the herniated disc, which frequently lies between the L5 and S1 or L4 and L5 vertebrae.

The initial treatment of a herniated disc in a teenager or adult is bed rest and ibuprofen (up to 400 to 800 mg every 6 hours). A short course of

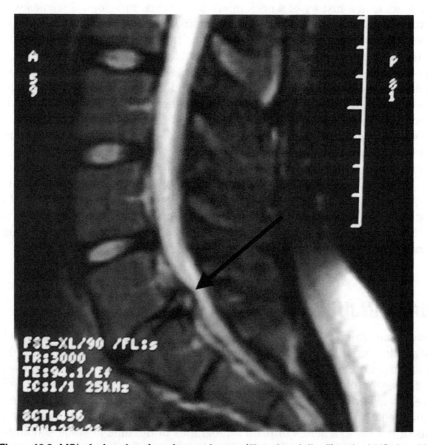

Figure 12.3 MRI of a **herniated nucleus pulposus** ("herniated disc") at the L5/S1 level in a 14-year old adolescent female with lower back pain radiating down the right leg.
(Courtesy of Howard Seigerman, MD, and Eliot Lerner, MD, The Valley Hospital.)

a corticosteroid (prednisone, 60 mg per day for 5 days) is sometimes prescribed. An opiate analgesic is sometimes needed to relieve severe pain. After 1 to 2 weeks, light exercise such as walking is recommended. Heavy lifting must be avoided, and the patient should be taught to bend at the knees when stooping to tie shoes or pick up objects. If the pain continues to be severe despite these measures or if neurological symptoms such as foot drop persist, it may be necessary to remove the disc fragment surgically. The results of surgery in adolescents and children have not been extensively evaluated but are generally good according to one study (10).

Unexplained back pain

Persistent back pain that is not attributable to trauma suggests a potentially serious problem. Depending on the location of the pain and any abnormal neurological findings, MRI of either the lumbar or thoracic spine should be ordered. If MRI of the spine is normal, a renal or abdominal lesion should be excluded by appropriate imaging studies. Ankylosing spondylitis, other autoimmune disorders, and some infectious diseases also may present with back pain. Laboratory studies including rheumatoid factor, erythrocyte sedimentation rate, Lyme titer, and HLA B27 antigen should be ordered.

PERIPHERAL NERVE INJURIES

The diagnosis of an injury to a peripheral nerve initially relies on the clinical findings. Electromyography (EMG) (see following section, Electrical Tests of Muscle and Nerve Function) is primarily used to support but not make the diagnosis and may not yield a positive result for up to several weeks after a nerve injury. In the great majority of pediatric cases, dysfunction of a single nerve (*mononeuropathy*) is caused by trauma. If there is no history of trauma, the physician should consider a hereditary, metabolic, infectious, or immunological cause and look for evidence of tumor compressing the nerve.

Adult patients with *radial nerve palsy* often have slept in a chair with hard armrests ("Saturday night palsy"), awakening to find that they are *unable to extend (dorsiflex) the hand and fingers*. This syndrome is uncommon in childhood, when radial nerve palsy is more often the result of a fracture of the humerus. Sensory loss and paresthesias are not reported in cases of radial nerve palsy since the radial nerve does not carry sensory fibers. The hand is held in a limp-wristed position, and the patient can offer little resistance to flexion of his wrist and fingers. The brachioradialis reflex is absent. The other deep tendon reflexes in the upper extremity, and all other movements of the arm, wrist, hand, and fingers are unaffected. Treatment consists of splinting the hand and occupational therapy. Recovery takes weeks to months.

Median nerve palsy is usually caused by a serious injury to the elbow, usually a fracture of the distal humerus. Symptoms include *weakness of flexion of the thumb, index, and middle finger* and *sensory loss over the thenar portion of the palm and the palmar surface of the first three digits.* The fingers may be held in the "position of benediction," which is extension of the thumb, index, and middle finger. Treatment consists of splinting and rest, and occupational therapy may be helpful. In some cases, surgical decompression of the nerve at the elbow is necessary.

Carpal tunnel syndrome is caused by intermittent compression of the median nerve at the wrist. The usual symptoms are *pain, numbness, or paresthesias* in the thenar area of the palm and the first three digits. Symptoms often can be provoked by tapping the wrist over the nerve (*Tinel sign*) or pressing the dorsal surfaces of the hands together (*Phalen sign*). *Splinting the wrist* is the standard treatment for mild cases of carpal tunnel syndrome. Corticosteroid injections and surgery are reserved for patients with refractory symptoms.

Ulnar neuropathy is usually caused by a traumatic injury to the elbow, in many cases a fracture of the distal humerus. Patients present with weakness of the ring finger, fifth digit, and the intrinsic hand muscles, resulting in a "claw hand." Sensory loss over the hypothenar eminence accompanies the motor deficits. Surgery is performed in some cases of fracture or when the nerve has been dislocated at the elbow.

Peroneal neuropathy results when the peroneal nerve is compressed against the head of the fibula. The most common cause is sleeping on a hard surface. Peroneal neuropathy presents as *foot drop*, causing a disturbance of gait. The patient cannot heel walk or dorsiflex the foot. All other lower extremity muscle groups, the deep tendon reflexes, and sensation in the lower extremity are unaffected. Treatment consists of physical therapy and an ankle-foot orthosis. Recovery occurs over weeks to months.

Meralgia paresthetica is caused by compression of the lateral cutaneous nerve of the thigh. The patient typically complains of sensory loss or paresthesias over the external part of the thigh. The cause is variously described as wearing tight belts or tight pants or excessive walking. If these possible causes are addressed, the symptoms usually disappear.

Nerve regeneration and nerve grafting

A damaged nerve spontaneously regenerates along the basal lamina of the dead nerve segment. One millimeter per day is the usual rate of regrowth. Nerves transected at a more proximal point along their course obviously take the longest to regenerate. In many cases, function is largely eventually restored, but in some cases, the regenerating nerve encounters a scar (neuroma) or other obstacle preventing regrowth.

Nerve grafting is performed in cases of nerve transection or when a neuroma has prevented regeneration. The most common techniques are direct grafting of the remaining nerve trunks and interposition of a graft taken from another, less important nerve (usually the sural nerve) to connect the nerve trunks. In cases of *nerve avulsion*, when a nerve root has been torn from the spinal cord, it is not possible to regraft the nerve to its point of origin. A nerve leading to another muscle group can often be rerouted to supply the damaged nerve. The patient must learn to "think" about moving the muscle originally supplied by the rerouted nerve in order to move the muscle that it now supplies.

Electrical tests of muscle and nerve function

EMG is a procedure in which a thin recording needle is inserted into the belly of a muscle. The electrical activity of the muscle is displayed on an electronic screen. EMG is useful in the diagnosis of traumatic nerve injuries, nontraumatic neuropathy, diseases of the neuromuscular junction (e.g., botulism, myasthenia gravis), and diseases of muscle. Abnormal electrical activity is first noted about three weeks after an injury to the nerve supplying a muscle.

A *nerve conduction study* (*NCS*), often performed with the EMG, measures the amplitude and velocity of an electrical impulse traveling within a peripheral nerve. A mild electric shock is delivered over the proximal part of the nerve and recorded at one or more distal locations. In cases of *axonal injury*, the *amplitude* of the impulse is diminished, whereas in cases of *demyelination*, the *conduction velocity* is slowed. In cases of transection or severe demyelination, EMG may suggest evidence of *conduction block*. In cases of demyelinating disease such as Guillain-Barré syndrome (see Chapter 13), *delayed F-waves* recorded during the NCS are diagnostically important.

EMG is a somewhat painful procedure that may be poorly tolerated by young children. NCS is less traumatic and often suffices in cases of nerve injury.

REFERENCES

1. Quality Standards Subcommittee of the American Academy of Neurology. The management of concussion in sports (practice parameter). *Neurology.* 1997;48:581–585.
2. Plum F, Posner J. *The Diagnosis of Stupor and Coma.* Philadelphia: FA Davis; 1980.
3. Jennett B, Teasdale G, Braakman R, et al. Prognosis of patients with severe head injury. *Neurosurgery.* 1979;4:283–289.
4. Brust JCM. Coma. In: Rowland LP, ed. *Merritt's Textbook of Neurology.* Baltimore: Williams and Wilkins; 1995:26.
5. Hurlbert RJ. The role of steroids in acute spinal cord injury: an evidence-based analysis. *Spine.* 2001;26(24 suppl):S39–S46.
6. Ditunno JF Jr. New spinal cord injury standards, 1992. Clinical assessment following acute cervical spine injury. The section on disorders of the spine and peripheral nerves of the American Association of Neurological Surgeons and the Congress of Neurological Surgeons. Sept 20, 2001. http://www.spineuniverse.com/pdf/traumaguide/3.pdf

7. Richter M, Ferrari R, Otte D, et al. Correlation of clinical findings, collision parameters, and psychological factors in the outcome of whiplash associated disorders. *J Neurol Neurosurg Psychiatry.* 2004;75:758–764.

8. Gun RT, Osti OL, O'Riordon A, et al. Risk factors for prolonged disability after whiplash injury: a prospective study. *Spine.* 2005;30:386–391.

9. Pobereskin LH. Whiplash following rear end collisions: a prospective cohort study. *J Neurol Neurosurg Psychiatry.* 2005;76:1146–1151.

10. Savini R, Martucci E, Nardi S, et al. The herniated lumbar intervertebral disc in children and adolescents. Long-term follow-up of 101 cases treated by surgery. *Ital J Orthop Traumatol.* 1991;17:505–511.

13

STROKE, ACUTE PARAPARESIS, AND OTHER SERIOUS DISORDERS OF ACUTE AND SUBACUTE ONSET

STROKE IN CHILDHOOD AND ADOLESCENCE

Pediatric patients account for 1% of all cases of stroke. Stroke can be caused by ischemia (blockage of a cerebral artery) or bleeding in the brain (intracerebral hemorrhage). Acute monoparesis and hemiparesis are the most common manifestations of a stroke in a child. Aphasia, a visual field deficit, diplopia, and ataxia are less common in children than in adults. Physicians should remember that *transient* focal neurological deficits associated with a *headache* are a typical *migraine* manifestation. If the patient had a *focal seizure before the onset of hemiparesis*, his or her motor deficit is often a transient *Todd paralysis* (see Chapter 6).

Physical examination in the emergency room

The pediatric patient who has had a stroke must undergo a comprehensive medical and neurological evaluation. However, in the emergency room, specific aspects of the history and examination take precedence. First and foremost, it is essential to determine (a) if there is a prior history of seizure or migraine (either of which might cause a transient neurological deficit) and (b) the extent of the patient's deficits. The neurological examination should assess the patient's alertness, speech and comprehension, visual fields, extraocular movements, pupils, facial and tongue movements, gross and fine motor movements of all four extremities (the pronator drift test is often used here), deep tendon and plantar reflexes, sensation in all extremities (a brief initial examination is acceptable), and cerebellar function. Equally important is a *medical assessment* looking for *signs of an acute condition that might cause cerebral ischemia or bleeding* (e.g., severe hypertension, dehydration, meningitis, amphetamine toxicity, and cardiac arrhythmia) and that needs urgent attention.

Ischemia versus bleeding

The next step is generally to order a *noncontrast computed tomography (CT) scan of the brain* to exclude the possibility of intracerebral bleeding. The CT image will always reveal bleeding in the brain. Ischemic changes generally do not appear in a CT scan for at least 24 hours. Therefore, if the CT reveals no evidence of bleeding and the patient's clinical presentation suggests a stroke, an ischemic stroke becomes the working diagnosis.

Causes of ischemic stroke in pediatric patients

In the adult population, hypertension, diabetes mellitus, heart disease, and cerebrovascular disease are by far the most common causes of stroke. The list of possible causes of stroke in the pediatric population is much longer. Furthermore, even after a comprehensive battery of diagnostic tests has been completed, no cause is determined in many cases.

In children with *congenital heart disease or infectious endocarditis*, a cardiac embolus may cause a cerebral infarction. *Hypercoagulable states* caused by a congenital or acquired disorder (e.g., Factor V Leiden deficiency, homocysteinemia, protein C or S deficiency, and cardiolipin antibody syndrome) are sometimes identified. Patients with a history of *sickle cell anemia* are at risk for small- and large-vessel cerebral arterial infarction caused by damage to the vascular endothelium, predisposing to thrombosis (1). Oral *trauma* (such as falling with an ice cream stick in the mouth) can injure the carotid artery, leading to dissection and thrombosis. Carotid or vertebral artery dissection can also occur spontaneously. Patients with a *cerebral arterial malformation* (arteriovenous malformation, moya-moya syndrome, and other vascular anomalies) also are at risk for stroke (2). *Familial hypercholesterolemia* and *mitochondrial disorders* (see Chapter 14) are also possible causes of stroke in a young person. Finally, a stroke may occur as a complication of severe dehydration, meningitis, leukemia, thrombocythemia, anemia, or vasculitis.

Case 13.1

A 15-year-old adolescent male experiences sudden-onset severe weakness of the right leg while playing soccer and collapses to the ground. His right arm is also weak, and his speech is slurred. He is immediately transported to the emergency room.

The patient has no prior history of any medical problems. He has never had a migraine headache or a seizure, and he does not report a headache now. He takes no medication.

He presents as a frightened, healthy-appearing teenager. His blood pressure is 145/87. He does not have a fever. The neck is supple, and no carotid or cranial bruits are noted. The cardiac rhythm and heart sounds are normal. The patient's speech is slurred but intelligible, and he follows directions well. The visual fields are full to confrontation. The pupils are equal and reactive, and the extraocular movements are intact. Facial, tongue, and palatal movements are symmetrical. Motor examination reveals decreased tone on the right side, a positive pronator drift test, slow fine finger movements, 4/5 strength in the upper extremity, and 3/5 strength in the lower extremity. Motor examination of the left upper and left lower extremity is normal. The deep tendon reflexes are diminished on the right side, and the right toe does not move in response to plantar stimulation.

A CT scan of the head reveals no evidence of bleeding or any other intracranial abnormality.

Diagnosis: *Acute ischemic stroke.*

Outcome: Given the extent of the patient's neurological deficits, a decision was made to initiate treatment with tissue plasminogen activator (tPA). The family participated in the decision and was informed of the benefits and risks and of the fact that the Food and Drug Administration has not approved this drug for use in pediatric patients. The risks of no treatment were also discussed. An appropriate dosage, by weight, of intravenous tPA was administered over 1 hour beginning 2 hours after the onset of symptoms.

After tPA was given, diffusion-weighted MRI was performed and demonstrated an infarction in the region of the left hemisphere basal ganglia. Magnetic resonance angiography (MRA) revealed narrowing of the lumen of the left internal carotid artery suggesting dissection. The patient was admitted to the intensive care unit.

A pediatric hematologist and cardiologist were consulted. Routine blood tests, echocardiogram, Holter monitoring, plasma lipids, plasma lactic acid, plasma homocysteine, and an extensive series of tests for disorders of coagulation yielded normal results.

During the next several days, the patient made a noticeable recovery and, by discharge (10 days later), was able to walk with a cane and could use the right arm for simple tasks. His speech was still slightly slurred. He was prescribed warfarin by the hematologist and took this medication for the next 3 months. At the 6-month follow-up, his speech and gait were normal, although fine motor coordination of the right hand was still not quite back to baseline. A repeat MRI/MRA study showed a chronic left basal ganglionic infarct and a patent left carotid artery.

Diagnostic testing and treatment

As noted earlier, CT will always determine whether or not the patient's symptoms are a result of intracerebral bleeding, but CT does not reveal evidence of ischemia for at least 24 hours. *Diffusion-weighted magnetic resonance imaging (MRI)* is highly sensitive to ischemic changes and should be done as soon as possible (Fig. 13.1).

Tissue plasminogen activator (tPA) can be administered to adult patients within 3 hours of the onset of stroke symptoms. tPA can dramatically

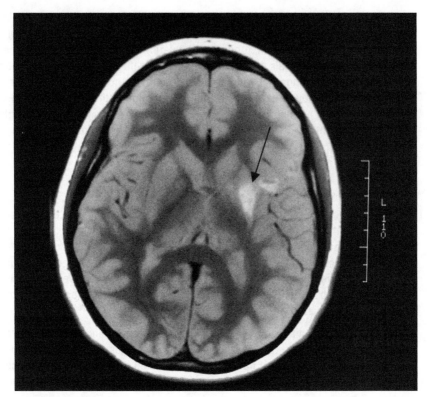

Figure 13.1 MRI of an **ischemic stroke** in the left basal ganglia of a 15-year-old adolescent male.
(Courtesy of Howard Seigerman, MD, and Eliot Lerner, MD, The Valley Hospital.)

improve the neurological deficits caused by an acute stroke and also has been shown to improve the long-term outcome following stroke in adults (3). No clinical studies of tPA in children have been conducted, although tPA has been given to pediatric patients with a good outcome (see Case 13.1, which is based on an actual patient).

tPA may cause *bleeding* in internal organs, including the brain. The incidence is 1% to 5% in adults. For this reason, tPA is not usually administered to adult stroke patients with relatively minor deficits (minimally slurred speech, mild hand incoordination, etc.). Given that young (<5 to 7 years old) children often make an excellent spontaneous recovery from stroke, it would seem prudent not to administer this drug to patients less than 8 to 10 years of age, regardless of the extent of their neurological deficits. In older children and adolescents, the risks and benefits must be carefully weighed and discussed with the family. Stroke can be a devastating condition, and the possibility of reversing an infarction or minimizing neurological damage may be worth the risks associated with tPA in some cases.

The patient should be admitted to the intensive care unit. Underlying conditions, such as infection, arrhythmia, or dehydration, should be aggressively treated. *Aspirin* and other *platelet aggregation–inhibiting drugs* (e.g., clopidogrel, dipyridamole) are routinely prescribed to adults with an ischemic stroke and are sometimes prescribed to children and adolescents, although they are not yet standard therapy. Antiplatelet drugs are administered to adults primarily for the purpose of preventing worsening of the infarction and preventing future strokes and are not expected to reverse a stroke that has already occurred. **These drugs are not given after tPA.** Corticosteroids play no role in the treatment of stroke.

Magnetic resonance angiography (MRA) of the carotid and vertebral arteries, the circle of Willis, and the cerebral vessels should be done with MRI of the brain to search for evidence of a vascular anomaly or arterial dissection. A cardiologist should be consulted. *Echocardiogram* and *Holter monitoring* are ordered to investigate the possibility of cardiac arrhythmia or an endocardial abnormality predisposing to thrombus formation. *Complete blood count (CBC), erythrocyte sedimentation rate, electrolyte panel, liver function tests, and urinalysis,* should be ordered. Other potentially informative tests include *sickle-cell preparation, prothrombin and partial thromboplastin times (PT and PTT), lipid profile, plasma homocysteine, lactic acid, protein C and S, antithrombin III, cardiolipin antibody, Factor V Leiden,* and additional studies to evaluate coagulation (generally recommended by a hematologist). If the results of all these tests are normal and no cause for the stroke has been discovered, *cerebral angiography* may be considered to exclude a vascular anomaly. Angiography is more sensitive than MRA and remains the "gold standard" for evaluating the cerebral vessels. However, angiography is itself associated with a small ($<1\%$) risk of a stroke and, consequently, is often deferred. *Lumbar puncture* (LP) may be appropriate if an intracranial infection causing the stroke is suspected or to obtain cerebrospinal fluid for another diagnostic purpose such as for seeking evidence of a mitochondrial disease (see Chapter 14).

Prognosis

Young patients (<5 to 7 years of age), as a rule, have the best outcome. It is by no means uncommon for a young child to make a remarkable recovery even after a large hemispheric infarction, although such an outcome cannot be guaranteed. In many cases, language skills, functional use of the arms and hands, and ability to ambulate recover within a year, in some cases completely. However, as is the case for neonates who have had a stroke (see Chapter 10), subtle cognitive deficits that affect academic performance may be noted over the long term. Children who have had a stroke should undergo neuropsychological testing during the course of recovery; should receive physical, occupational, or speech therapy; and should be closely followed for several years.

Older children and teenagers are more likely to have permanent disabilities such as hemiparesis or aphasia, although some functional recovery can be anticipated. Physical, occupational, or speech therapy is always prescribed. Deficits persisting longer than a year are likely to be permanent.

Any patient who has had a stroke that involved the cerebral cortex or temporal lobe is at increased risk for *focal seizures*.

INTRACEREBRAL HEMORRHAGE

An intracerebral hemorrhage (ICH) may occur as a result of a coagulation or platelet disorder, bleeding from an arteriovenous malformation or a hemangioma, or severe hypertension (which, in adolescents, may result from cocaine or amphetamine abuse) (Fig. 13.2). An ICH often presents with *focal neurological symptoms*, such as hemiparesis or aphasia, that are *unaccompanied by headache*. In comparison, a ruptured cerebral aneurysm causes a subarachnoid hemorrhage (SAH) (see Chapter 2) typically presenting with a *severe headache*.

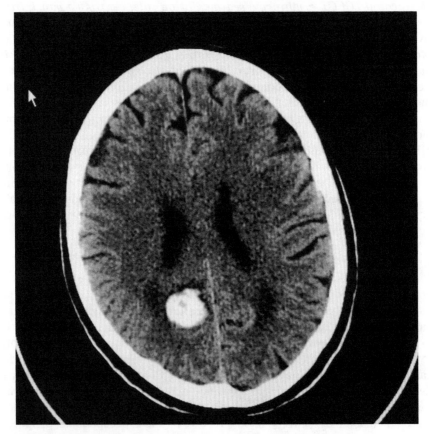

Figure 13.2 CT scan of a right parietal lobe **intracranial hemorrhage**. (Courtesy of Ajax George, MD, New York University School of Medicine.)

Urine toxicology screening, CBC, and coagulation studies should be ordered in cases of ICH. If there is an underlying bleeding diathesis, it is promptly addressed by administration of platelets or clotting factors. The cause of severe unexplained hypertension must be sought and appropriately treated. In the case of a large ICH, a neurosurgeon is often consulted.

ACUTE AND SUBACUTE ONSET OF DIFFICULTY WALKING

Physicians will sometimes need to evaluate a child or adolescent who has rapidly become *unable to walk* (Table 13.1). *Chronic or slowly progressive loss of the ability to walk* entails a different differential diagnosis (see Chapter 14).

TABLE 13.1

Common causes of acute and subacute gait disturbance in children

Disorder	Clinical features	Diagnostic tests
Transverse myelitis	Often asymmetrical lower extremity weakness, sensory level, urinary incontinence or retention, back pain; reflexes often absent; sometimes Babinski sign	MRI of spinal cord; LP; blood tests for infections, autoimmune disorders, other causes (see text); brain MRI to exclude acute demyelinating encephalomyelitis
Ruptured spinal arteriovenous malformation	As above; usually acute onset with severe back pain	MRI of spinal cord; LP if MRI normal
Spinal epidural abscess	Fever plus above	MRI of spinal cord
Spinal cord infarction	Hyperacute onset; otherwise as above	MRI of spinal cord; initial study often negative; may need to repeat MRI in 2–5 days
Cerebral infarction (stroke)	Acute onset of *unilateral* weakness, sometimes with visual or speech involvement	Head CT; diffusion-weighted MRI; see text for additional studies
Guillain-Barré syndrome	*Subacute* onset of progressive weakness in legs more than arms; variable sensory involvement without sensory level; usually absent	MRI of spinal cord often ordered to exclude myelopathy; LP and electromyography after 1 week; serology tests

(continued)

TABLE 13.1

(continued)

Disorder	Clinical features	Diagnostic tests
	deep tendon reflexes; no bowel/bladder symptoms	for Epstein-Barr virus and *Helicobacter*
Acute postinfectious cerebellar ataxia	Symmetrical ataxia affecting upper and lower extremities as well as trunk; no weakness of sensory symptoms; no bowel/bladder symptoms	No specific test; MRI sometimes ordered to exclude a brain lesion but not normally indicated
Toxic synovitis	Pain on ambulation (antalgic gait); no abnormal neurological findings; usually associated with a viral syndrome	None
Viral myositis	Pain in calves causing difficulty walking; no physical findings other than tenderness; usually history of concurrent or preceding viral illness (influenza or coxsackie)	Markedly elevated creatine phosphokinase that returns to normal in a few days to weeks
Psychogenic gait disorder	Often occurs in a particular setting, or onset was associated with an emotionally traumatic event; odd-appearing gait; patient never falls; inconsistent physical findings; no bowel/bladder complaints; normal reflexes	At discretion of physician; some testing generally ordered to exclude a neurological disorder

MRI, magnetic resonance imaging; LP, lumbar puncture; CT, computed tomography.

Paraparesis means weakness either of both arms or of both legs and, in practice, almost always refers to weakness of the lower extremities. Onset of paraparesis within *seconds to a few hours suggests an acute spinal cord syndrome (acute myelopathy)*. If paraparesis develops *subacutely* (over a period of a few days), *Guillain-Barré syndrome* is a more likely cause.

Spinal cord diseases often cause a *disturbance of bladder or bowel function* (e.g., urinary retention, constipation, or incontinence) and are characterized by a *sensory level*: a marked loss of sensation below a specific dermatome demonstrable by a careful sensory examination. In most cases of myelopathy, weakness in the lower extremities is somewhat *asymmetric*. The lower extremities are *hypotonic*, and *deep tendon reflexes* are diminished or absent in the legs; this is known as the syndrome of *spinal shock*. Since diseases of the peripheral nerves (i.e., Guillain-Barré syndrome) also cause diminished reflexes, *absence of reflexes is not a particularly useful physical finding when evaluating a patient with acute paraparesis*. Spasticity and hyperreflexia do not develop as the result of a spinal cord lesion for at least several weeks.

MRI of the spinal cord should be ordered in all cases of acute myelopathy. Important potential causes include transverse myelitis, spinal epidural abscess, spinal cord infarction, and arteriovenous malformation (AVM). A ruptured AVM is suggested if MRI demonstrates blood within the spinal cord or spinal canal. If the patient has a history of back pain and fever and MRI demonstrates an extramedullary fluid collection, the patient can be assumed to have a spinal epidural abscess. This condition requires prompt neurosurgical intervention (drainage or needle aspiration) as well as aggressive treatment with antibiotics and corticosteroids to prevent spinal cord infarction and permanent disability. Primary spinal cord infarction may be difficult to diagnose. The initial MRI study is often normal. Spinal cord edema often is demonstrable by MRI after 48 hours. A disorder of coagulation should be excluded if an infarction is suspected, as in cases of stroke.

Transverse myelitis

Transverse myelitis (TM) is an acute, segmental spinal cord syndrome that has generally been attributed to an inflammatory or infectious process. In many cases, no etiology is determined; the term *transverse myelopathy* may be more appropriate when LP reveals no evidence of inflammation. Typical symptoms and signs of TM include asymmetrical lower extremity weakness causing difficulty walking, urinary incontinence or retention, and dermatome-defined sensory loss (sensory level). Back pain is often reported. Patients with *TM and inflammation of the optic nerves* are said to have *Devic disease*, a syndrome that is more common in adults than children and is considered a form of multiple sclerosis.

Diagnostic studies

Diagnostic studies to evaluate the patient with suspected TM are suggested by the Transverse Myelitis Consortium Working Group (4). MRI is the most important test to order, typically revealing one or more areas of *abnormal signal within the spinal cord* (Fig. 13.3). These lesions may or may not enhance following the administration of intravenous contrast. LP should be performed in all cases of TM. Mild pleocytosis with a predominance of lymphocytes and monocytes, elevated protein, and normal glucose are typical findings and suggest an inflammatory process. Other commonly ordered spinal fluid studies include oligoclonal bands, immunoglobulin G, and polymerase chain reaction for herpes simplex virus. *MRI of the brain* should be ordered to look for evidence of acute disseminated encephalomyelitis

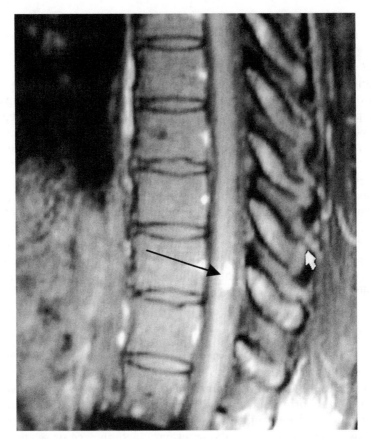

Figure 13.3 MRI of a thoracic spinal cord lesion in a case of **transverse myelitis**. (Courtesy of Howard Seigerman, MD, and Eliot Lerner, MD, The Valley Hospital.)

(see section on encephalitis). Blood tests, including CBC, erythrocyte sedimentation rate, antinuclear antibody, and Lyme, *Mycoplasma*, Epstein-Barr, and cytomegalovirus titers also are frequently ordered.

Treatment

It is common practice to prescribe a *corticosteroid* to patients with TM, although the benefits have not been carefully studied. Methylprednisone, at a high dosage comparable to that given for acute spinal cord trauma (see Chapter 12), is usually administered for several days, followed by a rapidly tapering oral regimen (prednisone 60 mg reduced daily by 10 mg). Patients who do not respond to a corticosteroid are sometimes treated empirically with immune globulin, plasmapheresis, or even cyclophosphamide or azathioprine. If an infectious cause is identified, it is treated, when possible, with an antibiotic or antiviral drug. The prognosis for patients with TM is variable, with some patients making a complete recovery and others left with significant residual disability. Recurrence of symptoms occasionally occurs and may respond to a second course of a corticosteroid or another one of the drugs previously mentioned.

Guillain-Barré syndrome

Guillain-Barré syndrome (GBS) is a subacute, immune-mediated disorder of the peripheral nerves and, sometimes, the autonomic nervous system. In most cases of GBS, peripheral neuropathy is caused by demyelination. A history of *weakness of the lower extremities that worsens over several days* is typical. In many cases, the weakness becomes severe enough that the patient loses the ability to walk. The disease often also causes weakness in the upper extremities. In severe cases respiratory failure results.

Motor involvement is more pronounced than sensory involvement in cases of GBS, although patients may report paresthesias in the distal lower extremities. Bowel and bladder control is not affected.

In the variant form of GBS known as *Miller-Fisher syndrome*, involvement of the *cranial nerves* causes diplopia, ophthalmoplegia, and difficulty swallowing in addition to lower extremity weakness.

Examination and diagnostic studies

The physical examination of the patient with GBS reveals *marked weakness in the lower extremities* and *trace to absent distal deep tendon reflexes*, especially the Achilles tendon reflex. A clear-cut sensory level is never a feature of GBS; if a "level" is demonstrated, the patient probably has TM or another form of myelopathy and not GBS. The patient may have a wide-based gait and appear ataxic, but finger–nose testing is not abnormal, and nystagmus and titubation are not noted, differentiating GBS from acute cerebellitis (see Chapter 7).

The diagnosis of GBS can be confirmed by a *nerve conduction study* (see Chapter 12), which is most likely to yield an abnormal result when performed at least 1 week after the onset of symptoms. The most classic early finding is a *diminished or absent F-wave* (an anterograde electrical impulse recorded following stimulation of a nerve at a distal point). LP may reveal elevated CSF protein *without* pleocytosis, a pattern referred to as *cytoalbuminologic dissociation*. In some cases, evidence for a preceding or concurrent Epstein-Barr, Lyme, or *Helicobacter pylori* infection is suggested by an elevated peripheral titer.

Treatment

Almost all GBS patients require hospitalization and, usually, admission to an intensive care unit. *Intravenous immune globulin* (0.4 g/kg for 5 days) remains the standard treatment for GBS. A 2-day course of treatment at the same dose appears to be equally effective (5). *Plasmapheresis* is also effective but is usually technically more difficult to administer than immune globulin (6). Corticosteroids are of no benefit (7). *Pulmonary function testing* should be performed at least daily during the first few days of hospitalization, and intubation and mechanical ventilation should be strongly considered if there is a decline in pulmonary function. Cardiac function should be monitored because autonomic nervous system disease can lead to arrhythmia.

Most patients begin to improve after 2 weeks and eventually make a full recovery. In a small percentage of cases, GBS results in permanent neurological deficits. Many of these patients are thought to have had a distinct form of GBS caused by immune-mediated damage to the nerve axon rather than to the myelin sheath.

Other causes of acute- and subacute-onset gait problems

Postviral cerebellar ataxia (see Chapter 7) presents as an acute gait disturbance. *Titubation, nystagmus, and ataxia of the upper extremities*, which are findings never associated with diseases of the spinal cord, nerve, or muscle, are typical findings in cases of cerebellar ataxia.

Viral myositis often causes difficulty walking. *Severe calf pain* is a common complaint. The neurological examination is normal other than eliciting a general reluctance to walk and calf tenderness. *Marked elevation of the plasma creatine phosphokinase (CPK)* level and a history of a preceding viral illness, usually influenza or Coxsackie virus, suggest this condition, which is self-limited. The CPK level should start to decline within a week.

Toxic synovitis is a nonneurological disorder occurring during childhood that causes pain in the lower extremities and refusal to ambulate. The pathogenesis is not well understood, but there is often a history of an associated viral illness. The child is usually unwilling to walk or exhibits an *antalgic gait* (see Chapter 1), but the neurological examination and laboratory studies are unremarkable. The condition is self-limited.

Malingering and various other behavioral causes of not walking should always be considered in the case of a child unwilling to walk and especially if the neurological examination and laboratory studies are normal. The patient often has an odd or "hysterical" gait (see Chapter 1). Signs of weakness on examination are inconsistent, reflexes are normal, and despite complaining of being unable to walk, the patient does not fall and hurt him or herself. If the motor examination suggests "weakness" in the supine position (complete inability to raise a lower extremity off the examination table) but the patient can support his or her weight, it is likely that the problem is psychogenic. Another way to investigate the possibility of a functional disorder, while the patient is in the supine position, is for the examiner to place a hand under the "strong" leg and ask the patient to try to raise the "weak" leg. If the patient does not exert pressure on the examiner's hand, the patient is not trying to raise the "weak" leg. Possible motivations for the behavior (e.g., staying out of school, attention seeking) should be discussed with the family. Psychotherapy is often appropriate.

ACUTE CHANGE IN MENTAL STATUS

Drug or toxin ingestion

When a child or adolescent appears disoriented, confused, or agitated or is brought to the emergency room obtunded or in a coma, the physician should always consider *medication overdose, drug abuse, or poisoning*. The *pupils* should be examined. Dilated pupils suggest that the patient may have taken an amphetamine, cocaine, marijuana, or lysergic acid diethylamide (LSD). Meiosis can result from an anticholinergic medication, a barbiturate or benzodiazepine, or an opiate-based drug. *Respiratory rate and heart rate* also may be clues to the cause of an altered mental status (e.g., tachycardia in cases of cocaine or amphetamine intoxication, tachypnea in cases of metabolic acidosis caused by a drug or toxin, or a decreased respiratory rate from a narcotic overdose). CBC, plasma electrolytes and glucose, urine drug screen, plasma acetaminophen and aspirin levels, arterial blood gas, liver function tests, and plasma ammonia level should be promptly ordered. The medicine cabinets and kitchen cabinets in the child's home should be checked for medications and open containers. Accidental poisoning is a subject too broad to be covered here, and the reader should consult a standard medical, pediatric, or emergency room textbook. In cases of deliberate ingestion, many adolescents will admit that they have taken a recreational drug or a deliberate overdose of a prescription or over-the-counter medication as a suicidal gesture. Hospitalization is required in most cases, and psychiatric consultation should be requested (Table 13.2).

TABLE 13.2

Causes of acute changes in mental status

Disorder	Clinical features	Diagnostic tests
Medication overdose/substance abuse/poisoning (also see Table 5.3)	Dilated or meiotic pupils; sometimes with decreased or increased heart rate or respirations; patient may be agitated, aggressive, anxious, paranoid; obtunded or comatose; focal signs are unusual	Urine toxicology, blood alcohol level, aspirin, and acetaminophen levels; CAREFUL HISTORY; CHECK MEDICINE CABINETS IN HOME; psychiatric consultation in cases of suspected drug abuse, suicide attempt
Encephalitis	Usually fever; obtundation; often nuchal rigidity; focal neurological deficits may be noted; physical	MRI of brain; LP sent for appropriate cultures/ serological tests and polymerase chain

(*continued*)

TABLE 13.2
(continued)

Disorder	Clinical features	Diagnostic tests
	examination or history often suggest a concurrent or recent infection such as pneumonia; check for herpetic skin/mucous membrane lesions; may have history of insect bite or outdoor exposure	reaction for herpes simplex virus; chest x-ray; peripheral titers as indicated; infectious disease consultation usually requested
Acute demyelinating encephalomyelitis	Variable: fever, seizures, obtundation, focal deficits	MRI of brain and spinal cord; LP; laboratory tests (see text)
Meningitis	In older child and adolescent: fever, headache, and nuchal rigidity; in infant and young child: lethargy, irritability, poor appetite, and fever	Prompt LP followed by a corticosteroid and antibiotic; see Chapter 2 for other recommendations
Shaken baby syndrome (infants)	Obtundation, occasionally seizures or focal deficits; preretinal hemorrhages on funduscopic examination	Head CT; plain films of long bones and ribs to look for evidence of abuse; neurosurgical consultation
Schizophrenia, manic episode, other psychiatric disorder	Patient may be agitated, delusional, paranoid, or withdrawn; examination should reveal no focal neurological features or unusual physical findings	MRI should be done if no history of previous psychiatric diagnosis; toxicology screening; consider LP; all medical diagnostic tests for possible causes of psychosis (see Chapter 5) should be normal

MRI, magnetic resonance imaging; LP, lumbar puncture; CT, computed tomography.

Encephalitis

Mycoplasma pneumoniae, cytomegalovirus, and herpes simplex, Epstein-Barr (EBV), varicella, and influenza viruses are among the more common causes of *encephalitis*, or inflammation of the brain parenchyma. Mumps and measles may cause encephalitis in nonvaccinated persons. Encephalitis virtually always causes an altered mental status (e.g., agitation, obtundation, or coma) and usually, but not invariably, fever. Focal seizures may occur. Other focal deficits are less common. A history of exposure to domestic or wild animals or of long periods of time spent outdoors raises the possibility of arbovirus infection and other insect-borne diseases that cause fever and obtundation, including Rocky Mountain spotted fever and tularemia.

The physical examination should include a careful search for any signs that may suggest the type of infection. A nonspecific viral exanthem or a characteristic rash suggesting varicella, measles, or Rocky Mountain spotted fever may be noted. The mouth, pharynx, eyes, and ears should be checked for herpetic lesions. A history of pneumonia or cough raises the possibility of *Mycoplasma* or influenza. Diarrhea suggests enterovirus infection. The examiner should also perform a funduscopic examination looking for papilledema, signifying elevated intracranial pressure (ICP). If the patient has a stiff neck, it is possible that he or she has meningitis (see Chapter 2).

If encephalitis is suspected and the examination does not reveal papilledema, LP is performed. CSF should be sent for oligoclonal bands, and immunoglobulin G; viral culture; and the polymerase chain reaction (PCR) test for herpes simplex. The LP typically reveals a mild lymphocytic pleocytosis and elevated protein, although in some cases of encephalitis, the CSF is normal. Infectious disease consultation should be requested. Plasma titers suggesting exposure to *Mycoplasma*, influenza viruses, enteroviruses, EBV, cytomegalovirus, arboviruses, *Rickettsia*, and other possible organisms suggested by the history should be checked. Contrast-enhanced MRI also should be ordered.

The patient with encephalitis should be admitted to the intensive care unit. Elevated ICP is treated (see Chapters 2 and 12). *It is assumed that herpes encephalitis is the cause of encephalitis until proven otherwise,* and an appropriate course of treatment (21 days) with acyclovir is prescribed. In many cases of herpes encephalitis, contrast-enhanced MRI reveals an enhancing lesion of the temporal lobe. The lesion is biopsied if the diagnosis remains unclear (i.e., if PCR and viral culture are negative). If *Mycoplasma* is suspected on the basis of a history of pneumonia or peripheral titers, an appropriate antibiotic (e.g., azithromycin, clarithromycin) is started.

Acute disseminated encephalomyelitis (ADEM) is an immune-mediated disorder characterized by inflammation of the brain, brainstem, and/or spinal cord. ADEM often follows a viral infection or a routine immunization. Patients typically present with altered mental status, seizures, or one or more focal neurological deficits and often fever. The diagnosis is suggested by *MRI, which reveals areas of abnormal-appearing cerebral white and occasionally gray matter* (Fig. 13.4). LP often shows a mild lymphocytic pleocytosis and elevated protein.

The same blood and CSF tests should be ordered as in cases of TM (see earlier section on TM). ADEM and TM may coexist, and these two conditions in many instances appear to result from the same immune-mediated process. Therefore, MRI of the brain should be ordered in cases of TM, and MRI of the spinal cord should be ordered in cases of ADEM.

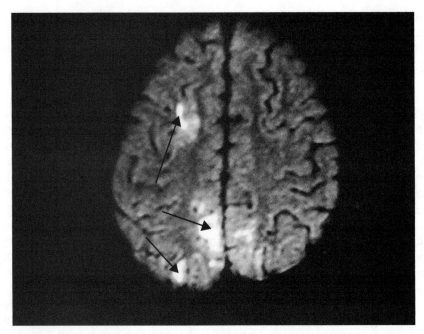

Figure 13.4 MRI showing areas of abnormal signal in the cerebral gray and white matter in a case of **acute demyelinating encephalomyelitis** in a 6-year-old girl. (Courtesy of Howard Seigerman, MD, and Eliot Lerner, MD, The Valley Hospital.)

The relationship of ADEM/TM to multiple sclerosis remains unclear, although recent studies (8,9) suggest that the two conditions are not the same. The presence of oligoclonal bands in the CSF is more typical of multiple sclerosis (8). Multiple sclerosis is uncommon in adolescents and very rare in children and does not present with fever, seizures, or a change in mental status. The diagnosis of multiple sclerosis relies on a history of *seemingly unrelated neurological symptoms appearing at different times,* for example, an episode of blurred vision lasting a few days followed, months later, by a complaint of paresthesias in the right arm. MRI reveals characteristic plaques in the cerebral, brainstem, or spinal white matter (Fig. 13.5) Unlike in ADEM, the gray matter is never involved.

ADEM is usually treated with a corticosteroid. A high dosage is often administered, as for patients with TM. Intravenous immune globulin, plasmapheresis, and cyclophosphamide are used in refractory cases. Many patients recover completely, but sequelae can also include permanent motor or cognitive deficits and seizures (9).

Meningitis in infants and young children

Fever, headache, and a stiff neck are classic symptoms of meningitis in an older child, adolescent, and adult (see Chapter 2). *Young children and infants are more likely to present with lethargy, irritability, anorexia, and*

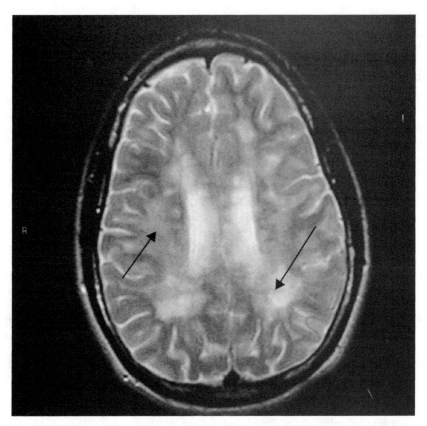

Figure 13.5 MRI showing diffuse white matter lesions in a 14-year-old adolescent male with **multiple sclerosis**.
(Courtesy of Howard Seigerman, MD, and Eliot Lerner, MD, The Valley Hospital.)

low-grade fever. Therefore, meningitis is an important possibility to consider when a very young patient presents with an altered mental status. LP must promptly be performed, and a corticosteroid and antibiotic should be started if meningitis is strongly suspected.

Other causes of acute change in mental status

Shaken baby syndrome should be also suspected when an infant is lethargic or unresponsive. The funduscopic examination classically demonstrates *pre-retinal hemorrhages* (which, however, also can result from accidental trauma or a bleeding diathesis). *CT of the head* reveals a subdural hematoma. Radiological studies of the chest and extremities may reveal fractures of varying age, suggesting abuse.

Adolescents with a history of an acute change in mental status that cannot be explained by diagnostic testing often have a *psychiatric disorder*. Schizophrenia, bipolar disease, and severe depression are possible etiologies (see Chapter 5). If one of these disorders is suspected and other causes have been excluded, a psychiatrist should be consulted.

REFERENCES

1. Steen RG, Xiong S, Langston J, et al. Brain injury in children with sickle cell disease: prevalence and etiology. *Ann Neurol.* 2003;54:564–572.
2. Ganesan V, Prengler M, McShane MA, et al. Investigation of risk factors in children with arterial ischemic stroke. *Ann Neurol.* 2003;53:167–173.
3. The National Institute of Neurological Disorders and Stroke rt-PA Stroke Study Group. Tissue plasminogen activator for acute ischemic stroke. *N Engl J Med.* 1995;333:1581–1588.
4. Transverse Myelitis Consortium Working Group. Proposed diagnostic criteria and nosology of acute transverse myelitis. *Neurology.* 2002;59:499–505.
5. Korinthenberg R, Schessl J, Kirschner J, et al. Intravenously administered immunoglobulin in the treat of childhood Guillain Barré syndrome: a randomized trial. *Pediatrics.* 2005;116:8–14.
6. Esperou H, Jars-Guincestre MC, Bolgert F, et al. Cost analysis of plasma-exchange therapy for the treatment of Guillain-Barre syndrome. *Intensive Care Med.* 2000;26:1094–1100.
7. Van Koningsveld R, Schmitz PI, Meche FG, et al. Effect of methylprednisolone when added to standard treatment with intravenous immunoglobulin for Guillain-Barré syndrome: randomized trial. *Lancet.* 2004;363:192–196.
8. Tenembaum S, Chamoles N, Fejerman N. Acute disseminated encephalomyelitis: a long-term follow-up study of 84 pediatric patients. *Neurology.* 2002;59: 1224–1231.
9. Brass SD, Caramanos Z, Santos C, et al. Multiple sclerosis vs acute disseminated encephalomyelitis in childhood. *Pediatr Neurol.* 2003;29:227–231.

14

OTHER IMPORTANT NEUROLOGICAL SYNDROMES

METABOLIC AND DEGENERATIVE DISORDERS

Hundreds of inherited errors of metabolism are described in the medical literature, and many of these disorders can damage the nervous system. Among the more common mechanisms of neurological injury are abnormal lysosomal storage in cerebral neurons, demyelination of the cerebral or spinal white matter, defects in aerobic or anaerobic metabolism, and the neurotoxic effect of compounds that cannot be metabolized because of an absence of a critical enzyme.

Metabolic diseases are often devastating. Patients' cognitive and motor skills typically regress, and behavior deteriorates. The senses may be impacted, leading to blindness or deafness. Spasticity or ataxia often develops. Intractable seizures are common. Stroke is caused by several metabolic disorders. Metabolic diseases also may damage other organs, including the heart, skeleton, bone marrow, lungs, liver, and kidneys.

Neurodegenerative disorders are diagnostically challenging. Many of these diseases are phenotypically similar. Any of thousands of enzymes involved in metabolic processes may be absent or produced in an inadequate quantity. More than one gene may be responsible for a given disease. The same disease may present differently depending on the patient's age or with different manifestations in patients of the same age. Therefore, the evaluation always entails a detailed history and physical examination and often requires a large number of blood and urine tests; lumbar puncture (LP); biopsies of skin, muscle, and other organs; repeated brain or spine imaging studies; ultrasonography; and genetic testing. Many of the specimens acquired for these tests must be sent to a specialized laboratory.

A lifetime of clinical and research experience is required to know these conditions well. Here we attempt to acquaint the reader with the most characteristic syndromes and suggest an approach to diagnostic testing.

When *not* to suspect a metabolic or degenerative disease

Many patients who should not be tested for a metabolic disease are subjected to an unnecessary work-up. The most common syndrome wrongly suspected to be degenerative is *mildly delayed gross and fine motor development* (see Chapter 8). In these cases, an undefined prenatal problem or constitutionally delayed maturation is a far more common cause of the delay in the infant's or child's development than a degenerative condition. Children who are continuing to make developmental progress, who have developed age-appropriate language skills, but who are a little clumsy or uncoordinated should not be worked up for a degenerative disorder. In other cases, a patient is already diagnosed with *a syndrome of congenital malformation*, yet additional testing is ordered to attempt to explain the patient's history of global developmental delay or low muscle tone. If an infant or child has been diagnosed with a specific congenital disorder (e.g., Down syndrome, fetal alcohol syndrome), it is not appropriate to order further tests to explain developmental delay or hypotonia, since these diseases are widely recognized to cause neurodevelopmental delays. Metabolic or degenerative disorders are also inappropriately tested for in otherwise unremarkable cases of attention-deficit hyperactivity disorder (ADHD), autism, learning disability (LD), and epilepsy.

How *not* to order metabolic tests

Physicians in training all too often develop the habit of ordering a stock "metabolic work-up" whenever they suspect a metabolic disease on the theory that this will "rule out" a metabolic disorder. The usual tests included are plasma quantitative amino acids, plasma ammonia, lactic acid and pyruvate levels, and urine organic acid assay from a 24-hour sample. The diagnostic yield of these tests is very low unless the patient's *clinical history* suggests a specific disorder associated with an elevation of one of these laboratory values. Collecting urine for 24 hours and the large amount of blood required for these tests is often difficult when the patient is an infant or toddler and is also traumatic for the patient and family. Borderline values often result, necessitating repeating the tests or ordering still more tests, whereas true-positive results are very unusual in the absence of clinical findings consistent with a degenerative disorder.

More importantly, the above battery of tests **does not detect many of the most common and important neurodegenerative conditions.** These tests do not yield an abnormal result in cases of leukodystrophy, mucopolysaccharidoses, Tay-Sachs and most other lysosomal storage diseases, ceroid lipofuscinosis, Friedreich ataxia, and ataxia-telangiectasia, to name only a few common inherited conditions.

There is no quick or easy way to "rule in" or "rule out" a metabolic disorder. Physicians must be aware of (a) the conditions that are unlikely to be caused by a metabolic disease, (b) the clinical syndromes that do suggest a degenerative

TABLE 14.1
Four syndromes suggesting a neurodegenerative disorder
Global developmental arrest or regression
Unexplained, acute symptoms in a neonate (especially intractable vomiting, coma, and seizures)
Myoclonic seizures accompanied by neurological deterioration
Unexplained progressive or intermittent ataxia
Also: be aware of signs of *mucopolysaccharidoses, mitochondrial disorders, and leukodystrophies*

process (Table 14.1), (c) features of specific disorders, and (d) the tests that are likely to yield diagnostically useful information in a particular case.

WHEN TO SUSPECT A DEGENERATIVE DISORDER: FOUR IMPORTANT SYNDROMES

Global (motor *and* cognitive) neurological regression or stagnation

For the clinician, the hallmark of many degenerative disorders is *neurological regression*. While other etiologies (e.g., brain tumor or congenitally acquired HIV infection) might produce developmental regression, a hereditary degenerative disease should *always* be considered in these cases. Degenerative diseases of the brain generally cause regression of both *motor and cognitive* function (global regression). If there is a history of *only loss of motor milestones*, a progressive *neuromuscular disease* is the most likely cause (see Chapter 8), although in very rare cases, a disease normally causing global regression primarily causes motor regression. If there is a history *only of loss of language skills, autism* (see Chapter 9) should be suspected.

In the case of a child older than 3 or 4 years of age, deterioration of gray matter (causing *regression with seizures*) or white matter (causing *regression with cognitive slowing and spasticity*) is often clinically obvious. In infants and young children, it is often a far more difficult task to recognize signs of a degenerative disease. Since the young nervous system may be experiencing *both maturation and destruction simultaneously, initially a degenerative process may present not as loss of function but as developmental delay or stagnation following normal development.*

Given the high prevalence of benign etiologies for developmental delay, recognizing these more serious cases may seem challenging. Several suggestions may be made here. First, in many cases of a degenerative disorder, the earliest developmental milestones were normally acquired, and the interval leading up to subsequent milestones *was unusually prolonged*. Second, in most cases of a degenerative disease, the *infant's behavior usually has changed* in terms of alertness, sleep pattern, and response to the environment. Third, *failure to thrive* is commonly reported. Fourth, *unusual physical and/or focal neurological findings* are often noted on careful examination (see following section on physical examination). Finally, *seizures* are much more typical of a degenerative disorder than of a static, benign condition.

The prototypical disorders causing neurologic regression are the *lysosomal storage diseases*. These diseases are each caused by a specific enzyme deficiency that leads to the *intracellular accumulation in lysosomes of material toxic to cerebral neurons*. Approximately 50 lysosomal storage diseases are recognized (1). *Tay-Sachs disease* is the best known of these conditions. Mucopolysaccharidoses, the Niemann-Pick diseases, GM1 gangliosidosis, Gaucher disease, and Fabry disease are other examples.

The age at which signs and symptoms are initially noted varies. During *early infancy, developmental delay, often accompanied by failure to thrive*, is often the initial complaint. *Older infants present with developmental arrest leading eventually to regression. Listlessness, irritability, deterioration of vision and hearing, and intractable seizures* are commonly reported. Cranial nerve palsies may be noted. Spasticity, opisthotonos, and dysphagia often develop. Motor and cognitive regression is typically noted when these diseases present in childhood or later. Ataxia, blindness, seizures, spasticity, and a variety of other serious neurological symptoms may also develop.

A macular *cherry-red spot*, resulting from the deterioration of retinal neurons, is often seen on funduscopic examination. An infant's *facial appearance* may be abnormal in some of these conditions (e.g., GM1 gangliosidosis). *Enlargement of the spleen and liver* is caused by many lysosomal storage diseases (e.g., GM1 gangliosidosis, Niemann-Pick disease, Gaucher disease types I and III). Fabry disease causes vascular pathology and stroke.

The diagnosis is primarily suggested by the clinical presentation. Routine blood test and MRI are often normal. Genetic testing identifies many of these diseases. In most cases, there is no cure or specific treatment for these diseases, which often eventually lead to death or survival in a vegetative state. Bone marrow biopsy is attempted in some cases.

Acute symptoms in the neonatal period that are unexplained by another disorder

A neonate who develops *intractable vomiting and becomes poorly responsive* after he or she is *first fed* may have an *aminoacidopathy, organic acidopathy*, or a *urea cycle disorder*. The cause is an absence or deficiency of an enzyme required for the metabolism of specific amino acids, organic acids, or compounds formed in the urea cycle. There are many such disorders; representative conditions are *isovaleric acidemia, methylmalonic acidemia, maple syrup urine disease, and ornithine transcarbamylase deficiency*.

Once first fed, these patients often become critically ill or comatose. Seizures may occur, and focal neurological deficits, such as disconjugate eye movements, may be noted on examination. Sometimes these infants have a characteristic odor that is a clue to a specific metabolic defect. Initial diagnostic tests include arterial blood gas, electrolyte panel, plasma glucose, complete blood count, liver function tests, quantitative plasma amino acid profile, plasma ammonia level, and urine organic acids. Metabolic *acidosis* is caused by many *organic- and aminoacidopathies*, whereas metabolic *alkalosis* is associated with *urea cycle disorders*. In cases of a urea cycle disorder, the *plasma ammonia level is markedly elevated.*

Mass neonatal screening identifies many of these diseases, but the number of conditions screened for varies from state to state (in the United States). The diagnosis also can sometimes be made on the basis of an abnormal elevation of one or more amino acids (in plasma) or organic acids (in urine), for example, markedly elevated plasma valine, leucine, and isoleucine levels in maple syrup urine disease and elevated methylmalonic acid in methylmalonic acidemia. The definitive diagnosis of a specific disorder usually requires enzyme assay from fibroblast culture or, if available, genetic testing.

The prognosis for many of these conditions, if untreated, is poor. Mental retardation, a cerebral palsy–like syndrome, survival in a vegetative state, or death often results. Fortunately, patients with several of these conditions can be effectively treated with a *specialized diet* eliminating the amino acids that cannot be metabolized. Protein restriction is also often helpful. Vitamin therapy (for example, vitamin B_{12} for methylmalonic acidemia and thiamine for maple syrup urine disease) is beneficial for patients with some disorders. During acute exacerbations, the patient may be given an antibiotic (neomycin) to reduce ammonia production by intestinal flora and lactulose to help the body metabolize excess ammonia.

Older children with a more quiescent form of one of these diseases often have a history of *marked general deterioration during an otherwise unremarkable illness* such as an upper respiratory infection. A history of a child inexplicably deteriorating during or after a seemingly routine viral infection should raise the possibility of an occult metabolic disorder.

Intractable neonatal seizures also suggest an inherited disorder. A more common cause should be excluded first (see Chapter 6). Diagnostic tests for neonates with unexplained seizures include electroencephalogram (EEG); magnetic resonance imaging (MRI); lactic acid, glycine, and pyruvic acid levels (CSF and blood); plasma amino acid, urine organic acid, and plasma ammonia level; biotin level; liver function tests; and genetic testing for any disorders suggested by the history and examination. A trial of *pyridoxine* should be administered intravenously while an EEG is recorded; if patient's seizures dramatically decrease in frequency and the EEG improves, the seizures were caused by *pyridoxine deficiency. Glycine encephalopathy, biotinidase deficiency, Alper syndrome, and Menkes syndrome* are rare causes of neonatal seizures.

Myoclonic seizures accompanied by neurological regression

This is known as *progressive myoclonic epilepsy*. The patient typically presents with *myoclonic seizures*, becomes ataxic, and cognitively deteriorates. The *neuronal ceroid lipofuscinoses* (NCLs), *Lafora body disease, mitochondrial encephalopathy with ragged red fibers* (MERRF), and *Unverricht-Lundborg syndrome* may present in this manner. NCLs, which are some of the most common degenerative disorders, often also cause *progressive blindness*. The diagnosis is suggested by characteristic inclusions, visible by electron microscope, in a skin or conjunctival biopsy specimen. During the last several years, the biochemical and genetic basis of the NCLs has been elucidated, leading to enzyme assays and genetic tests that are in the process of becoming available. Muscle biopsy and mitochondrial DNA mutation analysis are helpful in the diagnosis of MERRF. Lafora body disease is diagnosed on the basis of characteristic inclusions in skin and appendix biopsy specimens. Genetic testing may soon be available.

Unexplained ataxia

A history of *worsening cerebellar ataxia* suggests a *brain tumor*. If MRI does not reveal a tumor, a degenerative disorder may be the cause.

Friedreich ataxia manifests as progressive gait and limb ataxia, nystagmus, and dysarthria. Onset is during childhood or adolescence. The peripheral and central nervous system are involved; therefore, the deep tendon reflexes are diminished, sensory loss is demonstrable on examination, and nerve conduction studies are abnormal. Cardiac conduction defects and diabetes mellitus also occur. Friedreich ataxia can be diagnosed by means of a commercially available genetic test. There is no specific treatment for this devastating, ultimately fatal condition, although some benefit from coenzyme Q10 and vitamin E has been reported (2).

Ataxia telangiectasia presents in early childhood. Ataxia is the first manifestation. As the child grows older, ocular and facial *telangiectasias* appear. Decreased production of specific classes of immune globulin causes these patients to be susceptible to infection. Neoplasms are common and result in a life expectancy of 20 to 30 years.

Familial autosomal dominant ataxias, abetalipoproteinemia, Kearns-Sayre disease (see next section), *and leukodystrophies* (see Chapter 10) are some other possible hereditary causes of ataxia. Vitamin E deficiency, often caused by cystic fibrosis, should also be considered.

The *intermittent form of maple syrup urine disease* and *Hartnup disease* (see Chapter 7) may present with *intermittent episodes of ataxia* not explained by another process.

Mitochondrial diseases

Since mitochondria exist in most cells, *mitochondrial diseases* have many possible manifestations. All mitochondrial DNA is passed to the embryo *directly from the maternal ovum*. Therefore, these diseases are *inherited through the maternal lineage only*, and family members on the paternal side are unaffected. A history of maternal relatives with unexplained or unusual diseases supports the possibility of a mitochondrial disease.

Mitochondrial function is necessary for aerobic metabolism; therefore, mitochondrial diseases often cause a shift to *anaerobic* metabolism, resulting in an elevation of the plasma or cerebrospinal fluid *lactic acid* level. The plasma or CSF pyruvic acid level or the plasma alanine level is also sometimes elevated. *Muscle biopsy* is abnormal in cases of many of the mitochondrial diseases, with the classic finding being *ragged red fibers* following *modified Gomori trichrome staining*.

A history of *recurrent strokes in a child* suggests the syndrome of *mitochondrial encephalopathy with lactic acidosis and stroke-like symptoms* (MELAS). The diagnosis is suggested by the clinical presentation, brain MRI films showing recurrent infarction, and elevation of plasma or CSF lactic acid. Mitochondrial mutations associated with MELAS have been identified, and testing is available. *Homocystinuria*, a nonmitochondrial inherited disorder that may cause recurrent stroke, is diagnosed on the basis of an elevated plasma homocysteine level.

In cases of *Leigh syndrome*, which may be caused either by a mitochondrial DNA mutation or by a nonmitochondrial defect in pyruvate metabolism, MRI shows symmetrical white matter *lesions in the brainstem or thalamus*. The most common presentation is severe developmental delay during infancy, hypotonia, intractable seizures, cranial nerve palsies, and an abnormal respiratory pattern.

The mitochondrial disorder known as *Kearns-Sayre syndrome* results in progressive *cardiomyopathy, pigmentary retinopathy, and ataxia*. MERRF is described in the earlier section on ataxia.

There is no specific treatment for mitochondrial disorders, although the rate of deterioration is highly variable. Many of these disorders, especially the forms that present during infancy or affect cardiac function, can be fatal. A "mitochondrial cocktail" of coenzyme Q10, carnitine, vitamin B_{12}, and riboflavin is often prescribed because these enzymes and vitamins support aerobic metabolism and may enhance mitochondrial function.

Mucopolysaccharidoses

Cognitive impairment, "gargoyle-like" facial features, deafness, corneal opacities, bone and joint abnormalities, and organomegaly are suggestive of one of the *mucopolysaccharidoses* (MPSs). The MPSs are lysosomal storage diseases.

Each disease in this group is caused by a specific enzyme deficiency affecting the production of mucopolysaccharides (compounds found primarily in the ground substance of connective tissue). *Hurler syndrome* is the prototypical disease. Patients are noted to have dysmorphic facies, characteristic skeletal deformities (dysostosis multiplex), short stature, hepatosplenomegaly, heart disease, and corneal clouding. Several other MPSs, such as Hunter syndrome, present as somewhat milder variations of the Hurler phenotype. Hydrocephalus is a potential complication of several of the MPSs.

Although many of the MPSs cause mental retardation, Scheie, Morquio, and Maroteaux-Lamy syndromes are characterized by normal intelligence.

The finding of a high urine mucopolysaccharide level (*Berry spot test*) supports the diagnosis. Identification of a specific pattern of enzyme deficiency is accomplished by studies of cultured fibroblasts and, in some cases, can be confirmed by genetic testing. Enzyme replacement therapy is sometimes initiated to address nonneurological manifestations of these diseases. Corneal transplantation may help these patients' vision. Life expectancy is about 10 years in cases of Hurler syndrome but may be decades or even normal for patients with some of the milder diseases in this group.

Leukodystrophies

The *leukodystrophies*, which are covered in Chapter 10, include some of the most common neurodegenerative diseases. The cerebral white matter is primarily affected, and therefore, MRI is the best initial test.

Case 14.1

A 2-month-old male infant is brought for evaluation because of delayed development. He was born following an uncomplicated full-term pregnancy, weighed 6 pounds at birth, and had normal Apgar scores. His general health has been good, but he has not yet achieved head control. He occasionally smiles but seems less interactive, to his mother, than his older sister had been.

The physical examination reveals no unusual skin markings or facial features. The anterior fontanelle is open and flat. Head circumference is at the 25th percentile. Examination of the heart, lungs, and abdomen suggests no abnormality such as a murmur or organomegaly. Neurological examination make note of a somewhat lethargic infant who does not vocalize when stimulated. Pupils and extraocular movements are intact. Facial movements are symmetrical. Suck is strong. The baby lies in the frog-leg position. On pull-to-sit, there is marked head-lag, and the baby slips through the examiner's hands when held in the position of vertical suspension. Limbs are also hypotonic. Movements of the arms and legs are diminished but symmetrical. Deep tendon reflexes are obtainable. Primitive reflexes are normal for age.

Given a history of a marked delay in development and decreased alertness, a decision was made to initiate testing for a degenerative disorder. Complete blood count, plasma electrolytes, liver function tests, and ammonia level were in the normal range. The plasma lactic acid level was 10 times greater than normal range; this was confirmed with a second arterial blood sample. The pyruvate level was in the normal range.

Ophthalmological examination did not reveal corneal clouding or a cherry-red spot. MRI demonstrated symmetrical signal abnormalities in the brainstem and in the thalamus.

Diagnosis: *Leigh syndrome.*

Outcome: Mitochondrial genetic studies were negative. A muscle biopsy specimen was sent to a neuropathologist. No ragged red fibers, abnormal inclusions, or ultrastructural abnormalities were reported. Enzyme assay from a skin biopsy suggested a respiratory chain enzyme (pyruvate dehydrogenase) deficiency.

Subsequently, the baby made little developmental progress. At 6 months of age, myoclonic seizures started to occur that did not respond well to several antiepileptic drugs and required clonazepam for control. At 9 months of age, the infant's breathing pattern became irregular. The infant died at 11 months of age.

PHYSICAL EXAMINATION OF THE CHILD WITH A SUSPECTED NEURODEGENERATIVE DISEASE

The history will often suggest a degenerative process. The *family history* is also potentially valuable and may reveal unusual illnesses, children with unexplained diseases or deaths, or stillbirths. If the *parents are related other than by marriage* (a first-cousin marriage, for example), the likelihood of producing a child with an autosomal recessive disease is greatly increased. As noted, a history of unusual diseases on the maternal side of the family suggests a mitochondrial disease.

The physical examination will provide additional clues. *Progressive, postnatally acquired micro- or macrocephaly* should be noted. A thorough *eye examination*, in many cases requiring sedation and pupillary dilatation, may demonstrate cataracts, retinal pigmentary changes, macular degeneration, or optic atrophy. *Cherry-red spots* and *corneal clouding* in particular carry a high association with some of the lysosomal storage disorders and MPS. The child's *visual development* should also be assessed at regular intervals; unexplained, progressive blindness strongly suggests a degenerative process. *Hepatomegaly* is caused by several lysosomal storage diseases. Short stature and peculiar vertebral and other osseous maldevelopment (*dysostosis multiplex*) is often seen in cases of MPS.

The *skin* and *hair* should be carefully examined for coarse facies, eczema, alopecia, or abnormal hair growth and appearance. *Phenylketonuria* (PKU) is a slowly progressive aminoacidopathy associated with unusually fair skin and blond hair. *Biotinidase* deficiency causes alopecia, rashes, developmental delay, difficult to control seizures, blindness, and deafness.

Marked irritability or *excessive lethargy* in an infant may be an early clue to a degenerative disorder. A careful assessment of age-appropriate cognitive and motor milestones should, of course, always be a part of the examination. The neurological examination may reveal *hypotonia, opisthotonos, or hypertonicity*. Focal neurological signs, especially *cranial nerve palsies* and signs of *ataxia*, are always abnormal, although they are nonspecific.

APPROACH TO LABORATORY TESTING

Mass newborn screening has resulted in a dramatic decrease in morbidity from inherited disorders over the past 30 years. The results of standard screening should always be reviewed to make certain that any abnormal finding was reported.

In an increasing number of cases, the diagnosis of a degenerative disorder is made by *identification of the gene causing the disease*. The number of commercially available genetic tests has grown substantially during the last two decades as researchers have uncovered the genetic basis of diseases such as Friedreich ataxia, Rett syndrome, several of the leukodystrophies, and the NCLs. In cases of an inborn error of metabolism for which no genetic test yet exists, *enzyme assays* are often used. Leukocytes from whole blood or fibroblasts from a skin biopsy are cultured, and the amount of an enzyme required for a specific metabolic step is quantified. An absence or deficiency of an enzyme often identifies the disease.

If the physician strongly suspects a specific disorder on the basis of the history and examination (for example, in a case of Rett syndrome or spinal muscular atrophy), he or she may feel that it is appropriate to immediately order a genetic test. When the clinical diagnosis is less obvious, it is generally not appropriate to initially test for a specific genetic disorder given the high cost of these tests and the frequency of clinically similar disorders.

Other tests should be ordered, first and foremost, based on the patient's clinical presentation. As discussed earlier, a stock "metabolic work-up" is inadequate. Initial tests that are inexpensive and for which results are quickly available include *plasma glucose* (to exclude hypoglycemia, which is noted in many disorders of glucose utilization), *electrolytes* (anion gap; evidence of acidosis or alkalosis), *urinalysis* (ketones), *ammonia* (elevated in urea cycle disorders), and *lactic acid* (elevated in mitochondrial diseases and other disorders of aerobic metabolism).

The next step is to search for more definitive evidence of a specific class of metabolic disease. These tests are more expensive and frequently have turnover times ranging from days to weeks. The clinical picture should be strongly considered first. Examples are plasma and urine amino acids (aminoacidopathies), urine organic acids (organic acidurias, as well as some aminoacidopathies), plasma very long–chain fatty acids (peroxisomal disorders; see Chapter 8), and urine for mucopolysaccharides.

For some conditions (e.g., ceroid lipofuscinosis), a *skin biopsy* specimen may reveal characteristic inclusions when examined by electron microscopy. Diseases that cause degeneration of the cerebral white matter (e.g., Canavan disease, leukodystrophies) (see Fig. 10.3) or infarction (e.g., homocystinuria, mitochondrial disorders) are usually suspected on the basis of *abnormal brain MRI*. Degenerative diseases that affect muscle (e.g., mitochondrial diseases, glycogen storage diseases) cause changes visible on *muscle biopsy*.

Finally, as noted earlier, *testing for a specific DNA mutation* is becoming more and more useful in confirming the diagnosis of a degenerative disorder. In other cases, the definitive enzymatic determination is made from cell culture.

Genetic counseling

Genetic counseling should always be offered to the family because the possibility of having an additional child with a degenerative disorder may make them reconsider their plans. When additional children are desired and depending on the parent's feelings about the subject, genetic testing of future pregnancies may allow parents to have unaffected children. A genetic counselor may be helpful in these situations.

NEUROCUTANEOUS DISORDERS

The *neurocutaneous disorders* (phakomatoses) are identified by abnormalities of the *skin and nervous system,* which share a common embryonic origin (ectoderm). These disorders also may involve other organs including the heart, kidney, skeletal system, lungs, and eye.

Neurofibromatosis type I

Neurofibromatosis type I (NF1) is the most common neurocutaneous syndrome, with a prevalence of 1 in 3,000. *At least two* of the following findings are required for the diagnosis of NF1: (a) *six or more café-au-lait spots* >0.5 cm in diameter (1.5 cm in adolescents); (b) *inguinal or axillary freckling;* (c) *tumors (neurofibroma) of the spinal nerve roots or peripheral nerves;* (d) *iris hamartoma* (Lisch nodules); (e) an *optic nerve glioma;* (f) abnormalities of the *sphenoid or long bones;* or (g) a history of a *family member with diagnosed NF1.* The clinical manifestations of NF1 are highly variable. Although the disease is disfiguring or can result in serious neurological complications, in other cases the manifestations are mild and clinically unapparent.

NF1 is usually first suspected after a parent or doctor has noted café-au-lait spots (see Fig. 1.1). The physician should first make certain that these are, in fact, café-au-lait spots; a brown area of skin might be another kind of hyperpigmented lesion. The opinion of a dermatologist may be helpful. Café-au-lait spots are also noted in other disorders, such as McCune-Albright and Russell-Silver syndrome. These disorders can be differentiated from NF1 clinically.

If a child has more than five café-au-lait spots of appropriate size and a relative has been diagnosed with NF1, the child should also be assumed to have NF1. If there is no family history of NF1 and six or more café-au-lait spots are noted, a slit-lamp examination performed by an ophthalmologist has traditionally been the next step in diagnosis. However, Lisch nodules, which eventually occur in a large percentage of cases of NF1, typically *do not appear until adolescence*. Therefore, genetic testing is a more sensitive means of confirming the diagnosis of NF1 in a young patient. A gene linked to NF1 has been identified on chromosome 17 (3). Inheritance is usually autosomal dominant but can be sporadic. Genetic testing for NF1 has become increasingly sensitive and is *now recommended if the clinical diagnosis requires confirmation*. The family should be informed that the genetic test does not predict how severe the disease will be in a particular patient.

Many children with NF1 have learning disabilities (LD) and ADHD, and a substantial number are autistic. Special education is often required, and stimulant drugs and medications to manage behavioral problems are prescribed to many patients. Tumors of the nerve sheath (*neurofibroma*) develop in all patients, but the tumor load varies greatly. *Plexiform neuromas* can be disfiguring and may require surgical removal. Both tumors undergo malignant transformation in a small percentage of patients. Patients with NF1 are also at risk for developing *optic gliomas*, paraspinal neurofibroma, and other tumors of the central nervous system.

The routine care of a child with NF1 should include yearly neurological and ophthalmological screening. Patients should be specifically asked about changes in vision, headaches, and other symptoms that might suggest an intracranial tumor and also about radiating neck or back pain, sensory loss, parasthesias, and weakness of an arm or leg, which might be caused by a paraspinal tumor. The physician should not hesitate to order contrast-enhanced MRI of the brain or spine when a patient with NF1 mentions any of these symptoms. Screening MRI in the absence of symptoms is not recommended because a normal MRI result does not guarantee than a tumor will not develop in the future.

In most cases of NF1, MRI reveals small, unidentified bright objects (UBOs) in the cerebral white matter. These abnormalities are thought to represent hamartomas. A recent study suggests that the number of UBOs present roughly correlates with the degree of cognitive and behavioral impairment (4). A UBO should not enhance following the administration of intravenous contrast; if it enhances, it may be a malignant tumor.

Neurofibromatosis type II

Neurofibromatosis type II (NF2), with a prevalence of 1 in 40,000, is a much rarer disorder than NF1. To meet diagnostic criteria, patients must have *bilateral vestibular* (not auditory) *nerve schwannomas. Tumors of the spinal cord* (meningiomas, schwannomas, and ependymomas) are found in most cases. Intracranial meningiomas and peripheral nerve tumors also occur. Café-au-lait spots are *not* a sign and, if discovered, are irrelevant to the diagnosis of NF2. NF2 is inherited as an autosomal dominant trait (the gene is on chromosome 22) with complete penetrance. Genetic testing is available.

Hearing loss is the most common symptom of NF2. Other important manifestations of NF2 include difficulty maintaining equilibrium caused by a vestibular nerve schwannoma, cranial nerve palsies or ataxia caused by a neuroma compressing the brainstem or cerebellum, and hydrocephalus resulting from a tumor that obstructs the fourth ventricle. Contrast-enhanced MRI of the brain, *including images through the internal auditory canal*, should be ordered to evaluate these symptoms. Most vestibular nerve tumors can be successfully resected. Symptoms suggesting a spinal tumor (e.g., back pain, gait changes, paresthesias, incontinence) warrant special attention in these patients and should be investigated with contrast-enhanced MRI. Periodic brainstem auditory evoked response (BAER) testing is recommended for asymptomatic family members.

Tuberous sclerosis

The dermatological stigmata of *tuberous sclerosis* (TS) (Figs. 1.2 and 1.3) include *hypopigmented (ash-leaf) spots*, hypertrophied skin in the lumbar area *(shagreen patch)*, *periungal fibromata* around the fingernails, and small, fleshy growths *(adenoma sebaceum)* near the nasolabial folds. The prevalence of the disorder is 1 in 5,500 persons. Large *hamartomas in the cerebral cortex* ("tubers"; Fig. 14.1), *subependymal astrocytomas*, and other *brain tumors* occur in the great majority of cases. The tumors result in *symptomatic epilepsy* in most patients. *Infantile spasms* (see Chapter 6) may be the first sign of TS. Many patients eventually are diagnosed with Lennox-Gastaut syndrome. Mental retardation and autism are common. Nonneurological manifestations of TS include histologically benign but potentially clinically significant *tumors of the heart* (rhabdomyoma), *kidney*, and *lung* (angiomyolipoma). In a smaller percentage of patients, tumors of the retina, liver, gastrointestinal tract, and bone are discovered. Genetic testing is available but is usually unnecessary if a patient manifests characteristic

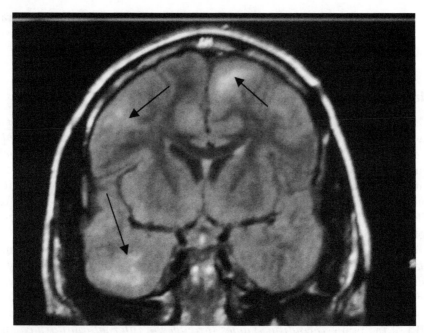

Figure 14.1 MRI of a cortical hamartoma ("tubers" shown by *arrows*) in a 15-year-old adolescent female with **tuberous sclerosis**.
(Courtesy of Ajax George, MD, New York University School of Medicine.)

clinical signs. Mutations linked to TS have been identified on chromosomes 9 and 16, as well as other genetic loci (5,6).

Most patients require multiple antiepileptic drugs to control their seizures. Many eventually undergo epilepsy surgery.

Special education is usually necessary. An echocardiogram and renal ultrasonography should be performed on a regular basis.

Sturge-Weber syndrome

Patients with *Sturge-Weber syndrome,* a congenital disorder with a non-genetic mode of inheritance (sporadic with an unknown prevalence) have a *facial hemangioma* (port wine stain) in the distribution of the ophthalmic branch of the trigeminal nerve. MRI shows a *venous angioma of the meninges* over the frontoparietal lobe on the same side. The angioma, which is often extensively calcified, is also visible by computed tomography (CT) and sometimes plain skull x-ray.

Patients with this disorder have *difficult to control focal seizures* originating in the abnormal hemisphere. Onset of the seizures is followed by the gradual development of *hemiparesis and cognitive regression* caused by progressive brain atrophy. Surgery, in many cases a radical cortical resection or even hemispherectomy, is often necessary (7). *Glaucoma* may occur in the ipsilateral eye, and the patient must be followed regularly by an ophthalmologist.

Rarer neurocutaneous disorders include *incontinentia pigmenti, hypomelanosis of Ito,* and *linear nevus sebaceous* syndrome.

GRADUAL ONSET OF PARAPARESIS

Spinal tumor

Persistent back pain *in the absence of a history of trauma* suggests a *spinal tumor*. Back pain that worsens at night is another warning sign. The patient's *gait* is usually affected. If the tumor is located within the cervical or thoracic spine, *upper motor neuron signs* (e.g., spasticity in the lower extremities, brisk reflexes, Babinski sign) develop over time (see Fig. 1.7). If the tumor is in the lumbar or sacral spine, it usually causes a *lower motor neuron syndrome* (weakness, hypotonia, and decreased reflexes) (see Fig. 1.8). Urinary sphincter dysfunction is common but varies with the location of the tumor (see section on bladder control).

MRI following contrast administration reveals the tumor, which may be located within a vertebral body (*extramedullary/extradural* tumor), the meninges or a nerve root (*extramedullary/intradural* tumor), or the spinal cord (*intramedullary* tumor). *Metastatic* spinal tumors (usually neuroblastoma in children) are generally extradural in location but may compress a nerve root or the spinal cord. A *neurofibroma*, often found in patients with NF1, is an extramedullary/intradural tumor that originates from a spinal nerve root and often causes pain and weakness in the distribution of the nerve (radiculopathy). A *meningioma* is an extramedullary/intradural tumor that, in pediatric patients, is usually a manifestation of NF2.

Spinal *ependymomas* are compact intramedullary tumors that typically arise in the sacral region. A spinal *astrocytoma* is usually a low-grade intramedullary neoplasm that may extend throughout much of the length of the spinal cord, creating an elongated cavity (*syrinx*) containing a small, contrast-enhancing mural nodule. In many cases of astrocytoma, symptoms of myelopathy develop very gradually. Scoliosis is often noted prior to the discovery of the lesion.

A *corticosteroid* is started at a high dosage if there is evidence of spinal cord compression (as in cases of spinal cord trauma; see Chapter 12). In cases of nerve root compression without spinal cord involvement, a lower dosage is more appropriate. Intramedullary tumors may not require a corticosteroid. Monitoring of *evoked potentials* during resection of intramedullary tumors helps the surgeon avoid noninvolved or critically important spinal cord tracts. Many intramedullary tumors can be completely resected and do not recur, and consequently, radiation therapy (RT) and chemotherapy (CHTX) are often not prescribed. The prognosis in these cases largely depends on the extent of preoperative disability.

Tethered cord

At birth, the caudal end of the spinal cord is situated at the level of the third lumbar vertebral body. As a result of normal skeletal growth, by adolescence, the tip of the spinal cord has ascended to the level of the first lumbar verte- bral body. When a *lipoma* or a *tight filum terminale* prevents this rostral movement, the lumbar segments of the spinal cord become slowly stretched, resulting in a progressive disorder of gait or, in some cases, urinary inconti- nence. This is known as a *tethered cord*. Tethered cord is a fairly common complication of spinal dysraphism (see Chapter 11). MRI of the lumbar spine (Fig. 14.2) reveals the adhesion. Surgery prevents further deterioration but does not reverse already existing neurological deficits.

Inflammatory diseases of muscle

A history of generalized weakness of insidious onset accompanied by fever or malaise suggests *polymyositis* (PM) or *dermatomyositis* (DM). Both are autoimmune disorders. PM and DM, like most diseases of muscle, cause *proximal* weakness, which should be contrasted with the distal weakness caused by diseases of the peripheral nerve. Complaints suggesting myopathy include easy fatigability, difficulty climbing stairs or arising from a chair, and

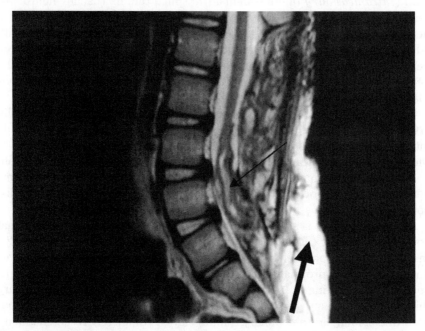

Figure 14.2 MRI showing a **tethered spinal cord** (*thin arrow*) with attached **lipoma** (*thick arrow*) in a 6-year-old boy.

(Courtesy Ajax George, MD, New York University School of Medicine.)

difficulty performing activities that require holding the arms above the head, such as brushing the hair. A *positive Gowers sign* often is elicited. In contrast to spinal cord lesions or neuropathies, muscle diseases *do not cause sensory loss, sphincter dysfunction, or loss of deep tendon reflexes.* Childhood DM is associated with *characteristic dermatological signs* (e.g., heliotrope discoloration of the eyelids, papular lesions over the joints of the fingers). DM is often associated with an occult carcinoma in adults, but the childhood form of DM is not associated with cancer.

Diagnostic testing

Electromyography (EMG) is often abnormal, confirming clinical suspicion of a muscle disease. The plasma creatine phosphokinase (CPK) level is often mildly elevated. Immunological tests including antinuclear antibody and anti-Jo antibody are often positive. In many cases, *muscle biopsy* is required to definitively diagnose PM and DM. In cases of DM, the muscle biopsy reveals evidence of *microvascular inflammation.* In cases of PM, infiltrating leukocytes are seen *within the muscle itself* and not the blood vessels. In some cases, there is also laboratory or clinical evidence of a second autoimmune disorder, such as thyroiditis or systemic lupus erythematosus.

Treatment

A *corticosteroid* is usually prescribed. A high dose of prednisone (1 to 2 mg/kg/day) is usually maintained for several weeks, followed by a gradual taper to a maintenance regimen (usually 10 to 15 mg every other day) that is continued for months to years. Plasmapheresis, immune globulin, antimalarial drugs, and immunosuppressive drugs (e.g., cyclophosphamide, cyclosporine) are used to treat refractory cases. Adverse effects of corticosteroids and other immunosuppressant medications, as well as the underlying diseases, result in significant morbidity.

NEUROLOGICAL CAUSES OF BLADDER CONTROL PROBLEMS

There are, essentially, three neurological systems involved in the control of micturition (Fig. 14.3):

1 *Parasympathetic* fibers originating from *sacral* spinal cord supply the *smooth muscle in the bladder wall* that *maintains bladder tone* during filling and *produces expulsion of urine* during micturition. Although this pathway can function autonomously, it is modulated by afferents from the brainstem and cerebrum.

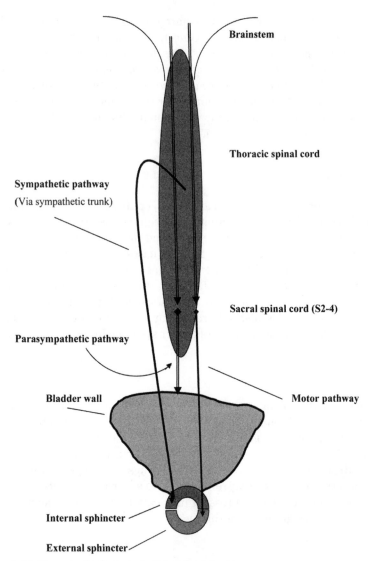

Figure 14.3 Neurological control of bladder function.

2 *Sympathetic* fibers supply the *internal urinary sphincter* that is respon-sible for *involuntary continence* (e.g., preventing micturition during sleep). Sympathetic fibers originate in the *thoracic spinal cord* and travel to the internal sphincter via the *sympathetic trunk*.

3 The *external urinary sphincter*, which allows for *voluntary control of micturition*, is supplied by *sacral spinal motor neurons at levels S2-4*.

A pathway from the brainstem and frontal lobes that provides for executive control of micturition projects to these sacral motor neurons.

Keeping these three pathways in mind, the following syndromes may be understood:

1 *Lumbosacral spine lesions* (e.g., myelomeningocele) typically result in a *flaccid bladder* due to *impaired parasympathetic function*. The *internal sphincter remains closed (intact sympathetic supply)*. The result is a flaccid bladder that expands passively as it fills with urine. When the bladder exceeds its mechanical capacity, urine leaks out through a closed sphincter (*overflow incontinence*). This syndrome is treated with regular bladder catheterizations and a procholinergic medication (bethanechol) that increases the tone of smooth muscle in the bladder wall.

2 In cases of a *thoracic spine lesion*, the opposite occurs: parasympathetic outflow to the bladder wall is not only spared, but it is *intensified* because the brain no longer modulates parasympathetic activity. However, the thoracic lesion *interrupts the sympathetic pathway*. The result is a *spastic bladder* that frequently reflexively empties through *a nonfunctioning internal sphincter*. Antispasmodic medications (e.g., oxybutynin) to diminish bladder contractions are used to treat these patients.

3 Brain- and brainstem-level structures and efferents modulate the parasympathetic outflow to the bladder and also supply the motor neurons controlling external sphincter. When these systems do not function optimally, the bladder tends to empty more frequently, and the external sphincter functions less effectively. Therefore, many children whose behavior is characterized by *poor executive function* (for example, children with ADHD, mental retardation, or autism) often *wet the bed* or have a daytime continence problem. Imipramine is sometimes prescribed to these patients. There is often improvement with age.

When urinary incontinence is *unlikely* to result from a spinal lesion

A spinal cord tumor or a tethered cord is often suspected when a child has a history of unexplained urinary incontinence. However, if no other neurological symptoms are reported and the neurological examination is normal, a spinal lesion is *unlikely* to be the cause. MRI should not be ordered as an initial test. Cervical spinal cord lesions typically cause *neck pain, flaccid weakness in the upper extremities and spastic weakness in the lower extremities, loss of sensation, and abnormal reflexes.* Thoracic spinal lesions give rise to *back pain, paraparesis, a sensory level, and abnormal reflexes.* Lumbar spinal lesions cause low *back pain, flaccid lower extremity weakness, diminished reflexes, and lower extremity sensory loss.* In rare cases (*cauda equina syndrome*), a sacral spinal lesion causes incontinence but no motor disturbance. However, as a general rule in cases of incontinence presenting without motor or sensory symptoms or abnormal signs, *a nonneurological cause of the problem should be sought* (i.e., consultation requested from a urologist) *before MRI of the spinal cord is ordered.*

COMMON CRANIAL NERVE DISORDERS

Bell palsy

When the facial nerve becomes inflamed, it swells and can be compressed if the surrounding facial canal is small in diameter. The result is *Bell palsy* (BP). Patients or their parents typically notice an asymmetrical smile, drooping of the face on one side, inability to keep food in the mouth, or an inability to close one eye. In some cases, involvement of the chorda tympani nerve, supplying taste fibers, results in a *loss of taste sensation on the anterior two thirds of the tongue*, and when a branch of the facial nerve supplying the tensor tympani muscle is involved, *excessive sensitivity to loud noise* on one side is reported. Involvement of facial nerve parasympathetic fibers results in *decreased lacrimation* and, often, a dry or irritated eye.

The physical examination of the patient with BP should reveal weakness of the muscles supplied by all divisions of the facial nerve, in other words, *all of the facial muscles on one side*. This is a key finding differentiating BP from stroke, which usually causes weakness in *only the lower half* of the face. The part of the brainstem facial nerve nucleus supplying the muscles of the *forehead* receives projections from *both* hemispheres of the brain, whereas the portion supplying the *lower half of the face receives only contralateral* projections. Therefore, a lesion in one *cerebral hemisphere* (e.g., stroke) causes weakness in the contralateral *lower face only*. In other words, a patient with only lower facial weakness should be suspected of having a stroke, whereas a patient with both upper and lower facial weakness almost always has BP. *Ability to raise the eyebrow* is a good measure of upper facial weakness.

Lyme disease is a common cause of BP. All patients with BP must be examined for the characteristic bulls-eye rash of Lyme disease and questioned about possible exposure to deer ticks. The serum Lyme titer should be checked. If the Lyme titer is positive and infection is confirmed by Western blot, the current recommendation for BP (8) is a 21- to 28-day course of an appropriate oral antibiotic (e.g., doxycycline). If the patient also has or later develops symptoms of headache and stiff neck, an LP is indicated. Pleocytosis accompanied by a positive Lyme titer suggests Lyme meningitis, which is treated with a 14- to 28-day course of an intravenous antibiotic (e.g., ceftriaxone or penicillin G).

Otitis media can involve the facial nerve and cause BP. The symptoms should improve following treatment with an antibiotic. A herpes simplex infection presenting with vesicles on the tympanic membrane (Ramsey Hunt syndrome) also can result in facial nerve inflammation. Patients are treated with oral acyclovir.

In many cases, no cause is found. A viral infection is presumed to be the etiology, although this is impossible to verify. Rare causes of facial nerve palsy such as sarcoidosis should not be routinely screened for in otherwise unremarkable cases. The yield of MRI of the brain and CT of the temporal bones is low, and these tests are also not necessary in typical cases (9).

Symptomatic treatment for BP includes a lubricant (saline solution, Natural Tears) for the affected eye and taping the upper lid shut to prevent injury to the cornea. If the patient is seen within 5 days of the onset of symptoms, a short corticosteroid course (Medrol Dosepak, Pharmacia/Upjohn; or prednisone 60 mg daily for 5 days) is often prescribed to hasten recovery. Studies demonstrate a modest clinical benefit (10). Some physicians also prescribe acyclovir to treat presumed herpes simplex infection. In the great majority of cases, the palsy completely resolves within a few weeks to a month, with or without corticosteroid or antimicrobial treatment. In rare cases, improvement is not complete. Nerve grafting is sometimes performed in cases of permanent facial palsy.

Facial palsy in the newborn

Facial palsy in a neonate may result from an injury to the facial nerve during a traumatic delivery or as a result of pressure from obstetric forceps. In either case, complete recovery almost always can be expected within a few months.

Asymmetrical movement of the *mouth* that is noted *only when a baby cries* is caused by underdevelopment of the depressor anguli oris muscle on one side. These patients are said to have the *syndrome of asymmetric crying facies*. The observer's impression is that there is weakness on the side of the mouth that droops when the baby cries. The "drooping" is actually the *normal* downward movement of the corner of the mouth. The *lack of movement of the other corner* is the abnormality. This condition usually spontaneously improves as the infant grows older (11).

Mobius syndrome refers to usually complete, bilateral nerve facial palsy caused by agenesis of the facial nerve nuclei in the brainstem. Other cranial nerve palsies and congenital malformations often are associated. Bilateral facial weakness can also be a sign of congenital myopathy, congenital myotonic dystrophy, and other *hereditary neuromuscular diseases*.

Facial sensory symptoms

Facial sensory loss, especially if accompanied by sensory loss in the ipsilateral arm, is an uncommon complaint in the pediatric population and should raise suspicion of a cerebral or brainstem lesion. Contrast-enhanced MRI should be ordered. Facial *pain* that is not caused by a dental problem or an oral infection may be a manifestation of *trigeminal neuralgia*. The pain of trigeminal neuralgia is usually severe, lancinating or burning, and exacerbated by mild sensory stimulation (e.g., light touch or a breeze). The pain may be localized to the forehead, maxillary, or mandibular region. Contrast-enhanced MRI should be ordered, with special attention paid to the brainstem and trigeminal nerve. Trigeminal neuralgia can be an early manifestation of *multiple sclerosis*, in which case areas of demyelination (plaques) in the white matter are usually visible. The pain can often be controlled with carbamazepine, oxcarbazepine, gabapentin, or valproate (see Chapter 6). Bouts of intractable pain are effectively treated with intravenous lidocaine.

Ptosis

Ptosis means a drooping eyelid. Unilateral ptosis that has remained constant over a long time period and that is not accompanied by other neurological abnormalities is usually *congenital*. In many such cases, the ptosis is also noticeable in *pictures taken at a younger age*. The ptosis often worsens slightly with fatigue. There is generally improvement during childhood.

Ptosis accompanied by blurred vision or double vision is cause for concern. Recent-onset ptosis should also be carefully evaluated. *Contrast-enhanced MRI* to look for a brainstem or orbital tumor should be ordered. *Horner syndrome* should be excluded clinically (see Chapter 10). MRI of the carotid arteries should be ordered if Horner syndrome is diagnosed.

Myasthenia gravis (MG) should be considered if ptosis *fluctuates markedly during the day*. MG is an autoimmune condition caused by antibodies directed against the acetylcholine receptor within the neuromuscular junction. In classic cases of MG, bouts of *generalized weakness* occur, but MG may also affect only the extraocular muscles (*ocular myasthenia*), causing intermittent ptosis or double vision.

The *anti-acetylcholine receptor antibody titer* is often ordered as an initial test for MG. If the titer is positive in the presence of signs and symptoms of MG, the diagnosis is confirmed. A high false-negative rate, especially in cases of ocular myasthenia, makes a negative result essentially meaningless. Therefore, patients with a negative result who are suspected of having MG should undergo edrophonium (*Tensilon*) testing. Edrophonium temporarily blocks the action of acetylcholinesterase, enhancing the effect of acetylcholine and producing a marked transient improvement of ptosis, diplopia, and weakness. The procedure is described elsewhere (12,13) and must be performed by an experienced neurologist. The diagnosis of myasthenia gravis can also be made by repetitive nerve stimulation during the electromyogram (EMG).

Patients with MG often undergo *thymectomy* (whether or not a thymoma is revealed by a chest x-ray). Treatments for generalized MG include anticholinesterase medications, corticosteroids, immune globulin, and plasmapheresis. Management is often challenging and should be directed by a neurologist experienced in the treatment of this disorder. In contrast, ocular MG may be a mild and self-limited disorder, and no treatment is often needed.

The condition previously called ophthalmoplegic migraine is discussed in Chapter 2. Rarely, ptosis in an infant or child is a manifestation of a hereditary *neuromuscular disorder* (see Chapter 8).

Nystagmus

Nystagmus is a type of involuntary eye movement. There are two forms: (a) *jerk nystagmus*, which is characterized by a rapid abducting movement of the eye followed by a slower return movement; and (b) *pendular nystagmus*, which is a symmetrical back-and-forth movement of the eye.

It is normal to observe one or two beats of jerk nystagmus when a patient's eyes are deviated to one side. *Gaze-evoked nystagmus* refers to *persistent* jerk nystagmus evoked by lateral gaze. *Medication*, especially antiepileptic drugs, barbiturates, and benzodiazepines, is *the most common cause* of gaze-evoked nystagmus. Gaze-evoked nystagmus is also a common finding in cases of *labyrinthitis* (see Chapter 7). Pseudotumor cerebri, hydrocephalus, and brainstem disease can also give rise to gaze-evoked nystagmus and should be suspected if the patient complains of headaches or if papilledema or one or more focal signs is noted on examination. Gaze-evoked nystagmus also may occur in the absence of an underlying cause.

The triad of *pendular nystagmus, head bobbing or nodding, and* (in some cases) *torticollis* is called *spasmus nutans*. The cause is unknown. Spasmus nutans is seen in infants and resolves spontaneously by age 3 years. Other causes of pendular nystagmus include many ophthalmological disorders, lesions of the posterior fossa, and neurodegenerative conditions (classically, Pelizaeus-Merzbacher disease). *MRI of the brain* should be ordered to evaluate pendular nystagmus.

Congenital nystagmus, which can be either jerk or pendular, is sometimes a sign of *blindness*. If the nystagmus *diminishes when the infant fixes on an object*, it is less likely that the infant is blind. An ophthalmologist should be consulted, regardless.

Double and triple vision

The physiological basis of double vision (diplopia) is *always* that the two eyes are not directed at the same point. The patient's eye movements may be obviously disconjugate, or in subtle cases, an *asymmetrical corneal light reflex* may be the only abnormal finding (see Chapter 1). *Contrast-enhanced MRI of the brain and orbits must be ordered to evaluate unexplained double vision.* Midbrain or pineal tumors typically result in *vertical* dissociation of images, whereas pontine tumors result in *horizontal* separation. Demyelinating diseases, MG, pseudotumor cerebri, hyperthyroidism leading to exophthalmos, and masses in the orbit are other possible causes of double vision.

Triple vision is virtually always a *factitious symptom* invented to get attention.

Extraocular palsies

A *palsy of the sixth cranial nerve* often accompanies or follows mononucleosis or another *viral infection*. The patient is unable to abduct one or both eyes. The condition usually resolves within 1 to 2 weeks. Sixth nerve palsy is also associated with hydrocephalus and pseudotumor cerebri (see Chapter 2).

Congenital sixth-nerve palsy is known as Duane syndrome, and congenital third-nerve palsy is called Brown syndrome. *Trochlear nerve palsy* is a delayed complication of head injury (see Chapter 12).

Eye rolling

Most doctors are aware that tonic eye deviation or upward eye rolling is often noted during a seizure. The eyes normally roll upward when the eyelids are closed (*Bell phenomenon*). Patients who are *very drowsy or sedated* may roll their eyes upward or their eye movements may briefly appear disconjugate. Upward eye rolling is also common during a *syncopal episode*. Eye rolling or eye deviation unaccompanied by other signs of a seizure is unlikely to be a seizure manifestation.

Stereotypic, intermittent eye movements (e.g., deviation, eye rolling) that occur while the patient is *awake and alert* and that can be *suppressed* are *tics* (see Chapter 4).

Loss of vision

A head injury, a migraine headache, or a seizure may cause a *transient loss of vision*. If visual loss is *nontransient* and restricted to one visual field, a cerebral hemispheric lesion should be suspected. A stroke is a possibility (see Chapter 13). If the symptom followed a head injury, a cerebral contusion may be the cause (see Chapter 12). Acute persistent loss of vision in *one eye* is usually caused by an ophthalmological problem.

Subacute-onset loss or dimming of vision, loss of color vision, and eye pain are symptoms of *optic neuritis*. *Papilledema* is often noted on examination. Contrast-enhanced MRI of the orbits may reveal abnormal signal in one or both optic nerves. If optic neuritis is diagnosed, MRI of the brain and spinal cord should also be done to search for evidence of demyelination elsewhere in the nervous system (see sections on acute disseminated encephalomyelitis and transverse myelitis in Chapter 13). LP sometimes reveals lymphocytic pleocytosis. An ophthalmologist should be consulted. Optic neuritis often responds well to a corticosteroid and may be self-limited. Possible causes, including Lyme disease, other infectious diseases, and autoimmune disorders, should be investigated.

Blindness can result from many *metabolic and degenerative diseases.* The NCLs (see earlier section, Myoclonic Seizures Accompanied by Neurological Regression), Leber hereditary optic atrophy, leukodystrophies, and mitochondrial diseases should be considered.

Unequal pupils (anisocoria)

A slight degree of pupillary inequality is a normal finding; a discrepancy of more than 1 mm (*anisocoria*) is not normal. The first step in the evaluation of anisocoria is to see whether both pupils dilate in the dark and constrict in response to bright light. These functions may be tested in a dark room with a flashlight.

If one pupil does not dilate in the dark, a disorder of the ipsilateral sympathetic pathway is suggested. The patient should be carefully examined for other signs of Horner syndrome (e.g., ptosis, anhidrosis). Horner syndrome requires evaluation with MRI and magnetic resonance angiography (MRA).

If one pupil does not constrict in response to light, the defect is in the parasympathetic supply to that pupil. Tonic (*Adie*) pupil is a congenital or acquired condition characterized by deficient parasympathetic enervation of the pupil. *A much rarer* cause, in children, of a persistently dilated pupil on one side is a posterior communicating artery aneurysm compressing the ophthalmic nerve.

Other common visual symptoms

A patient who is experiencing a *migraine headache* often reports seeing *flashing or colored lights or zigzag lines.* Similar visual illusions and distortions may characterize *partial seizures originating from the occipital lobe,* a cause that is more likely than migraine if the patient does not report headaches or nausea. *Blurred vision* is a side effect of many *drugs,* is a common *migraine* manifestation, and, in many cases, is caused by a primary *ophthalmological problem.* If one of these causes cannot be diagnosed, MRI should be ordered to search for a tumor compressing the optic chiasm or in an occipital lobe. The complaint of *nearby objects looking far away* (micropsia) is reported in cases of migraine, temporal lobe epilepsy, and anxiety.

Hearing loss and related complaints

Failure to acquire language skills (see Chapter 9) is a potential sign of congenital hearing loss, although in practice only a small percentage of language-delayed children are found to have a peripheral hearing problem. All young children with a history of delayed language acquisition should be sent for a *formal audiological evaluation.*

TABLE 14.2
Interpretation of bedside hearing tests

Rinne test result	Weber test result	Diagnosis
Same volume in both ears	Air conduction louder than bone conduction in both ears	Normal or (much less commonly) bilateral sensorineural hearing loss
Same volume in both ears	Bone conduction louder than air conduction in both ears	Bilateral conductive hearing loss
Sound diminished in one ear	Bone conduction louder than air conduction in affected ear	Conductive hearing loss in affected ear
Sound diminished in one ear	Air conduction louder than bone conduction in affected ear	Sensorineural hearing loss in affected ear

If an older child with previously normal hearing complains of hearing loss or tinnitus, a tuning fork may be used to better define the problem. First, the vibrating tuning fork is rested against the forehead at the glabella (between the eyebrows), and the patient is asked if the sound is equally loud in both ears (*Rinne test*). If the sound in one ear is noticeably softer, hearing loss on that side is suggested. Next, the vibrating tuning fork is held a few inches away from the ear affected by hearing loss and, after a few seconds, is rested against the mastoid process (*Weber test*). Normally, and in cases of sensorineural hearing loss, *air conduction is better than bone conduction*, and therefore, the tuning fork held in air is perceived as louder. The opposite finding (*better bone than air conduction*) is typical in cases of conductive hearing loss. Table 14.2 summarizes these tests and results. All patients with suspected hearing loss should have a formal evaluation by an audiologist and an ear, nose, and throat specialist. Hearing loss associated with other focal neurological symptoms or signs may suggest a brainstem or petrous bone tumor, and MRI should be ordered.

TREATMENT OF BRAIN TUMORS AND COMMON COMPLICATIONS OF TREATMENT

The diagnosis and initial management of pediatric brain tumors is reviewed in Chapter 2. This section further discusses imaging studies, newer treatment modalities, and treatment-associated adverse effects.

Diagnostic studies

Contrast-enhanced MRI is the imaging study of choice for the detection of brain tumors. MRI is always ultimately necessary if a tumor is suspected or can be visualized by CT. When a brain tumor is discovered, MRI of the spinal cord will often be ordered to look for evidence of tumor seeding ("drop metastases"). LP provides cytological evidence of cerebrospinal metastasis.

Genetic and chemical *tumor markers* from biopsy specimens (14) are increasingly used to help gauge the aggressiveness of the tumor and may suggest the susceptibility of the tumor to specific kinds of therapy.

Functional imaging modalities that are useful in the treatment of brain tumors include positron emission tomography (PET), single-photon emission tomography (SPECT), and magnetic resonance spectroscopy (MRS). These studies are primarily ordered to assess the metabolic activity and infer the malignancy of an abnormal-appearing area revealed by MRI. This information may be important in deciding whether or not surgery should be performed. Patients who have had prior neurosurgery or RT also are evaluated. For example, MRI often demonstrates a cavity where a tumor was resected or an area of necrosis where a tumor has been irradiated. Functional imaging, by revealing the metabolic activity of the area, will help the surgeon and neuro-oncologist judge whether or not there is residual tumor in the treated area.

Nonsurgical treatments

RT is often administered when a brain tumor cannot be completely resected. In other cases (e.g., ependymoma, astrocytoma, and medulloblastoma), RT is given even if an apparently complete resection has been achieved (15).

Unfortunately, irradiating the neuraxis of a young child often damages the cerebral white matter and consequently results in irreversible and often severe *deterioration of cognitive function*. The danger of cognitive regression may be reduced by *conformal radiation* (a more focused field), when a lower total dosage is administered, or when *proton-beam* rather than X-irradiation is used. *Neuropsychological testing* is administered prior to the initiation of RT and may be repeated after treatment. In addition to causing cognitive deterioration, RT can cause ototoxicity, myelopathy, and neuroendocrine dysfunction.

CHTX plays an increasingly important role in the treatment of medulloblastoma and oligodendroglioma and is being used experimentally for other tumors. Combining CHTX and RT may allow for a decrease in the dosage of radiation administered. Wafers containing CHTX compounds are sometimes placed within the surgical cavity to maximize the exposure of residual tumor. When CHTX is systemically administered, the drug used must be able to cross the blood–brain barrier; not all drugs can. CHTX agents frequently used to treat brain tumors include etoposide, platinum compounds, vincristine, nitrosourea compounds, and cyclophosphamide.

Adverse effects are potentially severe, including myelosuppression, renal insufficiency, peripheral neuropathy, ototoxicity, myelopathy, and seizures.

Postsurgical neurological syndromes

Cranial nerve palsies, hemiparesis, and ataxia may be noted after surgery to resect cerebellar and brainstem tumors. In some cases, these deficits are permanent. Other manifestations of *posterior fossa syndrome* are a labile affect and decreased speech (mutism). These two symptoms may improve after 1 to 2 months.

The *diencephalic syndrome* is noted in cases of a thalamic tumor or after thalamic surgery. It is characterized primarily by *somnolence*. Midbrain lesions often cause a similar syndrome. *Pituitary surgery* often is followed by diabetes insipidus, hypocortisolism, decreased production of reproductive hormones, or growth hormone deficiency. Many of these children exhibit signs of emotional lability, which is presumably a result of disruption of the limbic system.

REFERENCES

1. Lyon G, Adams RD, Kolodny EH. *Neurology of Hereditary Metabolic Diseases of Children.* New York: McGraw Hill; 1996.
2. Hart PE, Lodi R, Rajagopalan B, et al. Antioxidant treatment of patients with Friedreich's ataxia: four-year follow-up. *Arch Neurol.* 2005;62:621–626.
3. Barker D, Wright E, Nguyen K, et al. Gene for von Recklinghausen neurofibromatosis is in the pericentromeric region of chromosome 17. *Science.* 1987;236:1100–1102.
4. Feldmann R, Denecke J, Grenzeback M, et al. Neurofibromatosis type I: motor and cognitive function and T2-weighted MRI hyperintensities. *Neurology.* 2003;61:1725–1728.
5. Flodman P, Baumann R, Yoshiyama K, et al. Classification of tuberous sclerosis families based on linkage analysis with 9q34 and 11q22-11q23 markers. *Am J Hum Genet.* 1989;45:A139.
6. Kandt RS, Haines JL, Smith M, et al. Linkage of an important gene locus for tuberous sclerosis to a chromosome 16 marker for polycystic kidney disease. *Nat Genet.* 1992;2:37–41.
7. Kossoff EH, Buck C, Freeman JH. Outcomes of 32 hemispherectomies for Sturge-Weber syndrome worldwide. *Neurology.* 2002;59:1735–1738.
8. Pickering LK, ed. *2003 Red Book: Report of the Committee on Infectious Diseases.* 25th ed. Elk Grove Village, IL: American Academy of Pediatrics; 2003:407–411.
9. Gilden DH. Bell palsy. *New Engl J Med.* 2004;351:1323–1331.
10. Williamson IG, Whelan TR. The clinical problem of Bell palsy: is treatment with steroids effective? *Br J Gen Pract.* 1996;46:743–747.
11. Papadotos C, Alexiou D, Nicopoulos D. Congenital hypoplasia of depressor anguli oris muscle: a genetically determined condition? *Arch Dis Child.* 1974;51:891.

12. Fenichel G. *Clinical Pediatric Neurology*. Philadelphia: Saunders; 2001:157.
13. Spiro AJ. Disorders of the myoneural junction. In: Berg B, ed. *Principles of Child Neurology*. New York: McGraw Hill; 1995:1659.
14. Rickert CH. Prognosis-related molecular markers in pediatric central nervous system tumors. *J Neuropathol Exp Neurol*. 2004;63:1211–1224.
15. Halberg FE, Wara WM, Fippin LF, et al. Low-dose craniospinal radiation therapy for medulloblastoma. *Int J Radiat Oncol Biol Phys*. 1991;20:651–654.

Index

Page numbers followed by *f* indicate figures; those followed by *t* indicate tables.